29-50

FUNDAMENTALS OF
OPERATING DEPARTMENT PRACTICE

D1395806

1

n1L

8

19

DEDICATION

This book is dedicated to all non-medical theatre workers, without whose dedicated support, anaesthetic and surgical practice would not be possible.

FUNDAMENTALS OF OPERATING DEPARTMENT PRACTICE

Edited by

Ann Davey SRN, SCM, RCNT

Mersey ODP Assessment Centre Manager
John Moores University, Liverpool
Chairman of Proprius

Colin S. Ince MB ChB, FRCA

Consultant Anaesthetist, St Helens & Knowsley Hospitals Trust
Chairman Mersey ODP Assessment Centre
ODP External Verifier

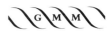

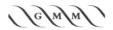

© 2000

GREENWICH MEDICAL MEDIA LTD
137 Euston Road
London
NW1 2AA

ISBN 1 900 151 189

First Published 2000

617.917 DAV
SMC

Distributed worldwide by
Oxford University Press

Typeset by Saxon Graphics Ltd, Derby
Printed by Ashford Colour Press Ltd, Hants

Contents

Chapter 19

Chapter 20

Chapter 21

Chapter 22

Chapter 23

Chapter 24

Chapter 25

Chapter 26

Chapter 27

Appendixes

Contributors

John Balance
MB ChB FRCA
CONSULTANT ANAESTHETIST
Hereford County Hospital

Paula Bolton-Maggs
FRCPP FRCPath FRCPCH
CONSULTANT PAEDIATRIC HAEMATOLOGIST AND HAEMOPHILIA
CENTRE DIRECTOR
Royal Liverpool Children's NHS Trust
Alder Hey, Liverpool

Peter D Booker
MBBS FRCA
SENIOR LECTURER IN PAEDIATRIC ANAESTHESIA
Royal Liverpool Children's NHS Trust
Alder Hey, Liverpool

Sheila Collins
SRN DipHE BA (Hons)
NATIONAL ODP ADVISER, CITY & GUILDS OF LONDON
INSTITUTE
Professional Training and Development Co-ordinator
Leighton Hospital, Crewe

Ann Davey
SRN SCM RCNT
ODP CENTRE MANAGER
John Moores University School of Health
Liverpool

Helen Davies
MB ChB FRCA
CONSULTANT ANAESTHETIST
St Helens & Knowsley Hospitals Trust
Prescot, Merseyside

Ann Dean
SRN RSCN DSCN NT BA (Hons)
SENIOR LECTURER IN VOCATIONAL STUDIES
John Moores University School of Health
Liverpool

Paul Duxbury
C&GLI 752
FORMER THEATRE MANAGER
St Helens & Knowsley Hospitals Trust
Prescot, Merseyside

Michael Greenall
C&GLI 752
SENIOR ODA
Fairfield Independent Hospitals
Crank, St Helens
Merseyside

George Grice
C&GLI 752
THEATRE CO-ORDINATOR
University Hospital Aintree
Liverpool

Terence M Hankin
BSc (Hons) MB ChB FRCA
CONSULTANT ANAESTHETIST
St Helens & Knowsley Hospitals Trust
Prescot, Merseyside

E Clare Howard
MB ChB FRCA
CONSULTANT ANAESTHETIST
University Hospital Aintree
Liverpool

Colin S Ince
MB ChB FRCA
CONSULTANT ANAESTHETIST
St Helens & Knowsley Hospitals Trust
Prescot, Merseyside

John A Kerry
PhD Cbiol MIBiol
BIOLOGICAL SERVICES MANAGER
University Hospital Aintree
Liverpool

Roger M King
BA CertED FIOT
SENIOR LECTURER
Department of Health & Science
Thames Valley University

Martin Maguire
RGN
RECOVERY TEAM LEADER
University Hospital Aintree
Liverpool

Robin R Macmillan
BSc MB ChB FRCA
CONSULTANT ANAESTHETIST
St Helens & Knowsley Hospitals Trust
Prescot, Merseyside

Vivienne Nelson
MB ChB FRCA
CONSULTANT ANAESTHETIST
St Helens & Knowsley Hospitals Trust
Prescot, Merseyside

Terry Ryan
MB ChB FRCA DRCOG DCH
CONSULTANT ANAESTHETIST
Liverpool Women's Hospital
Liverpool

Michael H Scott
FRCS ChM
CONSULTANT SURGEON
St Helens & Knowsley Hospitals Trust
Prescot, Merseyside

Andrew C Skinner
B Med SCI BM BS FRCA
CONSULTANT ANAESTHETIST
St Helens & Knowsley Hospitals Trust
Prescot, Merseyside

Edward Taft
C&GLI 752
ODP TRAINER
St Helens & Knowsley Hospitals Trust
Prescot, Merseyside

Richard Wenstone
MB ChB FRCA
CLINICAL DIRECTOR INTENSIVE CARE
Royal Liverpool University Hospital Trust
Liverpool

Thomas Williams
C&GLI 752
FORMER ODP TRAINER
Riyadh Al Kharj Hospital Programme
Riyadh
Kingdom of Saudi Arabia

Edmund Whelan
MB ChB FRCA
CONSULTANT ANAESTHETIST
St Helens & Knowsley Hospitals Trust
Prescot, Merseyside

Preface

Generally, textbooks are written for either nurses or anaesthetic assistants but this book seeks to embrace the knowledge needed for the generic theatre worker as envisaged in the Bevan Report. We seek to clarify the underlying principles needed for an understanding of anaesthetic *and* surgical practice and we do not intend to replace the readily available standard works, which should be used in conjunction with this text.

Fundamentals of Operating Department Practice defines the level of knowledge required for the ODP Level III qualification. It covers the practical aspects of operating department practice, where relevant.

Chapters do not follow the layout of the qualification structure but are grouped instead into areas of related knowledge. There is some intentional duplication to emphasise the importance of a particular subject, particularly when viewed from a somewhat different perspective.

National legislation, current at the time of writing, has been included but local policies and protocols have been used as illustrations. Drugs and other substances are referred to by their approved name wherever possible. Alternative names may be found by referring to the *British National Formulary* or a similar publication.

A. Davey
C. S. Ince
Liverpool, August 1999

Foreword

It was about twenty five years ago that I first managed a training school for Operating Department Assistants (ODAs). The two most difficult aspects of course planning were how much theory did the trainees actually need to know and to what level and depth should those theoretical subjects be taught.

This was a time of great change because ODAs were emerging as a new grade of staff within the theatre team and, for the first time, were undertaking formally approved training with a nationally recognized qualification. Although a syllabus and a final examination were identified, there was no guidance on curriculum development or learning objectives. As a result, course planning tended to vary in quality and relevance in different parts of the country.

Trainee ODAs would often be overwhelmed by the amount of theoretical knowledge it was thought they should acquire and even when fortunate enough to have access to comprehensive medical libraries, few text books were available that were directly relevant to their field of competence. Similarly, teachers from the wide range of disciplines with whom ODAs interacted in the clinical situation would sometimes have difficulty in setting their lectures at an appropriate level. This sometimes resulted in confusion or boredom on the part of the trainees and frustration or near despair on the part of the course managers.

Other qualified staff within the operating department often had great difficulty in accepting ODAs as professionals, partly because their role and qualification was poorly understood. The situation is now very different and it is greatly to the credit of the trainees of that time, their managers and a number of theatre specialists that Operating Department Practitioners (ODPs) have become such valued members of theatre teams today, being highly regarded as skilled and knowledgeable professionals.

One of the hallmarks of professionalism includes the ability to pass onto others skills and expertise. This has been achieved through the example of excellence in personal performance and by sharing knowledge, not only with one's peer group, but also with those from other disciplines. The publication of this book is there-fore a highly significant development in that some of the contributors are themselves former ODAs who are now in senior management and education. Nurses have also made a significant contribution and it is appropriate to mention the invaluable part many of them have played as training managers, work-based assessors and verifiers in supporting the development of the generic theatre practitioner of today.

Some of the authors are senior anaesthetists and it is right to acknowledge the enormous contribution that so many of their number have made to the development of ODPs as a professional group. Particular mention should be made of Dr Colin Ince who has masterminded the production of this book from inception to publication with the same dedication and enthusiasm with which he has supported the quality of operating department practice over a period of many years.

Theatre professionals no longer need to rely exclusively on texts primarily written for doctors, nurses and other medico-technical staff. This book, which is wholly relevant to the occupational standards of their qualification, also serves as a valuable resource for those wishing to access the National Vocational Qualification (NVQ) in Operating Department Practice. In addition it provides a good background to the advance practice units of the extended role (Additionally Accredited Units).

It should be remembered that operating department practitioners are not only the nursing and technical staff who provide non-medical assistance within the theatre team but they are also caring professionals in a wide range of clinical situations throughout the health-care setting. They currently have direct contact with patients in such areas as Recovery Units, Accident and Emergency Departments, Day Care Surgery Units, Intensive Therapy Wards and Resuscitation Teams. Good quality care should be available to all patients wherever they are found and operating department practice therefore incorporates those care standards, which already apply in nursing practice.

This is a weighty text, but every chapter has the merit of maintaining the essential link between theory, practice and clinical application. It complements rather than supplements existing books and the diversity of subject matter included reflects the wide range of background knowledge that is required to underpin the performance of an effective ODP.

This book will therefore be a valuable resource for many groups of health care professionals, such as trainee doctors, pre and post-graduate nurses, students of midwifery and medico-technical staff, working in a variety of high dependency fields. Operating department practitioners at all levels of experience and career development will find it an essential and comprehensive reference. It is worth quoting Dr Terry Ryan from Chapter 25 (Emergency and Obstetric Anaesthesia): "There is no doubt that the experience and training of the entire theatre team will have a major impact upon the outcome of any . . . operation. Without the necessary practical abilities theoretical knowledge is of little value."

This text addresses these issues across the whole spectrum of operating department practice and will help to support the maintenance of the highest standards of care, safety and treatment available to patients.

Kate Pittom
Training and Development Consultant to the NHS in
Operating Department Practice 1988 – 1996
National Verifier for the NVQ in Operating Department
Practice, City and Guilds 1991 – 1996

Acknowledgements

The idea for this book originated with Mr T. McCann, Principal Operating Department Assistant at Whiston Hospital, but the editors must also thank the publishers for suggesting that it should be written and for their support and help.

In addition, we are most grateful to Mrs S. Comer, Personal Assistant to Dr C. S. Ince, who patiently corrected the grammar and proof-read the text, and to Mrs K. Morton RGN, who is also an ODP, for ensuring that the text was understandable.

We are also grateful to our many colleagues who have given of their time and expertise, often at short notice and to St Helens and Knowsley Hospitals Trust for allowing us to reproduce the version of the consent form and information sheet as shown in Apendices 4a and 4b.

Mrs A. Davey
Dr C. S. Ince
Liverpool, August 1999

INTRODUCTION

C. S. Ince

Major advances in anaesthesia and surgery may only occur when the understanding of a principle or discovery is linked to its practical application and the potential usefulness of this development is realized. Even then, progress is limited by the technical ability of the time.

Thus, before the discovery of anaesthesia surgery was generally limited to amputations, the removal of bladder stones, the repair of fistulas and fairly superficial operations. Celcus, a Roman physician in AD 30, was probably the first to remove a bladder stone and the procedure changed little over 1800 years. This type of surgery was, however, made respectable when, in 1686, Charles François removed a stone from Louis XIV by cutting into the perineum.

The Massachusetts General Hospital in Boston only recorded 43 operations from 1821 to 1823 because the real prospect of death and the incredible pain suffered meant that only hopeless cases or patients in severe distress would consider the risk worthwhile. Surgeons therefore tried to introduce instruments into the bladder in order to crush these stones. Jean Civiale experimented on cadavers and on his own bladder stone. In 1823 he used forceps introduced through the urethra to hold his stone which was then drilled, causing it to break into pieces. His record showed that it was virtually painless.

Without anaesthesia, surgeons needed to practise with skill and speed. Susruta, an Indian physician in the 5th century AD, recorded the first operation for nasal reconstruction. A similar operation was performed on a bullock driver by a Mahratta surgeon, using a forehead skin flap modelled on a wax reconstruction of the nasal defect. This was first published in "The Gentleman's Magazine" in October 1794. Joseph Carpue, who trained at St George's Hospital London, researched the method and performed his first operation that lasted 37 minutes on October 23 1814.

Major developments in surgery only became possible with the discovery that inhaling certain chemical gases could produce insensitivity to pain. The possibility had existed for over 300 years because in 1540 Valerius Cordus used ether to successfully anaesthetize and then recover chickens. Joseph Priestly discovered nitrous oxide in 1772 and in 1800 Sir Humphry Davy used it to relieve the pain of an infected tooth.

On December 10 1844 Gardner Quincy Colton, a travelling lecturer in chemistry, demonstrated nitrous oxide inhalation at his 'laughing gas show' and Horace Wells, a Connecticut dentist, noticed that, while inhaling the gas, Samuel Cooley banged his shin but felt no pain. He realized its potential and on December 11 1844 Riggs, Wells' assistant, successfully extracted one of Wells' teeth under nitrous oxide administered by Colton. This was repeated on 15 patients in his practice and only two felt pain. On January 17 1845 he gave a demonstration at Harvard Medical School in the presence of John Collins Warren, a respected surgeon, but the patient felt pain and he was branded a fraud.

Meanwhile, Dr Crawford Long used ether to operate on the neck of James Venable on March 20 1842, having similarly observed that individuals engaged in "ether frolics" could injure themselves without experiencing pain. William T. G. Morton, an apprentice of Horace Wells, was present at the failed nitrous demonstration and gave the first recorded ether anaesthetic on October 16 1846 at the Massachusetts General Hospital, Boston, to Gilbert Abbott.

By December the news reached Dr Francis Boott who told Robert Liston, the Professor of Clinical Surgery at University College London. The technique was tried on a young woman undergoing dental extraction. On December 21 1846 an amputation performed by Robert Liston on Frederick Churchill was the first pain-free surgical procedure in England. Peter Squire gave the ether.

In 1847 Professor James Young Simpson introduced chloroform into obstetric practice. No mention was made, however, of James Waldie, the Liverpool chemist who suggested the method to Simpson and whose apothecary shop subsequently burned down.

In 1847 John Snow, the first full-time British anaesthetist, wrote 'On the Inhalation of Ether'. He realized that the common methods of ether and chloroform administration were faulty and developed both ether and chloroform inhalers. Snow gave chloroform to Queen Victoria during the birth of Prince Leopold. Although the first death from ether occurred in 1847 and from chloroform in 1848, Snow administered over 4000 anaesthetics without a death. Both ether and chloroform had significant disadvantages and newer agents (Cyclopropane 1930, Trichlorethylene 1941 and Halothane 1956) were introduced. The further development of vaporizers made administration more controllable.

Hewitt, McKesson and Boyle introduced anaesthetic machines from 1898 and in 1928 a circle circuit which incorporated carbon dioxide absorption using soda lime was developed by Brian Sword. (Joseph Priestly first described the absorption of carbon dioxide by alkalis in 1754 but it took nearly 200 years for this discovery to be utilized.)

The development of endotracheal anaesthesia allowed surgeons to perform more complicated procedures. Endotracheal insufflation was described in 1667 and in

1880 MacEwen passed a tube into the trachea using his fingers as a guide. Magill and Rowbotham further developed this concept in 1920, although cuffed tubes were not introduced until 1928. The first direct vision laryngoscope was used in 1896, with the Macintosh curved blade described in 1942.

Muscle relaxants made a great difference to surgical practice but were first used to control spontaneous ventilation rather than for paralysis. The South American arrow poison, curare, was described by Sir Walter Raleigh in 1596 but, although its physiological action was ascertained in 1850, it was first used as a full muscle relaxant on January 23 1942 by Griffith and Johnson in Montreal. Professor Gray and Dr Jackson Rees established its use in Britain and developed the Liverpool School of Anaesthesia using the triad of analgesia, muscle relaxation and narcosis. Suxamethonium was first used in Sweden and Italy in 1951 and still has an important place in anaesthesia. The development of newer muscle relaxants has been rapid but the ideal agent has still to be produced. Guedel and Treweek developed control of respiration by respiratory depression in 1934 and Crafoord used the first ventilator in 1940.

The ability to cannulate a blood vessel allowed the intravenous injection of anaesthetic agents and analgesics. Sir Christopher Wren gave the first intravenous injection of opium to a dog in 1657, using a bladder attached to a sharpened quill, but the first glass hypodermic syringe and needle were not developed until 1853. Chloral hydrate was used in 1874 to induce anaesthesia but, although barbitone was synthesized in 1903, it was not until 1927 that the first barbiturate was routinely used to induce anaesthesia. In 1934 Lundy introduced thiopentone which paved the way for many other intravenous anaesthetics.

The discovery of local anaesthetic agents permitted surgery to take place without general anaesthesia. Cocaine, which occurs in coca leaves, was isolated by Gaedicke in 1855 and was further purified by Nieman in 1860. It was Koller, however, in 1884 who demonstrated its use in the eye. In the same year Stewart Halsted performed a mandibular nerve block using cocaine and the following year an accidental subarachnoid injection of the drug produced regional analgesia. Lumbar puncture was shown to be a practical clinical procedure in 1891 and August Bier produced successful spinal analgesia in 1898, with extradural analgesia described in 1901. Cocaine was known to be toxic and the first alternative, tropocaine, preceded the development of procaine which was produced by Einhorn in 1903 and used by Braun two years later. Bier used this drug intravenously as an anal-

gesic in 1908. Nupercaine was introduced in 1929 and became popular as a spinal analgesic. Later, the spinal route was less used because of nerve damage resulting from phenol, which leaked into the anaesthetic ampoules from the sterilizing fluid. Spinal and epidural analgesia now have an established place in the anaesthetist's repertoire. (Harvey Cushing coined the term 'Regional anaesthesia' to describe pain relief resulting from a nerve block.) Lignocaine came into use in 1948 followed by prilocaine and bupivacaine.

One of the factors limiting major surgery was the ability to replace blood and fluid loss. Richard Lowther, in 1665, transfused the blood of one animal into another but the first attempt at fluid replacement was in 1832 when intravenous saline was used to treat the dehydration of cholera. Only after the discovery of ABO blood groups in 1900 by Landsteiner at the University of Vienna could major advances in blood transfusion occur and in 1914 Hustin used citrate in blood transfusion.

Although anaesthesia allowed surgical techniques to advance, large numbers of patients died from surgical wound fever. In February 1846 Ignaz Semmelweis, a Hungarian, became the assistant at the First Obstetrical Clinic in Vienna. In the 'lying in' section of the Vienna General Hospital 36 of the 208 mothers had died. Semmelweis discovered that, whereas 10% of mothers died in the ward where medical students were trained, only 1% died in the ward where midwives attended. The wards were next to each other in the same building.

At postmortem he found that these women had a picture of suppuration and inflammation throughout the body resembling surgical or wound fever. He and the medical students followed this with ward visits to carefully examine the mothers to try and find the cause. As a result the death rate increased but only on the days when women were admitted to the division attended by the doctors and medical students. Professor Kolletshka, who had given Semmelweis much support, died after being cut during a postmortem and at his own autopsy a similar pattern of suppuration was seen. Semmelweis then realized that examining patients after performing postmortems could be the cause.

On May 15 1847 Semmelweis made all doctors and students wash their hands in chlorine water before entering the maternity wards. Over the next month the mortality decreased from 12.34% to 3.04%. When this practice was extended to washing between examinations by the end of 1847, the death rate was 1.33%. Publications in 1847 and 1848 were met with derision by Semmelweis's professor who prevented him from further study, arranged for his removal from his post and abolished all his handwashing protocols.

Semmelweis left Vienna in 1848 and became a GP obstetrician in Budapest. On May 20 1851 he took the post of Honorary Head of Obstetrics at St Roch's Hospital in Budapest and over the next eight years reduced the mortality rate to less than 1%. On July 18 1855 he was appointed Professor of Obstetrics at Budapest University but his ideas were still rejected by the foremost obstetricians in Europe. Semmelweis died on August 14 1865 at the age of 47 of septicaemia following a cut at a postmortem, with his work largely unrecognized.

In 1863 Louis Pasteur discovered that microorganisms caused fermentation and putrefaction and that this process could be stopped by heat. Joseph Lister, who was Professor of Surgery at the University of Glasgow, read of this work and also that a Dr Crooks had eliminated the smell of the Carlisle drainage fields by treating the sewage with carbolic acid (phenol). Realizing the significance of the discovery, he introduced handwashing with carbolic and also soaked the dressings in this substance. His main argument was that the carbolic prevented germs from entering the clean wound. On June 17 1867 he performed a radical mastectomy on his sister without significant suppuration and the wound was healed in a few weeks. He also discovered that catgut ligatures, that were soaked for four hours in carbolic, did not cause suppuration and were absorbed by the body. These findings were presented to a sceptical audience at the British Medical Association's 35th annual meeting but Professor Simpson lead a vehement opposition, until his death in 1870. Although his ideas were widely implemented in Europe, it was not until the 1920s that 'Listerism' was accepted worldwide.

In the latter part of the 1870s a German doctor named Robert Koch identified rods and cocci under the microscope, observed them multiplying and used the organisms, which he named bacteria, to infect mice that subsequently died. He found ways of dyeing and photographing them and in this way identified the bacteria responsible for anthrax, cholera and tuberculosis.

Research soon showed that steam killed bacteria more efficiently than carbolic and Schimmelbusch and Terrier introduced the steam sterilization of instruments, sutures and dressings. Although it was known that bacteria collected under fingernails, rubber gloves were introduced by coincidence. John Halsted, the Professor of Surgery at Johns Hopkins Medical School, had a nurse assistant who developed severe eczema due to handwashing in carbolic. In 1890 he

developed a thin rubber glove, which could be steam sterilized to protect her hands. When she became his wife and retired from work, his assistants took it in turns to use the gloves for surgical practice. Thus, not only were the causal agents of infection identified but also a means was found to protect the clean wound from contamination.

The final part of this introduction traces the evolution of theatre training, reviews the current position and looks forward to new developments that will lead to safer practice. As anaesthesia and surgery developed, so did the need for non-medical assistance. A dedicated assistant to the surgeon and the anaesthetist is now vital for the delivery of safe surgical and anaesthetic practice. Initially learning was by experience, the anaesthetist often pressing into service a 'Box Boy' or a friendly theatre porter, with this role later developing into that of the Theatre Technician. Some anaesthetic departments, however, preferred to employ informally trained nurses. At first, surgical assistants were, invariably nurses who were trained in a similar manner.

The City and Guilds of London Institute (CGLI) 752 examination was introduced in 1976 as part of the recommendations of the Lewin Report. During the course, which concluded with a final examination, there was a single practical assessment in both surgery and anaesthesia. The emphasis was on theory and all parts had to be passed within three attempts. Apart from the recovery of patients from anaesthesia, most surgical and anaesthetic topics were well covered in the syllabus. Thus, qualified Operating Department Assistants were able to assist both the surgeon and the anaesthetist, although generally employers did not take full advantage of the dual capability.

The Regional Health Authorities were responsible for coordinating the training through regionally based and funded training schools, with support from a local steering or management committee, which was charged with the implementation of the syllabus, and training standards that were identified by the National Health Service Training Authority (later to become the National Health Service Training Directorate NHSTD). The NHSTD approved training schools for periods of up to five years, using visits by Approval Panels. The day-to-day quality assurance was the responsibility of City and Guilds of London Institute.

Although this represented a great advance, there was undue emphasis on theory. Students whose performance was poor under the pressures of formal examination conditions, although they may have been practically excellent, often fared badly. Similarly, practical ability was judged in a "one-off" situation in anaesthesia and surgery and students sometimes passed even though their overall performance did not justify this result.

Surgical assistants were either Registered General Nurses (RGNs) or State Enrolled Nurses (SENs). Theatre training was usually informal in the first instance but locally certificated awards were introduced in the late 1950s. In 1969 the Joint Board of Clinical Nursing Studies (JBCNS) was established with the aim of bringing uniformity and professional credibility to postregistration courses for nurses and midwives. In 1983 The English National Board for Nursing, Midwifery and Health Visiting (ENB) encompassed the JBCNS and additional courses were introduced. Although emphasis was placed on ethical issues and research as well as the acquisition of practical skills, the courses have been shortened and are now considered by many inadequate to cover the range of skills required. The ENB 998 Teaching and Assessing course for RGNs and the CGLI 730 Teaching Course are available for postbasic study.

Prior to the introduction of the concept of the 'Theatre Person', there were five main non-medical staff groups working in theatre: ancillary staff; surgical nurses; operating department assistants (ODAs) and anaesthetic and recovery nurses. Traditionally, nurses usually assisted the surgeon while anaesthetic nurses and ODAs (despite being multiskilled) supported the anaesthetist. ODAs were not permitted to have responsibility for controlled and scheduled drugs and therefore nurses had a much greater responsibility in postoperative recovery areas. This inflexibility reduced the efficiency of operating departments.

The Department of Health asked Professor P. G. Bevan to carry out a detailed study of the management of operating theatres. He recommended that the ENB and the NHSTD should look at the possibility of developing a common training for those involved in theatre work and that levels of competence should be defined for anaesthetic and surgical support personnel. Thus developed the concept of the "Operating Department Practitioner" (ODP), who would supersede but not replace the traditional roles of the nurse and the ODA and would have the knowledge and ability to practise in all theatre situations. (It must be stressed that this is only a generic definition describing somebody that practises in theatre and should not be confused with (Health Care) Operating Department Practice Level 3, which is a qualification.)

Meanwhile, the Department of Health proposed that National Vocational Qualifications (NVQs) should be developed for theatre staff as soon as it was practically possible. The Government set up the National Council for Vocational Qualifications (NCVQ) in

1986: together with the Scottish Vocational Education Council (SCOTVEC), it was responsible for approving all vocational qualifications.

The Lead Industry Body, the Care Sector Consortium, now known as the Occupational Standards Council, analysed the work practices which were required by the employer and which should be included in the award. After developing draft standards, determining the evidence requirements and developing an assessment system, the draft proposals were piloted within operating theatres. The Awarding Body was identified as the 'Joint Awarding Body' (JAB) with the CGLI being the active member and the award was submitted to the NCVQ for approval. This award, known as "Health Care: Operating Department Practice Level 3", is available to all personnel who wish to practise as the equivalent of assistants to the anaesthetist and/or surgeon or who wish to work in the recovery area. It has now replaced the CGLI 752 qualification but in no way disadvantages holders of this or any ENB certificate.

A vocational qualification is based on the achievement of competence. Defined as "the ability to perform the practical skills of the occupation", it encompasses everything a person should be able to do at work if they are to be effective in their job, including the necessary background knowledge (theory) and understanding to produce a safe practitioner. The NVQ framework currently has five levels of work practice, based on the complexity of the activities performed in the work area and the ODP qualification is at Level 2 for the support worker and at Level 3 for the assistant to the surgeon and/or the anaesthetist.

NVQ training differs from the more traditional methods in the following important ways: there must be open access for students of any sex, sexual orientation, race, religion or creed and training must not be 'Time Banded'. This means that no limit may be placed on the length of time taken to qualify but, in practice, the employing authorities limit this by Training Contracts. Access to Health Care: ODP Level 3 is through clearly defined entry criteria.

The qualification is divided into major parts known as Units, each of which deals with a specific area of experience, and these are further subdivided into Elements. Each Element has its own Performance Criteria and the range of clinical settings over which these apply. Sections of Elements and Units are completed as and when competence is consistently established and this is formally documented. On completion of all Units, the student may apply for the qualification but, should the student so wish, Units may be individually certificated.

Work experience takes place in the local hospital under the guidance of Work-Based Trainers and Assessors and the underpinning knowledge is taught within the hospital and at approved Assessment Centres. Work-Based Assessors (WBAs) are responsible for ensuring that the student generates sufficient and relevant evidence of competence, both practically and at a theoretical level. The Local Assessment Coordinator, who is competent in all areas of the qualification, collates and evaluates evidence from many different sources.

ODP Level 3 must be creditable to the Awarding Body and to the employer. The Assessment (Training) Centres, which consist of the schools and the related hospitals, are subject to a rigorous quality assurance process coordinated by the Awarding Bodies using External Verifiers, both at initial approval and at regular intervals throughout the year. It is possible, therefore, for centre approval to be withdrawn at any time.

Internal Verifiers, usually senior theatre staff, are responsible for the internal quality assurance relating to the National Standards of the qualification. An award can only be as creditable as those who are responsible for its administration and assessment. Thus the JAB places great emphasis on the training of WBAs, Internal and External Verifiers. Assessment Centres are responsible for the training of WBAs and Internal Verifiers and the JAB trains its External Verifiers and continuing appointment is dependent on satisfactory performance. These assessors must be seen to be competent and, therefore, the Training Development Lead Body (TDLB) has provided National Standards, which lead to a range of assessing awards. All verifiers and assessors must have achieved this award within 12 months of taking up their post.

Existing theatre staff who wish to obtain this ODP Level 3 award may be assessed against the National Standards or demonstrate their current competence and underpinning knowledge using witness statements from their employers. This is known as "Accreditation of Prior Learning or Experience" (APE or APL) and allows assessment of competence without the need for formal practical evaluation. No Unit may be totally acquired through APL.

In order to develop further the role of the theatre practitioner a series of Additionally Accredited Units (AAUs) have been introduced. The content relates to the high levels of skill and responsibility appropriate to the practitioners. The AAUs are intended to cover skills not specified by the standards contained within existing levels. Areas that have been assessed in Level 3 are only repeated if it is considered essential. These free-standing Units may be separately certificated and candidates may not have achieved the ODP 3 award prior to accessing the AAUs. In order to maintain the highest standards set by ODP Level 3, performance has been structured to ensure that candidates reach an equivalent level of competence before they are awarded unit recognition.

The AAUs are divided into two main groups. The seven Clinical Specialisms cover performance within the specific surgical and anaesthetic areas of ophthalmology, plastic surgery and burns, cardiothoracic surgery, vascular surgery, orthopaedic surgery, maxillofacial surgery and the neurosciences. The Generic Skill Units have been developed for those areas of technical ability which are applicable within the Extended ODP Role wherever this is perceived to be relevant by the candidate or the employer. This may not always relate to theatre practice. The units cover the following skills: venepuncture and intravenous cannulation; the administration of drugs; intubation and extubation; and basic and advanced cardiac life support.

Although there have already been great changes, this does not mean that the qualification in its current form is without fault. The need for modification was identified early on and a first revision is currently in place. During 1996-7 a fundamental review of the award has been carried out to make it more relevant to today's requirements. An additional AAU for surgical assistance will also be introduced and others are under consideration.

In these days of frequent litigation a nationally recognized qualification such as ODP Level 3, which is hopefully supported by the medical Royal Colleges and hopefully, in the near future, by professional registration for the ODA and the ODP, must give the same credibility to the non-medical practitioner as the medical profession has possessed for many years.

RECOMMENDED READING

Lee J, Alfred J. Atkinson, R.S. 1992 *A Synopsis of Anaesthesia*: Bristol: John Wright

Ince C.S. 1995 *The Training of non-medical theatre personnel*: Health Trends **27**(3):80.)

1

THE OPERATING DEPARTMENT PRACTITIONER, THE PATIENT AND THE LAW

J. Ballance & P. Duxbury

INTRODUCTION

Each patient passing through an operating department has a right to be dealt with in a sympathetic and professional manner. This care extends throughout the perioperative period, a term that describes the time around and including surgery and anaesthesia. Theatre professionals are becoming involved at all stages of this process and in some hospitals only operating department staff look after the day-case patients. Management of this care is discussed in Chapter 3 and many individuals are involved in what may be a lengthy process.

It is, however, important that care meets the highest moral, ethical and legal standards that have been introduced to protect not only the patient and the patient's rights but also those of the theatre worker. This chapter seeks to clarify some of this legislation but also tries to explain why it was introduced in the first place. Some of these topics are dealt with in greater detail elsewhere in the book and will only be mentioned in passing. It is important for the reader to understand that this section deals with English Law and must only be interpreted in this context.

THE LAW AND ETHICS

A principle may be defined as a theoretical base which can and must apply to all people in order to maintain a stable society. There are four main principles guiding the actions of the health-care worker:

1. Autonomy – the right to self-determination.
2. Beneficence – to act in a way to do good.
3. Non-maleficence – to act in a way to do no harm.
4. Justice – to be fair to all individuals.

Ignoring these principles may not necessarily be illegal because breaking the law and breaking an ethical code are not the same and it is for this reason that codes of practice have been introduced by the professional organizations. It is not illegal for a doctor to divulge confidential information about a patient, without that patient's consent, to a person not involved with their medical management but it does break the medical code of practice. If this action came to light the doctor would be disciplined and, depending on the seriousness of the complaint, may be suspended from practice. Examples include revealing a diagnosis such as HIV to a patient's relative or friend and informing the parent of a 17-year-old that she was taking the contraceptive pill.

In Britain we are all presumed to know the law and ignorance of the law is no excuse for breaking it. It is therefore most important that the health worker is aware of actions or omissions that may have legal consequences and that individuals may well be required to account for their actions in a court of law. This also applies to the professional organizations such as the General Medical Council and the UKCC because legal judgements take precedence over any professional disciplinary matter.

DOCTRINE OF JUDICIAL PRECEDENT

The Doctrine of Judicial Precedent states that cases must be decided in the same way when the material facts are the same. How, then, does this affect the health-care worker? Unfortunately or perhaps fortunately, the law is not a static function but its interpretation may change as it is tested by the courts.

One of the best examples of this is the 'Neighbour Principle' that was formulated in the case of Donoghue v Stevenson in 1932. Lord Atkin had to make a judgement on what was considered to be the duty of care. He defined it as:

> 'You must take reasonable care to avoid acts or omissions which you can reasonably foresee would be likely to injure your neighbour. Who is then my neighbour? The answer seems to be persons who are so closely and directly affected by my acts that I ought reasonably to have them in my contemplation as being affected when I am directing my mind to the acts or omission which are called in question.'

Until that judgement, there may have been some doubt as to what the duty of care meant but this is no longer the case and this statement now forms a yardstick by which all actions are judged. It is a definition that every health-care worker would do well to learn and always keep in mind.

RIGHTS AND OBLIGATIONS

The rights of an individual may be defined as 'that to which a person has a just or lawful claim' and it is an interest which will be recognized and protected by a rule of law. There are therefore some rights that each of us should expect and some which the State or an employer has a duty to provide. Examples include the following.

- Basic goods and services such as clean water, housing and food.
- Voting rights.
- An employer must provide a safe and healthy environment for their workers. This should be physically, psychologically, emotionally and spiritually sound.
- Employees have a right to be protected and to feel safe.

- The right of the individual to have an equal opportunity in any aspect of life (employment, training, facilities, etc.) is a fundamental right for everybody, irrespective of race, creed, gender, sexual persuasion or physical disability.

THE RIGHTS OF THE PATIENT

The health-care professional has a duty to care for the patient and the patient has a right to be cared for. Duty of Care may only centre round an individual patient or it may include the much broader concept of the whole caring environment. The basic rights that are relevant to health care are discussed below.

Health care and treatment were defined in the National Health Service Act 1947, which gives every patient the right to have medical treatment that is free at the point of delivery.

The right to choose, e.g. the choice of a doctor, hospital, carer or treatment although in practice this is a limited concept within the NHS.

The right to know is not always enforced. For example, a terminally ill patient may not wish to know the true facts. In this context the skill of the carer is paramount in trying to decide what the patient really wants, but it is very easy to make the wrong decision.

To be informed relates particularly to consent and the different effects of available treatments to which the patient may be subjected.

Patients have a right to be treated but also have the fundamental right.

To refuse treatment, both surgical and therapeutic. The patient does not, however, have the right to demand a certain method of treatment. Sometimes there may be a choice between an expensive drug, which may be marginally better, and a cheap drug and this may be very controversial. Equally controversial is the right of a Jehovah's Witness to refuse blood and blood products in a life-threatening situation. They do have this right but this does not apply to their children who are below the age of consent.

To take one's own discharge is a right but it must be clearly established that the patient has the mental capacity to understand the consequences of that action.

The right to life deals with issues such as protection of the unborn child but also raises such questions as 'When does a fetus become viable?'

Children also have the right of protection under the Children Act and this may potentially bring the carer into conflict with the parent(s). Thus there are clearly defined guidelines relating to the management of suspected child abuse.

The right of the patient to privacy may sometimes be difficult to implement in an open ward and the interpretation of what is meant by privacy may also lead to potential patient/carer conflict.

Perhaps the right of confidentiality is one of the most difficult to deal with. If a carer is given information that will affect the treatment of a patient but is sworn to secrecy, should they reveal it to the appropriate person? A patient who is about to have an operation but has concealed the diagnosis of HIV may put the safety of the theatre staff at risk and these individuals also have rights. This subject will be discussed in more detail later in this chapter.

Both patients and carers have the right of protection from harm. This includes such things as protection from infection (the Department of Health has ruled that all staff working in an environment that potentially exposes them to hepatitis B must be vaccinated) and the Control of Substances Hazardous to Health (COSHH – see Chapters 2 and 4 relating to the Safety at Work Act).

OBLIGATIONS

An obligation is a duty, usually legal or moral, arising from one's choosing to undertake a course of action. If this obligation is legal it is known as a contract and is legally binding. Contracts may be oral, written or implied and arise from the assumed intentions of the parties concerned. Compensation is the payment for loss or injury sustained and is part of common law – the Law of Tort (an evil wrong independent of contract), which allows for unqualified damages (compensation) to be paid if a contract is broken.

Compensation may be awarded for:

- Trespass, which also involves issues around consent.
- Defamation, which is the publishing of statements tending to lower a person in the estimation of right-thinking members of society. Every patient is entitled to protection against defamatory remarks but if the remark is true the patient has not been defamed. Slander is spoken defamation and the plaintiff must prove that special damage has occurred before guilt is established. It is therefore important that the care worker is discreet at all times. Communication in good faith for the benefit of the patient is permissible but gossip is not.
- Negligence, which will be dealt with later in the chapter.

CONSENT TO INVASIVE TREATMENT OR SURGERY

THE RIGHTS OF THE PATIENT

With regard to the consent of patients for invasive clinical procedures, ethical and legal points must be considered as these have a bearing on the professional judgements made in consent.

There are six main legal points that influence the obtaining of consent.

1. Under Common Law, a doctor may only administer treatment when a patient gives consent.
2. Under the Law of Trespass, a doctor who proceeds to act in the absence of consent will be liable for trespass, assault or battery.
3. For the consent to be legally valid, the patient must know in broad terms what is involved in the clinical treatment. English law imposes the higher obligation of providing information if the suggested procedure has any potentially significant risks or side effects.
4. Under the Law of Negligence, there is a similar obligation to provide information with the identification of potentially significant risks or side effects (breach of the duty of care).
5. Patient autonomy is a guiding principle of medical law.
6. The principle of self-determination will, in most circumstances, overrule the medicolegal principle of the sanctity of life. This principle entitles a competent adult to reject a specific treatment or select an alternative even at the risk of death, for reasons which may be rational, irrational, unknown or non-existent.

Informed consent to operation has three components as judged by the Thorpe Test (after Lord Thorpe):

1. Understanding and retaining information.
2. Believing the information.
3. The ability to weigh up and decide on the basis of that information.

Patients are entitled to receive sufficient information in a way that they can understand about the proposed treatments, the possible alternatives and any substantial risks so that they can make a balanced judgement. In some circumstances an interpreter may be needed. Patients must be allowed to decide whether they agree to treatment and may refuse or withdraw consent at any time. Guidance on the amount of information and warnings of risk to be given to patients can be found in the judgement of the House of Lords – Sideway v Gov. of Bethlem Royal Hospital (1985).

Patient autonomy is sacrosanct in law but the problem doctors and other carers face is what to tell patients: how much, how little or exactly what? In this regard, perhaps the following should be considered when providing information to the patient:

- The reasons for the procedure.
- The nature of that procedure including such things as the anaesthetic, duration of stay and physical/mental incapacity.
- The benefits.
- The discomforts.
- The substantial risks.
- The alternatives.
- The consequences of not having the procedure.

It is for this reason that NHS Trusts are now producing specific information sheets for the most common operative procedures and these include the main complications of the operation. The Clinical Negligence Scheme for Trusts (CNST) has replaced the now removed Crown Immunity and is the current standard for indemnification within Trusts. It has advised that only doctors who are capable of performing a procedure should explain that procedure to the patient and subsequently obtain the consent. In practice, the phrase 'by an appropriately qualified and experienced person' is more commonly used. This has radically changed the way that many surgical departments function because traditionally the houseman and not the surgeon was the individual charged with completing the consent form. Patients who are now admitted on the day of surgery often do not receive premedication because consent may not be obtained if the patient is under the influence of drugs.

The wishes of the patient should always be respected and this is particularly important when patients may be involved in the training of clinical students. Although information is sent out to the patient prior to admission, further explanation is often necessary. It should, however, be made clear that a patient may refuse to agree to a student being present without detriment to their care.

Unfortunately, it would appear that many patients are unaware of the nature of their operation or of the importance of informed consent. 'Ethical Issues in Anaesthesia' (see Recommended Reading) deals with this subject in detail and so we have only provided a few examples.

- Byrne et al (1988) – 45% of patients could not recall the basic details of the operation and 45% did not know the reason for their operation.
- Askew et al (1990) – 40% of patients could not name one risk or complication of the procedure.

- Cassileth (1990) – 69% of patients signed the consent form without reading it and, after the procedure was explained to them, 40% failed to understand the information.

Education, the medical condition and care in reading the form all contribute to this failure of recall. Indeed, some patients thought that the consent form merely protected the doctor.

What, then, do we mean by risk and what should be considered as a clinical risk? We could look at this either as the chance of the risk occurring (risk rate) or as the consequence of that risk on the patient as a whole. *Health Trends 1996* identified risk rates as follows:

- High risk: greater than 1:100 (1%).
- Moderate risk: 1:10 000 (0.01%) to 1:100 (1%).
- Low risk: 1:10 0000 (0.001%) to 1:10 000 (0.01%).

The effect on the patient as a whole may be categorized as follows.

- Severe: Death or total irrevocable loss of an organ, limb, major tissue or function leading to severe and probably permanent disability, which is likely to significantly modify the patient's future life.
- Moderate: Permanent or semi-permanent dysfunction of organ, limb or major tissue, which results in a disability requiring support, treatment or medication, possibly causing a modification of the patient's future life.
- Slight: Fully or almost fully recoverable dysfunction to organ, limb or major tissue with minimal impact on the patient's future life.

This is further complicated by the need to identify the risk arising from the procedure alone in a fit, normal patient and the risk resulting from pre-existing disease. Thus, a total gastrectomy has a much greater risk in a patient who is a hypertensive diabetic and in heart failure than in a physiologically normal individual. There is a need for the clinician to identify the nature of the risk, its rate and the impact that it will have on that particular patient.

The theatre practitioner is perhaps the last of four or five individuals who will check the consent form but one of the authors has seen a patient arrive into the anaesthetic room before the mistake was identified by the ODP. It is most important that the patient volunteers the information needed and that it is not assumed solely by inspection of the identification band and the case sheet.

Finally, an invasive procedure must include treatments that could conceivably lead the patient or parent to assume that an indecent act had occurred. It is not only unwise but also very foolish to insert vaginal pessaries or rectal analgesics without prior warning and this has been the subject of litigation.

OBTAINING CONSENT

Consent to treatment may be described as implied or express. In many cases patients do not explicitly give express consent but their agreement may be implied by their actions, e.g. the offering of an arm for taking blood (Clinton v Jones Arkansas 1991). Express consent is given when a patient confirms their agreement in clear and explicit terms, either orally or in writing.

Oral consent may be sufficient for the vast majority of contacts with patients by doctors, nurses and other health professionals. Written consent should be obtained for any procedure or treatment carrying substantial risk or side effect. If the patient is capable, written consent should always be obtained for general anaesthesia, surgery and certain forms of drug therapy. Oral or written consent should be recorded in the patient's case notes with relevant details of the health professional's explanation.

Consent should be obtained during preparation for the proposed procedure but, as previously stated, before any sedation or premedication is given. Consent to one procedure does not give automatic right to another procedure. A doctor may, however, undertake further treatment if the circumstances are such that a patient's consent cannot be requested and provided the treatment is immediately necessary and the patient has not indicated that further treatment is unacceptable. No alterations should be made to the consent form after the patient has signed it and, if there is a change to the planned procedure, the patient must be consulted and fresh consent sought.

OBTAINING CONSENT IN SPECIAL CIRCUMSTANCES

There are occasions when a patient is incapable of giving informed consent, including:

- Children under the age of 16 years.
- Children over the age of 16 but under 18 years.
- Refusal of parental consent to urgent or life-saving treatment.
- Adult or competent young person refusing treatment.
- Patients suffering from a mental disorder.

Where a child under the age of 16 achieves a sufficient understanding of what is proposed, that child may give consent to a doctor or other health professional making an examination and giving treatment. This is known as

'Gillick Competence'. The doctor or health professional must, however, be absolutely satisfied that the child has sufficient understanding of the procedure proposed. In most cases the parents will accompany these children but, if this is not the case, the child should be persuaded to have the parents informed unless it is clearly not in the best interests of the child. It is important to document all the factors taken into account when assessing a child's capacity to give valid consent. Parental consent should be obtained where a child does not have sufficient understanding, except in an emergency where there is no time to obtain it.

Section 8 of the Family Law Reform Act (1969) identifies that the consent of a young person who has attained the age of 16 years to any surgical, medical or dental treatment is sufficient in itself and it is not necessary to obtain consent of the parents or guardian. If a child is over 16 years and not competent to give valid consent, the consent of parents or guardians must be sought but this power extends only to the age of 18 years.

When a parent or guardian refuses to consent to urgent or life-saving treatment and time permits, court action may be taken to obtain consent from a judge. Otherwise hospital authorities should rely on the clinical judgement of the doctors and in such a case the doctor should obtain a written supporting opinion from a medical colleague that the patient's life is in danger. This should be discussed with the parents or guardian in the presence of the witness. The discussion should be recorded in the notes and countersigned by the witness. Some adults or competent young persons will wish to refuse some or all of the proposed treatment, e.g. on religious grounds. Whatever the reason, the patient should receive a detailed explanation of the nature of their illness and the need for treatment. They should also be warned that the doctor might properly decline to modify the procedure or treatment and the possible consequences if the procedure or treatment is not carried out. If the patient refuses to agree and they are competent, then the refusal must be respected. The doctor must record this in the notes and, where possible, have it witnessed.

The presence of mental disorder does not of itself imply incapacity, nor does detention under the Mental Health Act. Each patient's capability for giving consent has to be judged individually in the light of the nature of the decision required and the mental state of the patient at the time. The Mental Health Act (1983) took a major step forward in providing for mentally disordered people, detained in hospital under the powers of the act, to be given treatment for mental disorders without their consent where they are incapable of giving consent. Certain procedures and safeguards are laid down in relation to specific groups of treatment, including the need for multidisciplinary discussion and the agreement of doctors appointed to give a second opinion. It is not permissible to subject to compulsory treatment, patients who were voluntarily admitted to a mental institution. Before this treatment can be carried out the admission status of the patient must be changed, i.e. the patient has to be compulsorily admitted under the Mental Health Act. This is of more than theoretical interest to theatre workers as anaesthetists are involved in anaesthesia for electroconvulsive therapy.

The Act, however, does not contain provisions to enable treatment of physical disorders without consent, either for detained patients or those who may be suffering from mental disorder but not detained under the Mental Health Act. A House of Lords decision in 1989 helped to clarify the common law in relation to the general medical and surgical treatment of people who lack the capacity to give consent. No-one may give consent on behalf of an adult but the substantive law is that a proposed operation or treatment is lawful if it is in the best interest of the patient and unlawful if it is not.

In cases involving anaesthesia and surgery or where the treatment carries substantial or unusual risk, it would be advisable to record in the patient's notes that the patient is incapable of giving consent to treatment. It should also state that the doctor in charge of the patient's treatment is of the opinion that the treatment proposed should be given and that this is in the patient's best interest. The consent form must be signed by the clinician and witnessed by another clinician. The Law Commission was requested to look at the area of mental incapacity, which is currently a grey area under the Act. A Parliamentary Bill was scheduled for 1995 but this was postponed. The present government is about to review the situation.

EXAMINATION OR TREATMENT WITHOUT PATIENT CONSENT

The following are examples of occasions when examination or treatment may proceed without obtaining the patient's consent:

- For life-saving procedures where the patient is unconscious and cannot indicate their wishes.
- Where there is a statutory power requiring the examination of a patient, e.g. under the Public Health (Control of Disease) Act 1984.
- In cases where a minor is a ward of court and the court decides that a specific treatment is in the best interest of the child.

- Treatment for the mental disorder of a patient liable to be detained in hospital under the Mental Health Act 1983 (see below).
- Treatment for a physical disorder where the patient is incapable of giving consent by reason of mental disorder and the treatment is in the patient's best interest.

Because issues relating to consent are so complex it is not surprising that health professionals may potentially come into conflict with the law and the only solution is scrupulous attention to detail in all matters.

Examples of a consent form and a patient information leaflet are included in Appendix 4a and Appendix 4b.

CONFIDENTIALITY

Confidentiality may be defined as the imparting of knowledge with reliance on secrecy. In a 1998 court case, J. Rose stated '... preservation of confidentiality is the only way of securing public health ... patients will not come forward if doctors are going to squeal on them'. Thus, information is given in the knowledge that it will not enter the public domain and may only be passed on to others if the patient gives express or implied consent.

Confidentiality may be broken on the principle of Beneficence, which has already been mentioned. This involves the duty to care, the duty to do good and the duty of advocacy (protecting the right of the vulnerable and weak) and may be summarized by the maxim 'do unto others as you would have them do unto you'. The statement that best sums this up is that a health professional '... owes a duty of care not only to his patient but also a duty to the public'. It is in relation to the latter that the role of the law, which can enforce disclosure, must be considered. If confidentiality is broken the practitioner must be able to clearly justify that decision.

MEDICAL NEGLIGENCE

A charge of medical negligence may well be the reason why non-medical theatre workers find themselves in court, even though they may be innocent of all charges. It is for this reason that an understanding of the principles of negligence is so important.

There are two principles that underpin any claim for negligence: the patient must agree to be treated and treatment must be carried out with proper skill and care.

There are four main elements of medical negligence:

1. Existence of a legal duty of care.
2. Breach of that duty of care.
3. Injury or damage resulting from the defendant's acts or omissions.
4. Failure to note reasonable foreseeability of harm.

A LEGAL DUTY OF CARE

This was defined in R v Bateman (1925) thus: 'If a person holds himself out as possessing special skill and knowledge, ... undertakes ... treatment ... he owes a duty to use diligence, care, knowledge, skill and caution in administering the treatment'. In our discussion of 'Neighbour Principle' we have already mentioned, to whom this duty of care is owed (see above) and it covers not only treatment and procedures but also diagnosis and advice.

BREACH OF DUTY OF CARE

It is very easy to state that the duty of care fell below the expected standard but how do we measure this? J. McNair defined this in the case of Bolam v Friern Hospital Management Committee in 1958. This is now called the Bolam Test and, because of its importance, we will quote it fully.

'The test is not the test of a man on the top of a Clapham omnibus, because he has not got this special skill. The test is the standard of the ordinary skilled man exercising and professing to have that special skill. A man need not possess the highest expert skill: it is well-established law that it is sufficient if he exercises the ordinary skill of an ordinary competent man exercising that particular art ... (A doctor) is not guilty of negligence if he has acted in accordance with a practice accepted as proper by a responsible body of medical men skilled in that particular art.'

The duty of care is a legal statute but the standard of that care is determined by medical judgement. If there are two or more schools of thought:

'It is not enough to show that there is a body of competent medical opinion, which considers that the defendant doctor's decision was a wrong decision if there also exists a body of professional opinion, equally competent, which supports the decision as reasonable in the circumstances.'

The duty of care relates to the post that the person occupied and the law requires a junior to give the same standard of care as a more senior colleague. Both medical and non-medical professionals should therefore seek help if the duty that they have to perform is outside their scope or experience. Never be afraid to ask – advice is free.

INJURY OR DAMAGE AS A RESULT OF THE DEFENDANT'S ACTS OR OMISSIONS

The test is whether the damage would have occurred but for this breach of duty. The plaintiff must prove on the balance of probability that the negligence in question caused the injuries; In other words, what actually happened and what would have happened if the defendant had not been negligent.

REASONABLE FORESEEABILITY OF DAMAGE

The charge could only be proved if the damage were reasonably foreseeable at the time at which it occurred. 'We must not look at a 1947 accident with 1954 glasses' (Denning in Roe v Minister of Health). Complications of a treatment are not in themselves negligent but the course of action following a complication may be. Thus, it is not negligent for a practitioner to puncture an artery when preparing to give an intravenous injection but it is negligent for that person to inject the drug knowing that the vessel was an artery.

THE MANAGEMENT OF RISK IN THE THEATRE ENVIRONMENT

Theatre workers must always be aware of the legal repercussions that may follow unacceptable professional practice or a mishap to the patient. The practitioner may not necessarily be at fault but there are a number of ways in which this risk of a mishap may be decreased. Broadly speaking, they can be divided into the identification of the patient in theatre and the way that the patient is managed thereafter.

PATIENT IDENTIFICATION

The identification label should be fitted to the patient immediately on admission to the hospital (including day cases and unconscious patients) and should be childproof. If it has to be removed, e.g. while establishing an intravenous infusion, it should be resited immediately. The label should contain the patient's full name, date of birth and hospital number.

The name and hospital number should only be used when sending for a patient and the porter is usually given a card which contains the patient's name, ward of origin and the theatre number in which the operation will be performed. The nurse should check the details of the patient before leaving the ward and this should be recorded and signed on a check sheet. In addition, the correct notes, any necessary investigation results and the consent form should accompany the patient.

Operating lists should be typewritten and retyped if the order is changed. Fingers should be identified as thumb, index, middle, ring and little while toes should be numbered 2–5 except the first, which is either the great toe or the hallux.

When the patient arrives in theatre they should be asked, 'What is your name? What operation are you having? Which side is your operation?'. One of the authors has seen a patient almost have the wrong operation because she was scared to tell the anaesthetist that her name was not 'Mrs Smith' and that she was not having 'a breast operation'.

It is the responsibility of the surgeon and anaesthetist to identify the correct patient and the correct procedure before anaesthesia but we all work as a team and the earlier potential errors are identified, the better. It is very easy to confuse the site of the operation, especially if the operating list is handwritten or abbreviations are used. (Use only left or right and not l (L) or r (R) to identify the site.)

Allergies to lotions and drugs are important and failure to avoid a particular drug may result in a fatal reaction. It is, however, necessary to elicit what the patient really means by allergy. To some, allergy is feeling sick or unwell and a common allergy to antibiotics is the development of 'thrush' (a fungal infection and not an allergy).

CONDUCT IN THEATRE

Anaesthetic accidents are still much more common than they should be. Although the anaesthetist has the legal responsibility for ensuring that anaesthetic equipment is safe and in working order, the assistant to the anaesthetist is the first person to formally check this equipment. The use of minimal monitoring standards and pre-anaesthetic equipment checklists is clearly laid down by the Association of Anaesthetists and must be followed. Unfortunately, there are some anaesthetists who will readily blame ODPs for any problem resulting from equipment failure. In order to avoid criticism by the Coroner at best and litigation at worst, make sure that all the anaesthetic equipment is properly checked and that the appropriate documentation is completed before the start of an anaesthetic. The positioning of the patient and the management of instruments, needles and swabs are dealt with elsewhere but perhaps the greatest risk occurs when teams change over in the middle of a procedure. If this is done there must be scrupulous attention to the detailed checks before anyone leaves the operating table.

The use of tourniquets is fraught with potential danger. Although the anaesthetist or the anaesthetic assistant inflates the tourniquet, in law the safe use of the device is the responsibility of the surgeon. This includes the inflation pressure (not greater than 100 mmHg above systolic blood pressure) and the continuous inflation time (normally not longer than 90 minutes but there is some variation between the arm and the leg). Perhaps even more dangerous is the use of a digital tourniquet and the digit should be formally checked after the procedure to ensure that the tourniquet has been removed.

This list is by no means exhaustive but merely serves to illustrate ways in which the risk of litigation may be minimized.

THE HOSPITAL COMPLAINTS PROCEDURE ACT 1985

Recent governments have placed great store by the way that complaints are handled and the Patient's Charter has set many of the standards on which these complaints are based. Unfortunately, some members of the legal profession actively encourage patients to sue health authorities in general and doctors in particular. It is therefore important that health professionals are proactive when it comes to the management of complaints by ensuring that standards are met, as far as is possible, and that if there is a complaint, it is dealt with quickly and professionally. Patients are less likely to proceed with litigation if they are given a full explanation and an apology if this is indicated.

The more common types of complaint are listed below.

- Excessive waiting times, e.g. accident and emergency, outpatient clinics, before operations.
- Rudeness or indifference of staff.
- Lack or conflict of information.
- Unexpected death or discharge.
- Negligence or trespass.
- Loss or damage to property.

Patients may complain through a number of different routes:

- NHS Trust.
- Health Authority.
- Community Health Council.

The 'key test' for regulation of a group within the Act is whether there is a "potential for harm arising either from invasive procedures or the application of unsupervised judgement by the professional". ODPs now have the status of true health professionals, having fulfilled the criteria of the 'key test'.

Previously, the members of the Council for Professions Supplementary to Medicine (CPSM) all possessed a recognizable qualification based on an examination. ODPs do not have such an examination but the NVQ route to the qualification has put in place a potentially superior method of continuous assessment with regular testing throughout the qualifying period, thus ensuring a uniform level of achievement. Increasingly, training schools are now associated with a university or college of further education, thus linking the NVQ/SVQ award to a Certificate of Higher Education, which includes not only an examination but also research. The supplementation of theoretical knowledge by regular supervision from professionals in the workplace ensures the acquisition of a qualification entirely appropriate to the needs of a modern health service.

It is the implicit aim of the Consultation Group that the NHS will employ State Registered Professionals in the future. As ODPs take over more roles traditionally undertaken by nurses, managers and other health-care workers, state registration will thus ensure correct regulation. Previously, members of staff from different professional backgrounds and possessing different skills were involved in the perioperative care of the patient but it is inherent in the training of an ODP that they are able to manage all aspects of patient care within the theatre environment. It is for this reason that many nurses and ODAs are now seeking to achieve the ODP qualification and to extend their skills through Additionally Accredited Units. There are some problems, however, not least being the handling of controlled drugs in the operating theatre and beyond but these can and must be addressed by the prospect of both registration and a change in the Misuse of Drugs Regulations.

THE CONTROL OF DRUGS

With this in mind, let us now review the handling of drugs within the hospital environment and determine how the current legislation attempts to protect the patient and carer alike. Unfortunately, drug misuse still occurs within hospitals and both medical and non-medical staff have been implicated. It is important that all theatre workers have a working knowledge of the legislation on drug misuse because sooner or later they may become involved and, as previously stated, ignorance of the law is no defence.

Legally, there must be compliance with the Medicines Act 1968, the Misuse of Drugs Act 1971, the Misuse of Drugs (Safe Custody) Regulations 1973 and the Misuse of Drugs Regulations 1985.

THE MEDICINES ACT 1968

This act controls all aspects of the manufacture and distribution of medicinal products through the Medicines Control Agency. It issues a Product Licence when it is satisfied that the product is inherently safe and that it is produced to an acceptable standard of quality. The licence will also state in what circumstances the product may be used.

A manufacturer is granted a Manufacturer's Licence if they are able to produce a product to an acceptable standard of safety, quality and efficacy and the manufacturer may be a drug company or an NHS hospital. If a product does not have a product licence but has been made by the holder of a manufacturer's licence to the order of a medical practitioner, it is known as a 'Special'. A Prepared Medicine is one that does not have a product licence and has been prepared by somebody not possessing a manufacturer's licence. Usually this is under the supervision of a hospital or retail pharmacist. If a medical practitioner dilutes the drug they are responsible for ensuring the quality of the procedure.

The production of prefilled syringes for patient-controlled analgesia illustrates these differences. Morphine has a product licence for analgesic use but when diluted and used to fill a syringe, it may be either a Special or a Prepared Medicine. The Association of Anaesthetists recommends the following order of preference for prefilled syringes and devices used for patient-controlled analgesia:

1. A licensed medicinal product.
2. A Special produced in a licensed facility.
3. A Prepared Medicine.

The Misuse of Drugs Act 1971 contains three sets of regulations.

1. The Misuse of Drugs Regulations 1985 define five schedules of drugs: Schedule 1 contains drugs deemed to have no medicinal use which are subject to very tight control. This includes raw opium, cannabis and the hallucinogens. Schedule 2 is the most important for operating department practice and covers all the commonly used pharmaceutical opioids and amphetamines. Schedule 3 includes the barbiturates and some slimming preparations. Schedule 4 relates to the benzodiazepines. Schedule 5 deals with products containing Schedule 2 drugs but in much lower concentrations.
2. The Safe Custody Regulation 1973 and the recent amendments deal with drugs in Schedules 2 and 3.
3. The Misuse of Drugs (Notification of a Supply to Addicts).

Existing regulations cover the handling of controlled drugs by pharmacists, medical practitioners and nursing staff but refer to no other personnel. They give specific authority to the sister or acting sister for the time being in charge of a theatre in a hospital or nursing home (or male equivalents) to order or requisition controlled drugs. The regulations also give specific authority to the sister or acting sister for the time being in charge of an operating theatre to possess controlled drugs. This person is also given specific authority to supply the drugs that they are allowed to possess for administration to a patient in theatre, in accordance with the directions of a doctor or dentist.

When these regulations were drawn up the running of operating departments was not in the hands of ODPs and consideration was therefore given to how these theatre workers could be licensed to handle controlled drugs. It must be stressed that the regulations did not specifically exclude ODAs but ignored them, as the need for them to handle controlled drugs was not recognized.

It would appear to be the interpretation of the Home Office that the regulations authorize the possession of controlled drugs by an ODA only where they are engaged in conveying them from one person to another. It is therefore currently legal for an ODA to convey controlled drugs from a theatre sister to an anaesthetist and vice versa (Duthie Report, paragraph 8.6).

In many operating departments, there may not be a "sister or acting sister" present in the department when controlled drugs are required. It is therefore clearly inadequate for an ODP to be authorized solely to convey controlled drugs when they may be the senior person in the department.

The regulations deal with ordering, possessing and supplying controlled drugs but do not mention the custody of keys to 'controlled' drug cabinets. It is, however, the opinion of the Home Office that the "sister or acting sister for the time being in charge of a theatre", having the authority to possess and supply these drugs, would be expected to be responsible for the keys to the controlled drugs cabinet.

In 1994 the Home Office felt that the problem of the handling of controlled drugs should be reviewed along with a new look at the 1985 regulations. A member of the Home Office was quoted as saying, 'We shall give careful consideration to the proposal that ODAs should be enabled to handle controlled drugs in order to take account of current staffing practice within some NHS operating theatres'. The rules governing the handling of controlled drugs within private hospitals are somewhat different but it would be surprising if these were not reviewed as well.

A working group established by the Royal Pharmaceutical Society is at present seeking evidence to assist in a review of guidelines on the safe and secure handling of medicines. This multidisciplinary expert group has been set up under the auspices of the Society's Hospital Pharmacists group to update the Duthie Report and is inviting individuals, groups and organizations to submit oral and/or written evidence for its consideration.

For various reasons the staffing of operating departments has changed in recent years. The rise in the numbers of ODPs has been reflected in the falling number of registered nurses seeking employment in operating theatres. It is not now uncommon for anaesthetic rooms, operating theatres, recovery units, high-dependency units and other key areas, including management, to be staffed by ODPs.

The Misuse of Drugs Regulations 1985 is causing a problem because it is now possible to have a working operating department where the overall theatre manager or the most senior person in the department at the time is a non-nurse. Responsibility for the safe custody and issue of controlled drugs rests with the most senior registered nurse on duty in the department but many units are now 'bending' the rules in order to cover the current situation, not envisaged when these regulations were drawn up.

Some operating departments have several theatres, each of which may have its own controlled drug cabinet. If controlled drugs are to be readily available without delay, control of access to the drugs cabinet may have to be delegated to another member of the team. It is sensible that the person assisting the anaesthetist (the one most likely to require controlled drugs) should be the person holding the key. This is increasingly an ODP and guidelines must therefore be drawn up, which must take account of local circumstances. The Association of Anaesthetists of Great Britain and Ireland (AAGBI), in its publication 'Controlled Drugs', identified some suggested guidelines for operating departments for the handling of controlled drugs. The AAGBI felt that local guidelines should:

• Recognize and adhere to the relevant legal requirements.
• Promote good safe practice.
• Take account of local staffing arrangements.
• Be understood and accepted by all staff.

While there is a great need for national guidelines on the handling of controlled drugs with particular reference to the ODA and ODP, it remains important to develop local guidelines. A recent survey by the AODP (formerly BAODA) looked into the ways in which various departments have solved the problem of drug custody. The solutions employed fell into five broad groups.

1. A locked cupboard is kept in each anaesthetic room with the senior theatre nurse holding the key.
2. A locked cupboard in the anaesthetic room as above but the keys are left available for the ODP or the anaesthetist to gain access.
3. The senior nurse on duty is in the possession of keys for a central controlled drug cupboard. This nurse then issues a stock of drugs to the ODP or anaesthetist sufficient to meet the anticipated needs of all the patients on the operating list. There is also a version of this solution where controlled drugs are checked out on a patient-by-patient basis.
4. A locked cupboard is situated in each anaesthetic room with the keys being handed out to the ODP, as deputy for the senior nurse on duty, at the beginning of the day or list and returned to the senior nurse at the end of the day or list.
5. A locked cupboard is present in each anaesthetic room and the anaesthetic assistant holds the keys. A daily stock check is conducted with a trained nurse.

Difficulties with the custody of controlled drugs are seen by some to flow from problems surrounding accountability. The role of the ODP should be complementary to that of the registered nurse in the operating theatre but at present this is not always possible. The registration of ODPs will, hopefully, circumvent the inequality brought about by the perceived difference in accountability. The current position, where an ODP is permitted in law only to convey drugs but not to order, possess and supply them, is unsatisfactory. Equally unsatisfactory is a system in place in some units where the anaesthetist 'deputizes' for the senior nurse. This practice is unsafe because the anaesthetist is then given extra, inappropriate duties.

The AAGBI is on record as stating that the misuse of drugs regulations 1985 should be amended so that, as well as a sister or acting sister, ODPs may also be specifically authorized and be responsible for possessing and issuing controlled drugs.

RECOMMENDED READING

Joint Sub-Committee of the Standing Medical Advisory Committee and the Standing Nursing Advisory Committee 1970. *The Organisation and Staffing of Operating Departments: A Report.* London: HMSO.

Scott WE, Vickers MD, Draper H eds 1994 *Ethical Issues in Anaesthesia.* Oxford: Butterworth Heinemann.

Association of Anaesthetists of Great Britain and Ireland 1981 London: AAGBI *Report of a Working Party on the use of Controlled Drugs in Operating Theatres.*

2

ASPECTS OF HEALTH AND SAFETY IN THE OPERATING DEPARTMENT

T. Williams

Amongst the wide range of procedures undertaken during an average working day in the operating theatre environment, many either have the potential for causing harm or involve the use of hazardous substances. The necessity for safe practice is obvious but as perception of the problem among theatre workers increases, the real potential degree of this risk becomes apparent.

CROWN IMMUNITY

Crown immunity may have resulted in a lack of awareness and action as, prior to April 1991, hospitals within the NHS had a somewhat optional approach to liability until the implementation of Health and Safety law. Because of this, staff in the clinical areas generally remained unaware of this important and increasingly essential piece of protective legislation. However, their opposite numbers within the industrial sector implemented and developed the intention of the law, which was to create a safe place of work and safe working practices. It is possible, therefore, that some hospital staff were exposed to potential dangers from which workers in the industrial sector were legally protected.

THE HEALTH AND SAFETY AT WORK ACT

All present Health and Safety regulations, codes of practice and guidance arise from the 1974 Health and Safety at Work Act (HASAWA). This Act represented a new concept in legislation intended to protect workers and others from risks at work as well as from dangers that might arise due to work situations. Prior to this act, for many years there had been a group of statutes covering certain industries and occupations, which were partly concerned with safety but were increasingly felt to be inadequate.

The 1972 Robens Report was commissioned to examine the effectiveness of existing legislation and make recommendations for change – hence the introduction of the HASAWA. This brought together the existing statutes while allowing for implementation of new ones, thus creating a uniformity of employee protection across the working population. As a result, approximately eight million more workers gained occupational protection under the law. The 1974 legislation is an "enabling" act, allowing for the relevant government minister, i.e. Minister/Secretary of State for Employment, to add new pieces of safety legislation as and when required, without going through the lengthy process of parliamentary statute law.

Such new proposals are put forward by the Health and Safety Commission (HSC), which is the administrative and policy-making body of the HASAWA. It is composed of representatives from both sides of industry, i.e. The Confederation of British Industry (CBI) and The Trades Union Congress (TUC), in addition to local authority and independent members.

Enforcement is mainly by the Health and Safety Executive (HSE) with additional responsibilities also taken by local and fire authorities. HSE inspectors have wide powers of enforcement of the law by means of Improvement and Prohibition notices backed up by recourse to court action involving fines and/or imprisonment.

An Improvement Notice requires improvement of a potentially dangerous situation within a set timescale, whereas a Prohibition Notice becomes effective immediately and so halts a system or process with serious risk potential.

Staff often wrongly equate or refer to Quality Assurance (QA) and Health and Safety (H&S) as one and the same but for simplicity, QA mostly covers the issues involving service delivery to patients, whereas H&S oversees staff welfare.

H&S law, encompassing regulations, codes of practice and guidance notes, is to some extent a set of common-sense, yet research-based guidelines and ground rules which can aid local policymaking. However, the annually escalating number of work-related accidents and injuries reveals the need for enforcement via legislation, as previously poor safety records have proved that common sense sometimes needs to be enforced when it comes to occupational activity. HASAWA places a legal responsibility on both employers and employees.

Every organization with five or more employees is legally obliged to have a written safety policy and a stated structure for implementing that policy combined with a commitment to convey the policy contents to all staff. Employers must also establish H&S representatives, preferably in each separate work area, giving time for training and monitoring duties. Upon request from these representatives, management must establish a Health and Safety Committee with a functional network for effective communication and liaison.

Many hospitals are now appointing H&S Officers or delegating these duties to a specific person. Traditionally, the Personnel Department held this responsibility through a designated officer who also functioned as chairman of the Safety Committee, liaising with the Safety Representatives and other related committees and departments, i.e. Theatre Users, Infection Control, Medical Physics Laboratories, etc. as well as QA. More recently, the appointment of Risk Managers has become popular. Depending on hospital size, this post can be specific or form part of a Safety Officer's duties. The role involves seeking out practices and areas of potential risk via the system of "Risk Assessment" and in so doing, attempting to prevent accidents before they happen. This contrasts with traditional safety committee procedure, which retrospectively discusses accidents and makes attempts to prevent reoccurrence.

Risk Management is defined by the Medical Defence Union as " an approach designed to identify, assess and reduce risks to patients, staff and visitors with the aim of preventing the expenditure of funds on litigation and so enabling them to be used instead for the improvement of patient care". Carrying out Risk Assessment is also a responsibility of departmental managers. Initially many found this a new and difficult task but reference to various manufacturer and supplier guidelines in the form of "Hazard Data Sheets" has assisted in this responsibility becoming common practice.

H&S management, then, is about the effective control of risk while H&S itself simply involves the creation of safe places, systems and practices within the workplace and, therefore, increasing safety awareness with its benefits and implementation. In the five years since H&S law became compulsory within hospitals, implementation, enforcement and awareness of H&S issues generally have only slowly been adopted in hospital practice. Prior to this a few areas such as kitchens and workshops had already implemented the requirements of the law. There was an understanding with the Department of Health (DOH) that the spirit of the Act would be complied with, but the only remedy open to the HSE was to report serious offenders to the DOH.

Although the original intention of the HASAWA was to control safety and health hazards in specific work areas such as factories and offices, hospitals are no different from many large factories. They encompass diverse systems and processes and therefore possess their own inherent potential for hazard, risk and harm. Safety systems had been in place for some time in certain areas, e.g. X-ray departments, where the post of Radiation Protection Officer has existed for many years. Many hospitals attempted to create similar posts in the more hazardous workplaces such as pathology laboratories, works departments and theatres but until 1991 action was patchy. Even at senior management level, safety committees usually existed on a District basis with very few at the level of local departments.

However, there are positive and welcome signs and theatres appear to be amongst the more progressive departments recognizing the potential for harm in many areas of everyday practice once viewed as risk free. There are very few hospital-based work activities that create such a broad range of potential H&S risks as theatre work, including lifting and handling, exposure to toxic substances, allergic reactions such as latex sensitivity and infection control. The potential for harm is considerable.

Many of the potentially harmful substances used regularly in theatre would be subject to strict controls if and when used in industry and this also applies to the use of stipulated protective clothing and equipment. Similarly, theatre practices, if used in industry, would require intensive sampling and monitoring strategies. The everyday use of chemicals such as glutaraldehyde, atmospheric pollution caused by several suspected harmful anaesthetic gases and agents, contact with potentially dangerous and sensitizing drugs and exposure to the known problems inherent in the use of X-rays and lasers are but a few aspects which serve to highlight this point.

Maybe, in addition to Crown immunity, it was to some extent this industrial image of H&S that prevented its acceptance but no matter how different or exceptional hospital staff perceive their particular roles and situations to be, many duties and procedures equate with industrial practice. Below is a sample of regulations from the HASAWA that could directly apply to theatre work:

- The Ionising Radiation Regulations (1985).
- The Manual Handling Operations Regulations (1992).
- The Personal Protective Equipment Regulations (1992).
- The Provision and Use of Work Equipment Regulations (1992).
- The Health and Safety (Display Screen Equipment) Regulations (1992).
- The Safety Signs Regulations (1980).
- Workplace (Health, Safety and Welfare) Regulations (1992).
- The Management of Health and Safety at Work Regulations (1992).
- The Control of Substances Hazardous to Health Regulations (1988 and 1994).

COSHH is of particular importance to theatre staff as it deals with the control of so many substances used in theatre on a daily basis, e.g. disinfectants and sterilizing agents, hazardous patient waste, diathermy and laser emission, drugs and anaesthetic gases. Staff need to be aware of the addictive, inhalational and contact dangers of some anaesthetic agents as well as the potential harm of creating drug aerosols, so common when drugs are being prepared and drawn up, and alive to the need for Health and Safety implementation in operating theatres. Thus education and training are key aspects of the compulsory Health and Safety policy.

The COSHH regulations require a 'Risk Assessment' of all potentially hazardous substances to be carried out and a statement of the measures taken to control their use, either via substitution, prohibition or the provision of protective equipment. If there is any possible danger of inhalation the assessment should also include atmospheric monitoring, e.g. of anaesthetic gases and glutaraldehyde and solvents, all of which have an inhalational and contact danger.

Risks such as those associated with the use of autoclaves, lifting and handling patients and equipment, working in a continually air-conditioned, temperature-controlled environment and under conditions of artificial and strong lighting also have an applicable regulation/code under the HASAWA. Many larger departments now have their own photocopiers and computer banks but how many staff and managers are aware of the proven dangers, necessary controls and recommendations under the HASAWA? Footwear may be purchased with an eye to fashion as well as anti-static properties but the consequences of dropping objects and 'sharps' onto open-toed sandals may not always be fully appreciated.

The content and intention of the Act are very broad and only a few examples are listed here. The reader is encouraged to carry out their own research for further information so that both trainees and staff may become familiar with potential risks and their control measures. The importance of an early appreciation of health and safety issues is emphasized by the frequency with which the HASAWA is referred to in the National Standards relating to the ODP qualification.

All theatres must aim to have a trained H&S representative who should be a member of or at least report to the Theatre Users Committee. Risk-assessment, monitoring and surveillance of all potentially hazardous substances as well as the provision of ongoing education and training should be as normal and routine as damp-dusting, drug checking and the drill for checking an anaesthetic machine.

The Health and Safety Executive is a most influential body and, following regular hospital inspections, has the authority to close down a department if it considers that there is a significant risk to the well-being of the staff. If it is obvious that a hospital has identified the problem and has developed a remedial strategy, there is likely to be a greater measure of patience in order to see if the problem may be resolved. Such leeway will be in conjunction with a strict timetable and follow-up visits and if the problem is not resolved, departmental closure might be inevitable. In these days of financial stringency the ability to meet the deadlines might be very difficult. Examples of potential problem areas within the theatre complex include glutaraldehyde fume cabinets and the failure to use washing machines for the cleaning of surgical instruments. The HSE works closely with other agencies within and without the hospital. Thus, the recent changes in the law governing the use of sterilizers and the great financial investment needed to bring the hospital to the required standard may actually prevent some trusts from sterilizing their own instruments.

One of the fundamental issues that the HSE will investigate is the induction and ongoing training of the whole workforce. Doctors often think that they know what is needed already but this is no longer acceptable. All the staff must not only be aware of all the relevant safety policies but must also know where that policy may be found and how to carry it out. In fact, it is very likely that future HSE visits will concentrate on the staff who may be potentially ignorant and this certainly includes the medical personnel.

In the current era of litigation, trusts need to be as proactive as possible in minimizing the threat of legal action. One way in which this may be accomplished is by means of the Clinical Negligence Scheme for Trusts (CNST). The CNST has a number of different levels of achievement, with Level 1 accreditation being the easiest. Risk management and health and safety issues feature very strongly in this accreditation process.

Listed below are some of the more important issues that will be investigated during an HSE inspection.

- The roles, responsibilities and accountability of the various risk management and health and safety committees, including relationships to other relevant committees such as the Control of Infection Committee.
- Availability and situation of documentation relating to policies and procedures.
- Awareness by all staff of the situation and content of these policies and procedures.
- Protocols and mechanisms for managing and recording accidents to the workforce and the patient, e.g. needle stick injuries.
- Induction and training for all staff, including doctors, and the methods for recording this.

- Potential hazards within the working environment, identified by staff members or by direct inspection.

In summary, health and safety is a very wide and diverse field but if applicable H&S guidelines form the basis of departmental policies and procedures, high-quality, effective, safe and legal practice will minimize injuries to staff and reduce the possibility of litigation.

RECOMMENDED READING

Chard C. 1993 *Health and Safety for Nurses*. London: Chapman and Hall

Dewis, M. 1995 *Tolley's Health and Safety at Work Handbook*. Croydon:Tolley.

Health Services Advisory Committee. 1995 *Anaesthetic Agents: Controlling Exposure Under COSHH*. Sheffield: HSC.

Health and Safety Executive. 1995 *EH.40: Occupational Exposure Limits*. Sheffield: HSE

Holt A.,1993 *Principles of Health and Safety at Work*. Leicester: IOSHH.

Stranks, J. 1994 *Handbook Of Health and Safety Practice*. London: Pitman Publishing.

3

THE CARING PRACTITIONER

A. Davey

THE COMPLEXITIES OF CARE

Care may be defined as "providing for physical needs, help or comfort" (*Collins English Dictionary*) and carers may also be thought of as part of the framework of our human experience. Examples of both abound in our daily lives.

Care is partly instinctive but can be enhanced and developed by experience, education and effort. It is not and never has been the prerogative of one section of society, professional group or role holder and there are as many varieties of care and carers as there are people and situations.

Nevertheless, the research and theory underpinning modern concepts of care and their subsequent development into frameworks for practice have all originated from the nursing profession. Although much of the phraseology therefore inevitably refers to "nurses" or "nursing", this does not preclude the translation of the ideals, beliefs and values at its core to the practitioner's sphere of practice.

Care itself has many facets worth exploring but it should always be continuous, individualized, patient centred, needs-based and collaborative.

Perioperative care includes pre-, intra- and postoperative phases and involves every member of the multidisciplinary team (ideally this includes the patient) and must be planned, demonstrable and communicable.

In order to deliver care in a holistic way, carers need to be able to view those for whom they care as unique and complex beings whose goals and outcomes are ultimately determined by their individual needs and problems. It is also essential for carers to perceive, relate to and take account of the psychological and social aspects of problems as well as their more evident physical manifestations.

These requirements assume an ever-increasing importance in the current climate which affects our Health Service. Each Trust has a responsibility:

- To deliver an acceptable, affordable level of service;
- For strategies of Risk Management;
- For Clinical Audit.

All these are influenced by the impact of market forces, the Patient's Charter and the rising awareness and expectations of service users and purchasers. The political emphasis may change but the basic concepts will always be present.

THEORETICAL SOURCES AND CONCEPTUAL ORIGINS

It is one of the acknowledged marks of any profession that its senior members should evaluate current practice, explore prevailing methods and continually seek ways to improve what is done. This may be achieved through the development of new strategies and striving via evolving patterns of work to match the changing needs of their client group.

The application of such professional criteria prompted eminent nursing theorists to search for ways to define, describe and document the complex area of care and its delivery. To explain their conclusions they developed several theoretical models, which were then used to construct a conceptual framework upon which good practice could be designed and built. This may be compared to the way in which an architectural team produces a scaled-down model of a finished building in order to demonstrate the desired final outcome. In this way the prospective purchaser is able to understand the underpinning architectural ideas. Having produced the model the team then 'translates' the ideas into a conceptual framework, i.e. a detailed architectural plan from which the builders can accurately begin construction to predetermined specifications. From this emerges an end product, which everyone can understand and use.

MODELS OF CARE

The starting point for every care model is the perception of the patient as a unique and holistic individual who has specific care needs, which are based upon actual or potential problems. Actual problems include pain and loss of function or deformity while potential problems, such as postoperative vomiting, immobility and the fear of unconsciousness, may be compounded by one or more aspects of the human experience of life. These may be physical (pain), psychological (fear), social (absence from or inability to work) or spiritual (separation from loved ones).

Problems can rarely be confined to one category and are nearly always complex and interactive. Thus anxiety, though a common psychological problem, may be held to be socially unacceptable and its suppression may produce the physical effects of nausea, tension, sweating and pallor. Depending upon immediate circumstances the individual's character, culture, upbringing and current state of health assume greater or lesser importance and can thus be prioritized as these variables interchange.

The theorists expressed their ideas using three main types of model, which are described below.

DEVELOPMENTAL MODELS

Developmental models visualize an individual progressing along a line (or up a slope). As the most basic needs are met they can fulfil other 'higher' needs. In its simplest form, this is called the **Health Continuum** and is expressed as an uninterrupted line with illness at one end and well-being at the other (Fig 3.1.).

Slightly more complex is Maslow's Hierarchy of Needs, (Fig. 3.2) where basic requirements of life must be met before any of the more personal and developmental goals can be achieved.

INTERACTION MODELS

The Interaction Model deals with the effects of role expectation and role fulfilment on an individual's behaviour as they take part in the multiple interactions of daily life and the degree to which they can cope with these influences on their personality. This type of model is frequently utilized in the psychiatric field.

SYSTEMS MODELS

Systems Models focus on the interdependence of body systems and the interplay of the various 'stressors', defence mechanisms and resistance factors. 'Stressors' may penetrate to varying levels of the system, ultimately affecting the function of the whole.

A framework may be built using a combination of theoretical principles which then becomes an Eclectic Model, such as Orem's which has been adapted and amended to suit particular care settings.

THE CARE PROCESS

The Conceptual Framework emerging from the models of care described by the theorists was translated into action via a process approach. This inevitably became known as The Nursing Process but in fact process is a strategy employed in many other fields (e.g.

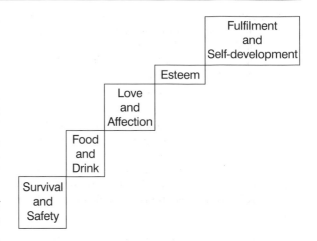

Figure 3.2   Maslow's hierarchy of needs

the learning process, the manufacturing process and the assessment process) involving as it does a systematic, cyclical approach through interdependent and sequential stages.

The care process can be visualized as a continuous cycle of assessing, planning, implementing and evaluating care with the patient always as the central focus of the cycle. Information recorded at each stage creates a vital link between the various stages and each leads the carer from the previous one to the next (Fig 3.3.).

This approach facilitates the use of information gathered from the evaluation of interventions (care actions) to inform future care delivery, thus encouraging the establishment of research-based practice. It

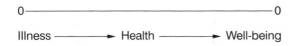

Figure 3.1   The health continuum.

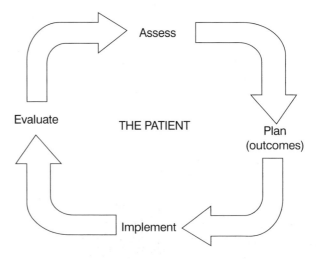

Figure 3.3   The process of care.

further fulfils the criteria for care mentioned earlier, i.e. individualized, continuous, patient centred, needs-based, collaborative and communicable. For care to be collaborative it must be communicable and therefore must be recorded clearly, concisely and in a form that is accessible to the whole team.

Despite traditional controversy, care has always been a function of operating theatre staff within the theatre suite and its practice has never been limited to the confines of Recovery Rooms and Reception Areas. However, this perception can be readily understood when we reflect that it is largely only in those areas that the recording of interventions is readily observable or routinely undertaken.

Only in exceptional cases is the systematic recording of a care process an integral part of the perioperative experience (scene). The recording of patients' problems (needs) has more frequently been fragmented and communicated only in a limited and somewhat haphazard way. This often amounts to not much more than a series of unconnected entries or checklists with reception, anaesthetic room, surgical and recovery staff all "ticking off" or filling in their respective documents which remain independent, incohesive and uncoordinated. Whilst each constitutes a valuable safeguard, such records hardly comprise a systematic approach to care.

THE STAGES OF THE PROCESS

ASSESSMENT

The starting point for any establishment of needs, without which planning can have no firm basis, involves high levels of communication skills such as active listening and attending. It requires an understanding of the conceptual framework provided by model theory, which will assist in the interpretation and prioritization of the individual needs and problems of each patient as well as the ability to view the patient holistically. Information about a patient may be gathered using a variety of sources and methods:

1. The patient.
2. The medical records or case sheet.
3. The ward care plan.
4. The relevant clinical personnel.
5. Patients' relatives and friends.

Much of the information gleaned will be in the familiar written or spoken format and is therefore easily accessed and recorded. Less obvious but equally potent can be all the nuances of non-verbal communication, which are particularly relevant to the usually anxiety-ridden preoperative period. The observation and interpretation of these clues are important skills to be developed by practitioners.

Whilst second-hand data about a patient may be gathered from records and staff, there can be no substitute for the detailed information about a patient's concerns, which can be collected and recorded in a preoperative visit or interview. This may be conducted by theatre staff in the days or hours preceding an operation and should be in a structured format designed to both give and receive information surrounding the patient, the procedures and outcomes.

Fundamental to the delivery of continued, patient-centred and collaborative care is this two-way information exchange. Its effectiveness in increasing patient satisfaction, reducing the length of hospital stay and improving relationships at all levels is well documented. This structured way of receiving information, being involved in discussing goals and outcomes and participating in the development of their own plan of care, is a proactive role well suited to allaying the anxieties and lowering stress levels of the preoperative patient.

The ideal would be a preoperative visit for every patient but this is not realistic because of the increased pressure of work within theatre suites, the decreasing time inpatients spend in hospital and the limited allocation of resources. Nevertheless, the benefits derived from and the skills developed by such strategies should not be discarded because they are too costly to constitute a significant part of daily routine. The promotion of good practice and the preservation of ideal standards of care should be actively pursued by professionals, especially in the guidance and preparation of future practitioners.

The information collected and recorded through the methods outlined above must be related to the priority of safety and survival, upon which the fulfilment of all other needs is dependent. Thus the presence of chronic obstructive airway disease (COAD) will be relatively more important than, for example, anxieties about appearance and the loss of dignity (no teeth, no make-up, strange clothing, etc.), although this may not be the perception of the patient.

A number of problems derive from the psychological aspect of inpatient (and possibly day-case) experiences. These include such things as strange surroundings, disrupted routines, the suspension of many of the normal rights and choices and strange and unknown people. Equally, the sense of vulnerability and loss of control, feelings of homesickness and loneliness due to separation at such a critical point are no less real for being almost universal. All these may cause anxiety, which is exacerbated in the very young, the elderly or in those with communication difficulties and may be especially hard to discern and express.

Similarly fear of outcomes, whether of a diagnostic, surgical or anaesthetic nature, will frequently remain undisclosed to all but the most skilled interviewer. Nevertheless, such fears are able to influence the emotional and psychological status of the patient at this difficult time. Giving the patient the opportunity to discover and describe problems, priorities and goals in partnership mobilizes their involvement with care delivery and encourages the development of the individual's personal coping mechanisms.

PLANNING

The information gathered from a preoperative visit or interview is used to determine the actions, preparations and/or conditions, which will be required during the intraoperative period in order to achieve an identified set of desired outcomes or goals based on the established priority of needs.

Because many potential problems are common to all patients undergoing anaesthesia and surgery they will be catered for by the routine arrangements designed to cope with or prevent such events. These strategies have become translated into the policies and procedures which underpin good practice in every operating department. Figure 3.4 briefly illustrates this point but the list is infinite.

However, there are many potential and actual problems/needs identified during the preoperative assessment which will require a more individualized approach to the planning of care activities. For example, due to a diminished response to hypoxia, the

patient with COAD would not be given the same oxygen therapy as a patient without respiratory disease. The planned action for this patient would ensure Controlled Oxygen Therapy. Similarly a patient's identified allergy might lead to an alteration to routine treatment or use of equipment. Cultural or religious influences may also have an effect on routine procedures.

The setting of goals and the design of actions to achieve them have implications for the collaborative and continued aspects of care delivery. In summary the plan should:

- Be communicable to all members of the multidisciplinary team in an
- Accessible, agreed format which will
- Coordinate the documentation of all relevant data about the individual episode of care but will
- Allow for the subsequent evaluation of the process and
- Provide a recorded proof of planned and delivered care.

IMPLEMENTATION AND EVALUATION

The complex nature of events within the intraoperative period has inevitably led to their traditional perception as a series of distinct procedural stages through which the patient progresses in sequence (reception, anaesthesia, surgery, recovery). The recording of care diminishes this fragmentary approach by using a structured format, which shares goals and increases team communication. An awareness of the scope, limitations and interdependence of roles within the multidisciplinary team is also heightened.

Potential problem	Action	Outcome
Infection of wound	*Aseptic technique* Panorama of cleaning and sterilizing procedures and policies to prevent cross infection	Clean uninfected wound. Healing without delay – minimal discomfort to patient
Secretions, blood, vomit, etc. occluding airway	Suction apparatus checked and to hand Head-down tilt available on trolley/table	Immediate clearance of fluid from airway No complications of occlusion or inhalation
Hypoxia following haemorrhage or respiratory depression	Oxygen is ready for administration	Return to and maintenance of normal O_2 and perfusion until homoeostasis is reestablished

Figure 3.4   Routine procedures for anaesthesia and surgery

Adjustments to the plan are made and recorded in response to changing patient needs by the relevant team members. This provides a foundation for estimating the effectiveness of the care delivered both immediately for the individual patient and for an eventual wider review to inform future practice through Audit.

Evaluative judgements are made throughout the implementation period (especially if the patient is conscious and able to contribute) and continue in the postoperative phase when physiological parameters are used to update the plan and monitor the patient's progress towards recovery from anaesthesia and/or surgery.

Records of observations, patient interaction and interventions, when recorded as part of the care plan, reinforce and demonstrate the continuity of care and facilitate a description of the total care delivered by the team when the patient is transferred to the care of the ward staff at handover. This structured information, together with details for the future management of the patient, enhances the coherence of care and encourages the development of cooperative management of the inpatient episode as a unified whole.

Final evaluation of the effectiveness of care delivered in the perioperative period can best be gained from a postoperative visit or interview. This allows feedback from the patient to be added to clinical data in order to give a valid appraisal of the degree to which the goals were achieved. Positive feedback from such an exercise is, of course, rewarding and reassuring but it is from the analysis of negative results that future practice can benefit, especially when the team approach to the setting and maintenance of standards of care is utilized effectively.

RECORDS OF CARE

The response to the tide of change within health-care practice is immensely variable and encompasses degrees of adaptation and development from simple amalgamation of a number of documents (checklists) to a radical reorganization of the whole approach to the management of every inpatient episode. Just as the most widely used model of care is likely to be an eclectic one, so care documents tend to develop and evolve and may emerge in one of the following styles.

STANDARD OR CORE THEATRE CARE PLANS

Standard or core theatre plans follow a checklist format and are designed to identify which of the potential problems common to all patients undergoing anaesthesia or surgery is applicable to an individual on a particular occasion. Standard care plans save time and are easy to use, but address neither the uniqueness of the patient nor the integral nature of the perioperative period within the wider inpatient experience. They can, however, readily be adapted to a more individualized approach by the provision of additional space for particularly relevant comments.

CARE PATHWAYS

Care pathways have been described by some writers as a multidisciplinary approach to the design, quality and delivery of care. In their purest form they are expressions of the anticipated pattern of care which would be given to a typical patient with a specific diagnosis (e.g. hip replacement) and may run from admission to discharge and on into return to community care (integrated care pathways). They seek to map out the expected interventions, treatment and outcomes for every discipline involved in the care of the patient in a seamless flow so that everyone, including the patient, knows what to expect and when. Care pathways provide for coordinated recording of every event as it occurs and deviations from the norm are marked as variances. It is from the analysis of these variances that the planning team will adjust or amend the common pathway.

There are many documented advantages to the employment of care pathways, not least of which is that their design, development and use bring members of the team together in strategies to define and maintain standards of care, whilst identifying and limiting costs. Working together and sharing documentation reduce duplication and fragmentation improve communication and understanding and raise awareness of quality issues. Despite the proclaimed and undeniable benefits of meticulous care documentation, it is important to keep in mind the importance of care itself over its recording. Whatever method is used and whichever documentary style adopted, cost effectiveness and ease of operation will be important factors in viability and survival.

The National Occupational Standards require the production of care records and the attendant rationale by every student practitioner. Good practice would seem to imply the continued application of acquired skills to the management of care within the perioperative period. This would be consistent with the improvement in standards and reduction of risks so relevant to current health developments. Examples of care documents can be found in Appendix 3.

4

STRATEGIES FOR INFECTION CONTROL IN THE OPERATING DEPARTMENT

A. Deane

PRINCIPLES OF INFECTION

We live in harmony with millions of microbes that exist in the environment, on our skin and in our alimentary tracts and mucous membranes. Very few of these microorganisms are pathogenic (cause disease) and infection will only occur if there is an imbalance between the environment, the human host and commensal (normal) microbes.

Individuals requiring surgery are particularly vulnerable to infection. In most cases, invasive surgery breaches the physical barriers to infection (skin and mucous membranes) and also causes stress to the body, both psychologically and physiologically. A high level of stress is known to suppress the immune system, thus increasing the likelihood of postoperative infection.

Endogenous (self-infection) infection occurs if microorganisms that normally exist harmlessly in one part of an individual's body transfer to another site on the same individual where they can become pathogenic. Exogenous (cross-infection) infections are caused by pathogens from a source other than an individual's own body. To prevent cross-infection in theatres, staff must be committed to the implementation of an infection control strategy that seeks to achieve three aims:

1. To control or remove the organism.
2. To eliminate methods of cross-infection.
3. To protect the population from infection.

THE CHAIN OF INFECTION

The series of components that must be present for infection to occur have been described as the chain of infection. There are five links in this 'chain':

1. Source of infection.
2. Reservoir.
3. Mode of transmission.
4. Individual at risk.
5. Portal of entry.

Infection control is based on disrupting or breaking one or more links in the chain.

SOURCES OF INFECTION

The invading organism or causative agent is a microbe that may be a bacterium, virus, fungus or parasite.

RESERVOIR

This is the environment in which the organism thrives.

There are three important reservoirs of infection within the operating department:

1. Humans (staff, patients and others).
2. Environment.
3. Equipment.

MODE OF TRANSMISSION

Micro-organisms can spread from one point to another via another agent or 'vehicle'. There are three ways in which infection can spread within theatres:

1. By direct or indirect contact.
2. Airborne.
3. Via a vector (e.g. glove powder).

Undoubtedly, the most important mode of microorganism spread is on the hands of theatre staff. Hands are the part of the body in most frequent contact with the environment and therefore the most likely to transmit infection.

INDIVIDUALS AT RISK

Infection following entry of microbes into the body will depend on many factors including general health, age, gender, immune status, the dosage and exposure of an infectious agent and inherent susceptibility. In recent years, infection control has focused on staff as well as patient protection, with particular emphasis on infection transmitted via blood and body fluids.

PORTAL OF ENTRY

Microorganisms may enter the body of a susceptible host through a natural orifice or a break in the skin or mucous membranes. Entry of microbes may occur following trauma or surgically invasive procedures.

THE PHYSICAL ENVIRONMENT

The operating department is designed to facilitate the movement of patients, personnel and materials as efficiently as possible to assist in the containment of infection. For this purpose, modern theatre complexes are divided into three distinctive zones that are usually located away from the general traffic and air movement within the hospital.

1. The *dirty zone* (unrestricted area) which often includes a central control area and access point for the removal of theatre waste. Normal clothing can be worn within this area.
2. The *clean/protective zone* (semirestricted area) which includes staff changing rooms, anaesthetic and

recovery rooms, storage areas for clean and sterile supplies, work areas for storage and processing of instruments and corridors to the restricted areas. Access to this zone is limited to authorized personnel and the patient. Both groups are normally required to wear approved theatre clothing.

3. The *sterile zone* (restricted area) includes the preparation rooms, operating theatres and scrub areas. Surgical attire, including hats and possibly masks, should be worn in this area at all times. (The value of wearing masks for patient protection remains a contentious issue.)

Theatre walls, ceiling and floor finishes should be impervious to bacteria and able to withstand frequent wet chemical cleaning. Curved joints between walls, ceilings and floors facilitate effective cleaning and drying.

Surface areas in theatres are normally damp dusted daily prior to the start of the first operating session. Cleaning solutions used for this purpose vary from hospital to hospital and therefore the theatre practitioner is advised to become familiar with the local damp dusting policy. If a sodium hypochlorite solution has been recommended, it should be remembered that because of the corrosive nature of this chemical, metal surfaces would need to be rinsed prior to drying. The undersurfaces of operating lights, which will be located directly above the open wound and often adjusted during procedures, require particular attention in order to keep them clean and dust free.

Effective ventilation minimizes the risk of airborne contamination within the theatre complex. Modern ventilation systems provide positive pressure ventilation and 25 filtered air changes per hour. Airflow is directed from clean to less clean areas. Ultraclean airflow canopies, which have the capacity to provide up to 400 air changes per hour, are frequently employed in orthopaedic theatres. Studies have shown that orthopaedic prostheses have a propensity to become infected, so an ultraclean environment is created to minimize the risk of airborne infection. Keeping theatre doors closed to prevent backflow of air into clean areas, restricting numbers of personnel within the operating theatre to essential staff and minimizing movement around the area also assist in reducing the risk of airborne infection.

The level of humidity is another environmental factor that can be controlled by theatre staff; it has been noted that humidified air levels of 50–60% suppress bacterial growth.

PERSONNEL PREPARATION

The operating department has been described as a high-risk environment because of the increased possibility of contact with blood and body fluids from splashing or aerosols and potential injury from needles, blades and sharp instruments. Therefore, staff training and regular updating on infection control and health and safety (see Chapter 2) are both important issues. Theatre staff and others who undertake exposure-prone procedures (EPP workers) must be immunized against hepatitis B. According to the Department of Health, those who refuse to comply will not be allowed to continue EPP work.

Attention to personal cleanliness and removal of all jewellery (which can harbour microbes) are important factors in the minimization of microorganisms within the theatre environment. When changing out of personal clothing into freshly laundered pantsuits (which cause less air disturbance than skirts), it is advisable to don a theatre cap or hood before the suit top. This sequence reduces the risk of carrying loose hairs on theatre clothing and subsequently shedding them in clean areas. The hair is commonly contaminated with *Staphylococcus aureus* and must therefore be completely covered by effective headgear. Designated, antistatic-soled theatre shoes should cover the toes to protect them from the risk of injury from dropped 'sharps'. The advantages of wearing autoclavable theatre shoes are now widely recognized.

Personnel with upper respiratory tract infections or weeping skin lesions should seek the advice of the Occupational Health Department before entering the theatre complex. Broken skin on exposed areas should be covered with occlusive waterproof dressings. Less obvious skin breaks on the hands are identified by using an alcohol skin disinfecting preparation because the resultant stinging sensation effectively locates areas of broken skin.

The value of wearing surgical facemasks is debatable. Some studies suggest that masks increase the shedding of *Staphylococcus aureus* from the cheeks and neck, while another hypothesis suggests that discarding masks causes contaminated nasal and oral droplets to atomize and remain airborne. It therefore appears that the primary reason for using facemasks is to protect the surgical team from infected blood. If worn, the facemask should fit snugly over nose and mouth. On removal, it should be handled by the tapes only and discarded directly into a waste container. Used masks should not be worn around the neck or screwed up and placed into the pockets of theatre clothing.

UNIVERSAL INFECTION CONTROL PRECAUTIONS WITHIN THE OPERATING DEPARTMENT

The hazards of human immunodeficiency virus (HIV) and the hepatitis viruses (HBV, HCV and more recently HGV) are well documented. The methods of preventing accidental exposure to these potentially serious infections are known as Universal Infection Control Precautions.

Universal precautions, also known as blood and body fluid precautions, were originally recommended when a patient was known to be or suspected to be infected with bloodborne pathogens. However, because we do not know which individuals may be infected, these standard infection control precautions should be consistently used for all patients. These safeguards protect both staff and patients.

HANDWASHING

Handwashing techniques are often inadequate. Studies have indicated that the cleaning product selected is less important than the quality of the handwashing and drying technique. The friction generated by thorough cleansing of all hand surface areas can remove the majority of resident and transient organisms on the skin. Use of an antiseptic detergent solution such as chlorhexidine will assist in reducing the number of remaining organisms. Due to the residual activity of chlorhexidine, it continues to inactivate microorganisms for some time after application and is therefore superior to soap and water. Handwashing takes place before and after patient contact, following removal of protective clothing, immediately following contamination with blood or body fluids and after handling contaminated or potentially contaminated articles.

PROTECTIVE CLOTHING

Once worn, items of protective clothing become vehicles of infection and must therefore be disposed of in accordance with local policy.

GLOVES

Intact, disposable gloves provide a physical barrier against pathogen transmission. Surgical gloves, however, do not protect the wearer from 'sharps' injury (e.g. scalpel blade, needles, etc.). Non-sterile latex gloves are worn by circulating staff in contact with contaminated and potentially contaminated materials such as specimens, body fluid spills, used swabs, linen, instruments and equipment. Although the effectiveness of latex as a barrier has been proved, manufacturers are developing non-latex products in response to increasing reports of latex allergy among wearers and patients who require frequent surgical intervention.

EYE PROTECTION

Scrub team members wear spectacles, goggles or visors to protect their eye membranes from infected splash or aerosol contaminants. Even in relatively bloodless procedures the goggles of team members may have obvious blood splashes on them. Other staff should also wear eye protection when there is a risk of contamination.

GOWNS

Disposable gowns made of material impermeable to bacteria and fluids afford staff the greatest protection. However, despite a wealth of literature that condemns the use of linen gowns in high-exposure areas, many operating departments are still routinely using linen products. (This may be due to the high cost of disposable materials.) It is common for these areas to have a separate policy that advocates the use of disposable gowns and drapes for the management of patients with a proven infection. Until universal precautions become truly universal, the linen gown wearers may protect their torsos from the blood and body fluids of patients by using plastic aprons underneath the gown.

SHARPS

Extreme care must be taken when handling and disposing of sharps because percutaneous (skin penetration) exposure to bloodborne pathogens carries a higher risk than that of mucocutaneous (involving mucous membranes and non-intact skin). Sharps must not be left lying around. Disposable sharps (e.g. needles, blades, electrosurgical tips and pins) should be discarded into a safe container immediately after use. Needles must not be bent, broken or resheathed. Whenever possible, the needle and syringe should be disposed of as one unit. Used suture needles and blades should be retained on magnetic, foam or sticky pads during surgical procedures and disposed of directly into a sharps container that conforms to British Standard 7320. Sharps bins should be sealed when three-quarters full, thus preventing possible injury from overflowing and protruding needles.

One American study suggests that sharps injuries can occur in as many as 7% of surgical procedures, so the scrub practitioner must take great care to avoid stab injury when handling sharp instruments. Some scrub staff have adopted an approach whereby scalpels and other small sharp instruments are passed to the surgeon in a receiver and returned to the scrub practitioner via the same route. The risk to non-immunized health-care workers following percutaneous exposure to hepatitis B virus from an infected patient is approximately 1:3. Although the risk to staff of becoming infected with HIV via the same route is 1:200, it should be remembered that as yet, there is no immunization or effective treatment available for those who subsequently develop AIDS. Theatre staff must be aware of the correct procedure to follow in the event of a needlestick or sharps injury and ensure all such injuries are reported to the senior person on duty. If an injury does occur the following sequence should be carried out.

1. Encourage the puncture wound to bleed under running water.
2. Wash the wound thoroughly with water and antiseptic detergent.
3. Cover the site with an occlusive waterproof dressing.
4. Note the patient's name.
5. Retain the sharp if possible.
6. Report to the departmental manager.
7. Complete an accident form.
8. Arrange for blood samples to be taken from yourself and from the patient.

WASTE DISPOSAL

Waste materials within the operating department can be classified as follows.

DOMESTIC

Non-clinical materials, which have not been in contact with blood or body fluids, e.g. paper, food remains. Domestic waste is placed into black plastic bags and, like normal household refuse, ends up at landfill sites.

CLINICAL

Any disposable material, other than 'sharps', which is contaminated with blood or body fluids, e.g. swabs, disposable gowns and drapes. These items are placed into yellow plastic bags and left for incineration according to local policy. Double bagging may be necessary.

Waste disposal bags should be no more than three-quarters full and the tops should be folded down and secured with plastic ties or clips. Securing bags by tying knots in them should be avoided to prevent one's hands from becoming contaminated.

BLOOD AND BODY FLUIDS

Whenever possible, the quantity and handling of these substances should be kept to a minimum, thereby reducing the risks from bloodborne infections. Blood and body fluids are normally collected in rigid, closed disposable suction units. Following use, these units are sealed and placed into specific containers which maintain the unit in an upright position. The containers, which are often provided by the unit manufacturers, are stored in designated areas until they are transported to the incinerator for disposal. Where reusable glass or plastic jar systems exist, the contents may be treated with a recommended sodium hypochlorite solution before being gently poured into the sluice. Care must be taken to avoid splashes and protective clothing, including eyewear, should be worn during this procedure. The jars may then be transported to the Sterile Services Department for cleaning and disinfecting. It should be remembered that suction tubing is also a potential infection hazard and therefore requires careful handling.

Spillage of blood and body fluid should be dealt with promptly. The wet area may be covered with disposable paper towels or treated with a sprinkling of sodium hypochlorite granules. Although both methods enable absorption of excess fluid to take place, sodium hypochlorite granules will also inactivate bloodborne viruses. If the spillage has dried, perhaps because it occurred in a location which was not immediately accessible, e.g. under the operating table, the area can be covered with disposable paper towels which have been soaked with a solution of sodium hypochlorite. Once the area has been rehydrated, the debris should be cleared up with gloved hands and treated as clinical waste.

When waste has been disposed of in the correct manner, attention to hand hygiene is of paramount importance in preventing cross-infection.

CONTROL OF SUBSTANCES HAZARDOUS TO HEALTH (COSHH)

In 1989, regulations involving COSHH became law. Regulation 6 requires that 'An employer shall not carry out any work which is liable to expose any employees to any substances hazardous to health unless he/she has made suitable and sufficient assessment of the risk . . . and of the steps to be taken'. As microorganisms, viruses and other infectious agents are included within the meaning of a substance hazardous to health, it is important that all staff working in high-risk areas have a full understanding of how to protect patients, colleagues and themselves within this clinical setting. Both employer and employee have a legal responsibility in this respect. Thus, if the employee does not take advantage of the protection provided, the employer may not be held responsible (see also Chapter 2).

ESTABLISHING AND MAINTAINING A STERILE FIELD

Members of the scrubbed team have a responsibility to provide and maintain a safe environment for the patient. Techniques employed by the practitioner to prepare for entry into the sterile field should be of the highest standard. Surgical hand hygiene, commonly referred to as 'scrubbing up', is performed prior to invasive surgery. Although local procedure will guide acceptable practice for each theatre department, the general principles of surgical hand hygiene are as follows.

1. Fingernails are kept short, clean and nail-varnish free, thus reducing the potential number of organisms.
2. Warm water is adjusted to a steady gentle flow to prevent wetting of theatre clothing or floor.
3. Hands are held higher than elbows at all times to prevent them becoming contaminated by water droplets from the arms.
4. Throughout the procedure care is taken to prevent touching taps or other contaminated articles.
5. Following thorough social washing from hands to elbows, rinsing begins at the fingertips and flows towards the elbows.
6. A sterile nail brush containing a measure of antiseptic detergent is used to scrub the nails only and is then discarded.
7. Systematic washing in antiseptic detergent from fingertips to elbows occurs for a minimum of two minutes.
8. Water is gently dispelled from elbows to sink and care is taken to prevent it from dripping onto the floor.

When the practitioner has completed thorough and effective surgical hand hygiene, they should don a sterile surgical gown and sterile gloves before entering the sterile field. To reduce the risk of contamination when gloving, it is recommended that a closed gloving technique be employed. Use of this method ensures that bare hands do not come in contact with the gown. Hands remain within the sleeves of the gown until the gloves have been manipulated over the cuff area. Wearing two pairs of sterile gloves (i.e. double gloving) may be recommended for some surgical procedures in accordance with local policy. For wearer comfort and ease of application, it is useful to select gloves which are one half size larger when donning a second pair. The integrity of gowns and gloves should be inspected before touching sterile equipment or the sterile field.

During movement from scrub area to instrument trolley, the practitioner's hands should remain within the 'sterile square', i.e. clasped above waist level. The shoulders, axillae and cuffed sections of the gown are areas of friction and should therefore be considered non-sterile. As it is not possible for the scrubbed practitioner to supervise the back of a surgical gown, this area should be considered contaminated. If it is necessary for adjacent members of the scrub team to change places during surgery, they should do so by moving back to back to prevent contact between sterile and contaminated areas of surgical gowns.

Surgical instruments, items and sterile equipment should be prepared just before use, thus minimizing the time of exposure to airborne contaminants. The circulating practitioner should inspect the outer packaging of sterile items for tears or moisture. If the integrity of outer wrapping is compromised, the item should be discarded. Expiry dates on packaging and lotions should also be checked before the contents are offered to the scrub practitioner.

When the patient has been positioned on the operating table, the scrub practitioner wheels the prepared instrument trolleys into the area, taking care not to place them too close to the undraped patient or any object which may contaminate them.

The incision site is cleaned with an antiseptic solution before the sterile drapes are positioned over the patient. Drapes require minimal handling and should not cause undue disturbance of airborne particles. Once the drapes have been secured, the scrub practitioner should draw the instrument trolleys into an accessible position within the sterile field. Scrubbed members of the team function within the sterile field. Non-scrubbed staff should remain outside this field. As additional sterile items are required, they are unwrapped by the circulating practitioner and passed to the scrub practitioner without contamination.

Heavy or sharp objects have the potential to penetrate protective barriers and must therefore be presented with care and opened on a separate sterile surface. Surgical instruments used on contaminated body tissues or substances e.g. inner surface of bowel or pus, should be isolated in a separate container following use.

If the scrub practitioner is familiar with the operative procedure he/she can accurately anticipate what is required for the patient at each stage during surgical intervention. A smooth and rapid surgical episode reduces undue exposure of an open wound to airborne contaminants and may therefore reduce the possibility of postoperative infection.

THE COST OF INFECTION

The cost of infection acquired within the operating department can be discussed at both human and financial levels. In human terms, the cost to the patient may include pain, suffering, prolonged hospital stay or worry about taking more time away from work, school or college. These stressful events may also have a disruptive effect on the lives of the patient's family who continue to visit their relative in hospital or on work colleagues who share the burden of the workload while the patient is absent. If a patient remains in hospital longer than would normally be expected, other patients may have their planned admissions cancelled because there are no beds for them.

The financial cost of hospital-acquired infection has an adverse effect on the health-care budget. Drugs, laboratory tests, further surgery, prolonged hospital stay or the need for care in the community, are expensive commodities which impact on already overstretched resources.

All theatre staff must understand the principles of infection control and consistently adhere to local policies and procedures. Preventing accidental transmission of infectious microorganisms in the operating department is a priority in ensuring a safe and healthy environment for patients, staff and others.

RECOMMENDED READING

Bowell B. 1993 Preventing Infection and its Spread, Surgical Nurse, 6(2), 5–12.

British Orthopaedic Association 1992 *Guidelines for the Prevention of Cross-Infection between Patients and Staff in Orthopaedic Operating Theatres with Special Reference to HIV and the Blood-borne Hepatitis Viruses*, 2nd ed. London: British Orthopaedic Association.

Fay M F. 1996 Hand Protection Against Viral Pathogens. *British Journal of Theatre Nursing*, 6(5), 5–9.

Health and Safety Executive 1988 *Control of Substances Hazardous to Health Regulations 1988 and Approved Codes of Practice*. London: HMSO.

Kalideen D, Edwards S. 1991 Dealing with HIV in the Operating Theatre. *Nursing*, 4(42), 18–22.

McCluskey F. 1996 Does Wearing a Face Mask Reduce Bacterial Wound Infection? A Literature Review *British Journal of Theatre Nursing*, 6(5), 18–20.

Mercier C. 1994 Reducing the incidence of sharps injuries. *British Journal of Nursing*, 3(17), 897–901.

Royal College of Nursing 1995 *Guidance on Infection Control in Hospitals*. London: RCN.

5

STERILIZATION, DECONTAMINATION AND THE SURGICAL FIELD

T. Kerry

INTRODUCTION

The provision of sterile surgical supplies is of paramount importance if such supplies are to be used with safety in the treatment of patients. The failure to follow recognized guidelines for the sterilization, disinfection and cleaning of surgical supplies and instruments renders the patient liable to infection, which could result in an increased hospital stay or in certain cases cause infections that are serious enough to bring about a fatality.

The complexity of modern materials used in the manufacture of medical and surgical equipment means that no single sterilization process is adequate to meet the needs of this changing environment. Flexible fibreoptic endoscopes are easily damaged by heat, as are specialist catheters and these materials require specialist sterilization methods. These range from chemical sterilizing agents and the use of toxic gases such as ethylene oxide to the more recent gas plasma systems, which utilize peracetic acid or hydrogen peroxide as the sterilant in conjunction with a radio frequency energy source.

Public awareness of the human immunodeficiency virus (HIV) and other viruses such as hepatitis B has highlighted the need for staff working within the Sterile Supply Department to pay scrupulous attention to the decontamination procedures in use. In addition, procedures should be in place to constantly monitor all aspects of the process. These include the maintenance of the equipment used in the decontamination process, microbiological monitoring and the storage and handling of raw materials. High-profile media coverage relating to salmonella in eggs, Creutzfeldt Jakob disease (CJD) and bovine spongiform encephalopathy (BSE) has also fuelled the need to have systems in place to ensure the adequate decontamination of equipment and materials. However, it should be noted that when dealing with the viruses associated with CJD, BSE and scrapie (in sheep), specialist guidance relating to decontamination and sterilization should be sought from the Control of Infection Microbiologist or other qualified person.

TERMINOLOGY

The misuse of terminology when addressing the subject of sterilization and disinfection frequently occurs and it is important from the outset to establish the correct meanings associated with each term.

STERILIZATION

The term is an absolute one and implies the total inactivation of all forms of microbial life including bacterial spores, yeasts and viruses in terms of the organism's ability to reproduce. If a killing action is implied the suffix "cide" is added. Therefore, a bactericide would be used to kill bacteria. This term is used in contrast to bacteriostasis, which denotes that microorganisms are merely inhibited from growing, hence the use of the suffix "stasis". For all procedures that involve a break in the skin or mucous membranes, sterilized equipment is essential.

DISINFECTION

Disinfection describes a process whereby the number of viable organisms has been reduced but which has not necessarily inactivated bacterial spores or some viruses. Disinfection is usually adequate for gastroscopes and items such as anaesthetic masks where sterilization is not indicated.

For any sterilization or disinfection process to be effective, decontamination and cleaning are essential prerequisites if the system is not to be compromised. Cleaning is a soil-removing process requiring energy, which removes a high proportion of all microorganisms present, including bacterial spores. The commonest organisms implicated in infections are, in general, the easiest to kill. Hot water at a temperature of 55–60°C with a small volume of detergent will kill, dilute and clean away organic matter. Once clean, the equipment can be dried. Quality control needs to be exercised over the cleaning process and it is important to prepare the detergent or disinfectant in accordance with the manufacturer's instructions. Consider the case of an operative diluting a disinfectant for use in a bench cleaning exercise. The manufacturer's instructions indicate that a 1:1000 solution is required. How many people will measure 1 millilitre of disinfectant to 999 millilitres of water? It is more usual to "test" for the correct dilution by smell and if it smells satisfactory then it must be right! To compensate for this and other anomalies caused by incorrect dilutions, various microbiological tests have been devised which examine the efficacy of the disinfectant when in use. These range from the tests devised by Kelsey and Sykes to suspension and carrier test methods, which measure microbial activity.

FACTORS AFFECTING DISINFECTANT POTENCY

The effectiveness of any disinfectant relies to a great extent on the conditions under which it operates and the following factors need to be considered at all times.

DISINFECTANT CONCENTRATION

The ability of the disinfectant to function correctly within the given range of microbial activity is dependent on the correct dilution. When employed in lower concentrations, it can stimulate biological processes, giving adverse effects, and so it is important to ensure that correct dilutions have been made.

TIME

Marketing and advertising strategies would have us believe that all microorganisms are killed instantaneously. When exposed to a particular concentration of disinfectant there is a gradual decrease in the number of living cells with time. This time is variable and depends on manufacture and the type of compound used as well as other relevant factors, some of which are discussed below.

HYDROGEN ION CONCENTRATION (pH)

The acidity or alkalinity exerts its influence on the reaction by affecting both the bacteria and chemical agent.

TEMPERATURE

The destruction of microorganisms using disinfectants is very similar to other chemical reactions in that an increase in the reaction is observed with an increase in temperature. There are practical limits to the temperatures at which disinfectants should be used and the manufacturer's advice should always be observed when preparing the solutions.

PRESENCE OF ORGANIC MATTER

Organic matter, e.g. blood and pus, can dramatically influence the action of the disinfectant and can under certain circumstances render it inactive. The removal of all extraneous material is necessary before attempting to disinfect equipment or work surfaces.

THE ORGANISM ITSELF

The species of the organism, its make-up and the presence of structures such as spores and capsules exert reactions in the disinfectant, which may not be able to be quantified.

SURFACE TENSION

This is responsible for the "wetness" of a fluid and assists in the spreading of the solution. For example, mercury has a very high surface tension and the formation of small spheres can be seen if it is split onto a surface. Alcohol has a very low surface tension and many solutions used within medicine are alcohol based, e.g. 70% isopropyl alcohol swabs are used for skin preparation.

The selection of which disinfectant to use for a particular application should be carefully controlled using the Hospital Control of Infection Policy as a guide for the correct selection of disinfectant. This document should be used as a valuable reference source. This is particularly important as the random or indiscriminate use of disinfectants can cause microorganisms to become resistant to them.

MICROBIOLOGY AND THE STERILIZATION PROCESS

The diversity of microorganisms that exist in the various ecological niches around the world is enormous. Microorganisms can be found at the bottom of the deepest oceans as well as in the natural hot springs that erupt in various parts of the world. Temperatures that these microorganisms are able to tolerate range from near freezing point to near boiling point. However, most of the pathogenic bacteria that cause infections have a very limited tolerance to these extreme conditions and are unable to survive outside the living host.

CELL STRUCTURE

All organisms are composed of units called cells and these may be divided into unicellular and multicellular types. Cells are composed of protoplasm and are divided into a nucleus (or nuclear area) and cytoplasm. Both unicellular and multicellular types have a limiting membrane. The organelles are small bodies inside the cell and are bounded by a membrane. They consist of:

- A *nucleus*, which controls the life of the cell via the genetic material.
- A *nucleolus*, which contains ribonucleic acid and helps in the production of ribosomes.
- The *endoplasmic reticulum*, the channel for transport of materials.
- *Mitochondria* or energy bodies responsible for cell respiration.
- *Lysosomes*, which contain enzymes responsible for the destruction of worn-out organelles.
- *Centrosomes*, concerned with cell division.
- The *Golgi Body*, which secretes materials such as enzymes.

- *Ribosomes*, involved with protein synthesis.
- The *cell membrane*, concerned with the passage of substances to and from the cell.

Cells that contain membrane-bound organelles are called eukaryotic and these include animal, plant and fungal cells. Cells lacking membrane-bound organelles are called prokaryotic and these include bacteria and the blue-green algae. A number of prokaryotes are able to produce a capsule or slime layer which is a loose, more or less amorphous layer deposited outside the cell wall. The cell wall gives shape and may be homogenous or multilayered.

Bacteria are able to reproduce by the process of binary fission, (i.e. dividing in two) and this can take from about 20 minutes to over one hour. This means that bacteria that are able to divide and multiply within 20 minutes will reach in excess of one million organisms over a period of seven hours. All bacteria are able to exist in the vegetative form but some are also able to exist as spores. Spore production is almost entirely restricted to the genus *Clostridia*, which are anaerobic organisms, and the genus *Bacillus*, which are aerobic organisms. *Clostridium tetani* is the causative organism of the disease tetanus, found in soil, sewage and marine sediments, whilst *Clostridium perfringens* is a common cause of food poisoning. *Bacillus* spp. are present in the soil, decaying animal and vegetable matter and frequently cause disease in man as well as food spoilage.

BACTERIAL SPORES (ENDOSPORES)

Species such as *Clostridium* and *Bacillus* are able to develop a resting phase or endospore, which enables the organism to survive in a dormant state during adverse conditions, for example the limitation of nutrients. Each cell forms one spore only and it contains some nuclear material (Fig. 5.1). When the spore germinates, which may be after many years, a new single cell appears. The spores are oval or spherical and are resistant to heat, radiation and chemicals. The spore coat contains proteins which resist dissolving, effectively making an attack-proof shelter. Once this coat is synthesized it becomes refractile. Spores show no detectable metabolism but there are genetically determined enzymes present for germination. The position of the spore is used as an aid to identification and these may be central, terminal or subterminal. The importance of spores in any sterilization process lies in their ability to resist the process and make themselves much more difficult to kill than vegetative cells. In order to make the growth conditions more favourable

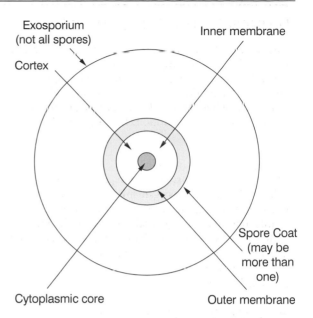

Figure 5.1   Components of a spore

and allow the spore to revert to the vegetative state, moisture is taken in. This has the effect of making the spore swell and rupturing the spore coat. The old spore wall is gradually discarded and a new vegetative cell is thus formed again.

GROWTH OF BACTERIA

The growth of bacteria is affected by several factors.

BACTERIAL NUTRITION

Sources of carbon, nitrogen and mineral salts are required for all bacteria to grow but some denitrifying bacteria are able to use very simple materials such as carbon dioxide as the source of carbon. However, most pathogenic bacteria need much more elaborate compounds such as carbohydrates and proteins.

MOISTURE

Moisture is essential for growth in combination with the other nutrients but the removal of moisture effectively stops the organism's ability to reproduce. However, in the absence of moisture certain organisms such as *Bacillus* spp. and *Clostridium* spp. are able to produce spores and can exist in this form for many years.

ENVIRONMENT

Bacteria that have the ability to grow in air are termed aerobes, in contrast to organisms which are able to flourish only in the absence of oxygen termed anaerobes. Others, termed facultative anaerobes, are able to grow in the presence or absence of air.

TEMPERATURE

The temperature of the human body is nominally 37°C and this provides optimum conditions for the growth of many pathogenic bacteria. Organisms able to reproduce within the temperature range 20–45 °C are termed mesophiles. The spores of the organism *Bacillus stearothermophilus* are extremely heat resistant and this organism is often used in the efficiency testing of sterilizers.

THE HYDROGEN ION CONCENTRATION OR pH

This is optimal for growth at around 7.4, although this does vary for differing organisms. A reduction in growth is apparent when the pH is made more acidic or alkaline.

As already stated, the spore-forming organisms present the greatest challenge to the sterilization process and to ensure that the chance of the recovery of a single such organism is not more than one in a million, the sterilization process has to be extremely rigorous. If spores are subjected to a thermal stress the rate at which they are destroyed can be illustrated graphically as shown in Figure 5.2. We can see from the graph that destruction of the bacterial population does not occur instantaneously but falls exponentially with increasing time. It is, however, more common to plot the graph as a semi-log curve, which results in a straight line (Fig. 5.3) and when this technique is applied to sterilization studies, the rate of destruction as the number of surviving organisms approaches zero is clearly seen.

STERILIZATION METHODS

Sterilization methods can be divided into three distinct groups.

1. The physical methods.
2. The physicochemical methods.
3. The chemical methods.

PHYSICAL METHODS

The physical methods are further subdivided below.

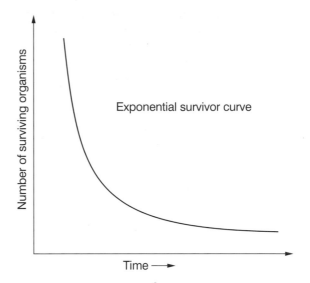

Figure 5.2   Destruction rate of spores subjected to thermal stress.

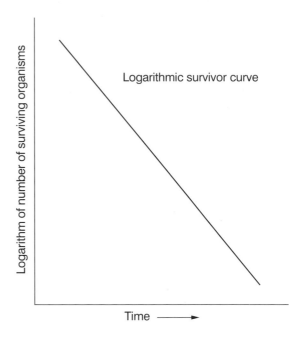

Figure 5.3   Destruction rate (semi-log curve).

Filtration uses membrane filters manufactured from cellulose nitrate or acetate. This system differs from the other methods of sterilization in that it is the removal and not the destruction of organisms that takes place.

Irradiation is a destructive process using γ rays or β particles from a linear accelerator. Because of the strict controls exercised when using this type of process, its use is confined to industrial plants.

Of all the methods of sterilization, heat is generally accepted as being the most reliable and wherever possible should always be the method of choice.

There are two destructive methods involving heat and their differing modes of action need to be fully understood before selecting a particular process. Dry heat sterilization, where the chief cause of destruction of the microorganism population is oxidation, is carried out in hot air ovens. The heat is transferred to the load by radiation, convection and, to a lesser extent, conduction. There are many difficulties in controlling the environment within the hot air oven and its use is primarily directed to the sterilization of powders and jellies, which are impervious to moisture. Long cycle times are unpopular in practice and its use in clinical areas is now rarely seen. The principle by which moist heat destroys microorganisms differs from that of dry heat. Above a particular temperature, moist heat, that may be hot or boiling water or steam under pressure, denatures and coagulates proteins. The temperature of this denaturation is dependent on the amount of moisture present. At a temperature of 80°C for 10 minutes, the vegetative form of all bacteria, yeast and fungi will be destroyed. The application of moist heat in the sterilization process is carried out in an autoclave, where steam under pressure is able to achieve temperatures in excess of 100°C, necessary for the destruction of spore-bearing organisms.

PHYSICOCHEMICAL METHODS

The physicochemical method of using low-temperature steam and formaldehyde at a temperature of approximately 73°C was introduced around 1966. There are many limitations to its use, particularly if liquid is formed during the cycle. This liquid, called formalin, is formaldehyde dissolved in water and is a dangerous poison if left in or on equipment. The cycle validation is achieved by the use of microbiological spore-forming organisms and a process challenge device termed a test helix, which is formed by a stainless steel tube and has a length-to-bore ratio of 1500:1. The cycle time plus the time to culture all the test organisms means that the load must be held in a bond store until satisfactory test results have been obtained. The popularity of this process has declined in recent years and it is now common to find only the low-temperature steam portion of the cycle being used for disinfection purposes and not sterilization.

CHEMICAL METHODS

The chemical methods currently available are popular because they offer a means of low-temperature sterilization. Equipment that would normally be damaged at the higher temperature offered by moist and dry heat processes is now able to tolerate the sterilization process at this reduced temperature without damage. The use of these substances is strictly controlled under Health and Safety legislation.

Glutaraldehyde at a concentration of 2% is commonly used in health-care settings to disinfect and sterilize heat-labile fibreoptic endoscopes. It is currently the only cold sterilizing solution effective against HIV and *Mycobacterium tuberculosis*. The control and use of this substance have to be meticulous as occupational asthma and respiratory problems are all too common if adequate containment is not achieved. Other health-associated problems includes headache, nausea, epistaxis and mucous membrane irritation. Adequate ventilation systems and environmental monitoring are essential where this substance is used.

Ethylene oxide is a gaseous process that was used for the first time in 1930 to sterilize spices. Ethylene oxide systems offer a means to sterilize items that are considered to be heat and/or moisture sensitive. Ethylene oxide is a highly diffusible gas, forming explosive mixtures with air, and for this reason it is generally mixed with carbon dioxide and freon. Any residual ethylene oxide and its associated by-products must always be reduced to a safe level after processing and adequate aeration times must always be met. Ethylene oxide is irritating to the skin and mucous membranes and excessive amounts must be avoided at all costs. Failure to achieve adequate aeration means that staff and patients could be subjected to serious chemical burns. The systems commonly operate at temperatures ranging from 37 to 55°C and therefore it is necessary to employ microbiological means to validate the process. Long cycle and microbiological testing times mean that its use is not generally accepted within the health-care setting and the process is more commonly found in an industrial environment.

New developments (which achieve rapid low-temperature, low-moisture sterilization) have been developed using plasma-based technology. Plasma is the fourth state of matter, consisting of a cloud of ions and electrons as well as atomic and molecular species, and it is naturally occurring. A typical plasma can be seen in a neon sign. The plasma is generated by a strong electric field and, together with the chemical precursors hydrogen peroxide or peracetic acid, free radicals are ultimately generated which interact with the cell membranes, enzymes or nucleic acids to disrupt the life functions of microorganisms.

Of all the sterilization methods available, moist heat using steam under pressure is by far the most suitable and generally accepted system in use within health-care premises today. Figure 5.2 shows us that if a population of living organisms is subjected to a lethal temperature, the number of survivors gradually falls as the exposure is prolonged. The time required to reduce a microbiological population by one log is termed the "D" or death value; it is the rate at which death occurs and this provides a quantitative relationship with time. If we start with a given microbiological population of 10^6 organisms and a death rate of 90%/minute then the numbers surviving after each minute will be 105, 104, 103, 102, etc. This geometric progression at equal time is called the exponential death rate. Given this information, we can now define the sterilization process in terms of time and temperature. The Hospital Technical Memorandum Number 2010, 1994 (Sterilization) defines the time temperature profiles for steam sterilization, as shown in Table 5.1. The use of a sterilization temperature of 134°C is the most common within health-care premises today.

Dihydrogen oxide (H_2O), in common with many other substances, can exist in three distinct states: a solid (ice), a liquid (water) or a gas (steam). Because steam is a very effective means of transferring heat energy and its temperature can be controlled very accurately, it is an ideal medium for sterilization by moist heat. A unit mass of ice, water or steam will contain the same number of molecules of H_2O and it is the amount of energy which these molecules possess that will determine their relative positions and hence the state in which they exist.

If heat energy is added to water the molecular movement increases and steam is formed when the molecules contain enough heat energy to overcome the pressure acting on the surface of the water. Heat is a form of energy and the basic SI Unit is termed the kilojoule (kJ).

STERILIZATION BY STEAM UNDER PRESSURE

In order to obtain the high temperatures necessary for sterilization, steam under pressure is used. Steam for the sterilization process can be obtained by two basic methods.

WET SATURATED STEAM

Transportable sterilizers utilize internal heating elements to heat water and thus produce steam. As the steam is in contact with the water from which it is produced, this is termed wet saturated steam.

DRY SATURATED STEAM

The large porous load or downward displacement autoclaves used within health-care premises are often supplied with steam generated at a central or satellite boiler house. Using appropriate distribution pipework, the steam is then carried direct to the sterilizer installation. Because of the methods used in the generation of steam, practically no moisture is left in suspension and this is termed dry saturated steam. Steam can be described as saturated when it is at a temperature corresponding to the liquid boiling point appropriate to its pressure. By plotting the saturated steam temperatures at differing pressures a phase diagram is obtained which shows the relationship between the two values (Fig. 5.4). Two considerations are thus possible:

1. Dry saturated steam that contains no water particles.
2. Wet saturated steam that is a mixture of steam and water particles.

Table 5.1 Time temperature profiles for steam sterilization (reproduced from Hospital Technical Memorandum 201)			
High Temperature Steam			
Sterilizing temperature (°)	115	121	126	134
Max. allowable temperature (°)	118	124	129	137
Minimum holding time (minutes)	30	15	10	3

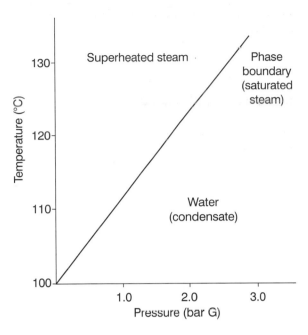

Figure 5.4   Saturated steam temperatures at differing pressures.

Because of the high pipework installation costs and steam distribution losses from the system, it is becoming increasingly common to provide a "steam generator" adjacent to the sterilizer. This is basically a sophisticated mini-boiler with the ability to control the steam quality very accurately. The heat energy within the steam is in two forms:

1. Sensible heat or enthalpy of saturated water causes a rise in temperature that can be sensed but is not a change in state.
2. Latent heat or enthalpy of evaporation causes a change in state without a rise in temperature. This refers to the additional heat energy needed to convert water at its boiling point to steam at the same temperature.

The specific heat capacity is the heat required to raise a substance of 1kg by 1°C and has the unit of kJ/kg/ °C. Therefore the amount of energy required to raise the temperature of water from freezing point to boiling point requires 419 kJ/kg of heat. At normal atmospheric pressure any further addition of heat to water at 100°C will not increase the temperature but will cause some of the water to boil into steam.

The dryness fraction is a measure of steam quality and indicates the moisture content and proportion of latent heat energy available. If dry saturated steam is further

heated, its temperature rises and the steam is said to be superheated. As such, its temperature and pressure are not related. Since this condition contains no moisture it cannot be used for moist heat sterilization (Fig. 5.5).

For efficient steam sterilizer performance, a steam supply of suitable quality must be obtained. This means a dryness fraction of approximately 0.95 is required. Too low a dryness fraction can result in "wet loads" but experience has shown that if this occurs it is generally attributed to improper wrappings or packing of the load. When saturated steam condenses it liberates all its latent heat immediately. This will occur whenever the steam touches a cool surface such as the load and this in turn will increase its temperature.

The presence of superheated steam, which contains no moisture, may result in a failure to sterilize and/or the scorching of textiles and papers. Superheat conditions within the load may result from one or more conditions.

Adiabatic expansion describes the condition that is usually produced by the excessive reduction in pressure through a reducing valve or partially closed

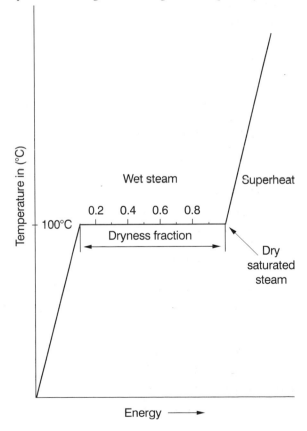

Figure 5.5   The dryness fraction

main steam valve. In practice, it is likely to be of significance in the circumstances normally encountered in the steam distribution system.

Exothermic superheating may occur as a result of rehydration of exceptionally dry material. This phenomenon is usually associated with certain textiles which have become excessively dry before sterilization. Autoclaves that incorporate a steam jacket around the chamber may produce similar effects if the jacket temperature is greater than that of the chamber.

STEAM STERILIZATION FAULTS

Pure saturated steam that does not contain air or any other non-condensable gases has a definitive temperature at a particular pressure. As air and other non-condensable gases can act as an insulator between load items and steam, their presence should be kept to a minimum. Dalton's Law of Partial Pressures shows that in a mixture of gases, the total pressure consists of the addition of the partial pressures of each gas. As air and steam expand by differing amounts when heated, the pressure/temperature relationship previously considered does not now hold. This discrepancy may be clearly seen if a comparison between the sterilizer temperature and pressure gauges is made. There is a difference between the terms gauge and absolute pressure (see Chapter 10) and these should be fully understood when observing sterilizing equipment indicators. The SI term for pressure is the bar and the appropriate value indicated on the sterilizer pressure gauge is termed the bar G (i.e. this is the gauge pressure above atmospheric). Absolute pressure (bar A) is the gauge pressure plus atmospheric pressure. Atmospheric pressure is approximately 1 bar, therefore 2.2 bar G is approximately equal to 3.2 bar A.

STEAM STERILIZER DESIGN

When steam under pressure is used as the sterilization medium, the equipment used is termed an autoclave. The physical size of the autoclave can vary from the small transportable units found in dental and chiropody clinics to the large systems found in an industrial setting. The simplest form of autoclave uses the principle of downward displacement to remove all the air. This is made possible by directing the steam flow to the top of the chamber and, as air is heavier than

steam, it will collect at the base of the chamber. Air removal is achieved by the use of an automatic steam trap fitted into the drain pipework, but in early equipment this function was achieved by the use of a hand valve. Temperature monitoring is carried out by means of a temperature detector fitted into the drain of the autoclave. During the venting period the mixture of steam and air will have a lower temperature than that of pure steam but as the air is removed the temperature will increase and this will be seen on the temperature indicator. This type of autoclave is only suitable for unwrapped instruments and bowls, but care must be taken to ensure that air is displaced from the load.

The fundamental differences between downward displacement and porous load autoclaves are:

1. The physical size of the chamber.
2. A pump is used for air removal.
3. A steam jacket is fitted to the porous load autoclave to reduce condensation.

Air detectors are fitted to all porous load autoclaves to ensure that the system will fail automatically where air is present in sufficient quantities to impair sterilization. Air is removed by use of a vacuum pump and a technique called multiple pulsing. Pulsing can and does take place above as well as below atmospheric pressure. This ensures that the temperature in the air detector corresponds closely to that in the load.

Inadequate air removal or air leaks from door seals or pipework will compromise the process and render sterilization incomplete and this must be detected by the control system and indicated accordingly.

AUTOMATIC CONTROLS

Modern steam sterilizers use sophisticated electronic control systems which are able to sense minute changes in temperatures and pressures. The use of computers to control, monitor and collect data is now commonplace. Automatic controls give a higher margin of safety and minimize the risks associated with inadequate air removal and incorrect temperatures, as well as controlling the safety functions fitted to the equipment, which protect the operator. These include the door-opening mechanisms and the admission of steam into the chamber.

6

THE FUNDAMENTALS OF CARDIOVASCULAR PHYSIOLOGY

R. M. King & C. S. Ince

WHAT IS THE CARDIOVASCULAR SYSTEM?

Before the practitioner can understand and treat the physiological and pathological changes that result from anaesthesia and surgery, she/he must have a working knowledge of cardiovascular physiology. This chapter is not intended to repeat standard anatomy and physiology texts but to provide a basic foundation on which to build a logical and practical approach to dealing with the management of cardiovascular problems within the theatre environment.

THE ANATOMY OF THE CARDIOVASCULAR SYSTEM

The cardiovascular system consists of a series of tubes or blood vessels containing blood, which is circulated around the body by a pump or 'more specifically' two pumps. One pump ensures that deoxygenated blood is transported to the respiratory system to facilitate the exchange of gases (*external respiration*). The second pump provides the means of delivering oxygen and nutrients to all the body tissues and at the same time removes carbon dioxide and other waste products of metabolism (*internal respiration*). Each pump consists of two chambers known as the atrium and the ventricle. The atrium receives blood from the great veins, after which the blood then enters the ventricle. This is mostly in a passive way although a small percentage is actively forced into the ventricle by contraction of the atrial muscle. The ventricle then pumps this blood into the arteries for distribution around the body. Because the muscular activity of the ventricle is much greater than that of the atrium, the ventricle has a much thicker and more muscular wall. In many animals, including man, these two pumps are combined as one organ, the heart. Thus, the heart is a four-chambered organ that pumps in a synchronized manner in order to deliver blood effectively to two distinct areas: the lungs and the tissues. The lungs receive blood from the pulmonary circulation while the systemic circulation supplies the other body tissues. This is illustrated diagrammatically in Figure 6.1.

THE PULMONARY CIRCULATION

Blood that has taken part in internal respiration requires replenishment with oxygen and also needs to release carbon dioxide. Deoxygenated blood from the tissues therefore returns to the right atrium via the inferior vena cava (from the lower part of the body) and the superior vena cava (the upper part of the body). This blood passes into the right ventricle, is then

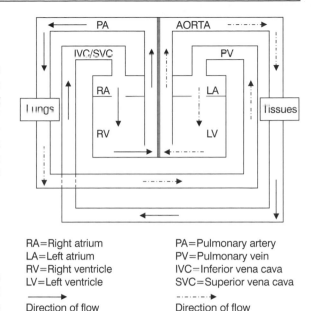

RA=Right atrium
LA=Left atrium
RV=Right ventricle
LV=Left ventricle

PA=Pulmonary artery
PV=Pulmonary vein
IVC=Inferior vena cava
SVC=Superior vena cava

Direction of flow
(Deoxygenated blood)

Direction of flow
(Oxygenated blood)

Figure 6.1   The heart and circulation.

pumped through the pulmonary artery to the lungs where it becomes oxygenated (see Chapter 7) and returned to the left atrium via the pulmonary vein. The tricuspid valve separates the left atrium from the ventricle and acts as a unidirectional valve, thus preventing blood regurgitating from the ventricle back into the atrium. Because the heart does not have to work so hard to pump blood through the pulmonary circulation, it generates less pressure. This explains why the pulmonary artery blood pressure is about 25 mmHg compared to a systemic pressure of about 120 mmHg and also why the right ventricle has a much thinner muscular wall than the left.

THE SYSTEMIC CIRCULATION

Oxygenated blood is pumped from the left ventricle into the aorta and thence to the body tissues. During its passage through the tissues it gives up oxygen and nutrients while at the same time the products of metabolism pass into the blood. This blood then returns to the right atrium as described above. The valve between the right atrium and right ventricle is called the mitral valve.

BLOOD VESSELS AND THE MOVEMENT OF FLUID

There are three types of blood vessels: arteries, veins and capillaries. All these vessels have an intimal or internal lining, composed of endothelium, and a layer of smooth muscle that is able to contract in response to stimulation of the vasomotor centre in the brainstem. Arteries conduct blood away from the heart, have a thick muscular wall and play an important role in the control of blood pressure. Small arteries are called arterioles and by constricting or dilating, they are able to selectively divert the blood flow. The skin is a good example of this. During cold weather the arterioles in the skin constrict and blood is diverted away from the superficial layers of the body in order to conserve heat. Because skin colour is due to the presence of blood within it, when the skin blood vessels constrict the skin has a pale or white appearance. A similar mechanism occurs during hypovolaemia in order to try and maintain the blood pressure. This is discussed in more detail later in this chapter. At any one moment, most of the blood is to be found in the veins and these vessels return the blood to the heart.

Capillaries are the smallest of the blood vessels and they are in direct contact with the cells of the body, e.g. lung alveoli, muscle cells and the renal tubular cells. The vessels may only be one layer of cells thick and it is through the capillaries that oxygen, nutrients and the products of metabolism enter and leave the body's cells. The capillary cell endothelium has 'pores' in it which allow the movement of water, electrolytes and glucose across the membrane.

Large molecules such as the proteins cannot normally pass through these pores and so remain within the capillary. The concentration of protein is therefore higher in the capillary than in the fluid outside the vessel. This sets up a concentration gradient and water will flow from an area of low concentration to an area of higher concentration in an effort to dilute the strong solution and restore equilibrium. This movement of

water across a semipermeable membrane along a concentration gradient is known as osmosis. Osmosis therefore draws water into the confines of the capillary and this force may be measured. It is known as the osmotic pressure of the solution and is equal to the pressure required to prevent osmosis occurring across the membrane. Osmotic pressure thus is the pressure with which a solution draws water across a semipermeable membrane. *Oncotic pressure* (colloid osmotic pressure) is the pressure exerted by proteins within plasma and is estimated to be about 25mmHg (3.3 kPa). There is an opposing force to this osmotic movement of water; the blood pressure. The blood pressure at the arterial end of capillaries has been estimated to be an average of 30–35 mmHg. One further factor in the equation is the net interstitial fluid pressure (interstitial oncotic pressure minus the physical pressure of the interstitial cells acting on the blood vessel), which is usually assumed to be between 0 and 2 mmHg. The net pressure (8mmHg) that facilitates the movement of fluid at the arterial end capillary is as follows: 30–35 mmHg blood pressure, –25 mmHg plasma protein osmotic pressure and –2 mmHg interstitial pressure. That is about 8 mmHg in favour of the movement of fluid from the capillary into the interstitial space.

At the venous end of the capillary, the situation is reversed. The figures are the same except that the venous pressure is about 14 mmHg. This means that the pressure gradient is effectively reversed and so fluid moves from the interstitial space back to the capillary. In fact, the volume of fluid moving out of the capillary at the arterial end is almost equal to the fluid returning to the capillary at the venous end. Any excess fluid remaining in the interstitial space and any proteins 'leaking' out of the capillary (no membrane is perfect) are reabsorbed back into the venous blood via the

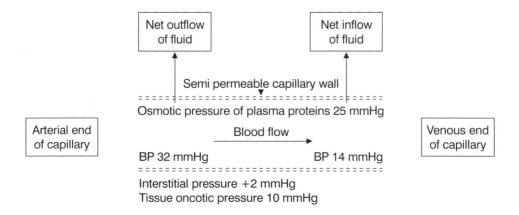

Figure 6.2   The movement of fluid across the capillary membrane.

lymphatic drainage system. This subject is discussed further elsewhere (Chapter 20) in relation to its implications for fluid and electrolyte balance.

THE PHYSIOLOGY OF THE HEART

Cardiac muscle is different from other muscle in two main ways.

1. Cardiac muscle has the property of rhythmicity. This means that the cells alternately contract and relax without being electrically stimulated by a nerve impulse.
2. Cardiac cells also have the ability to conduct electrical activity. Muscle cells are in close proximity to each other and therefore directly pass on the stimulus that causes contraction to the next cell. The collective result produces a wave of electrical excitement, closely followed by a wave of contraction and these waves spread rapidly through the cardiac muscle.

In amphibians, like the frog, the heartbeat originates in the sinous venosus, which is a chamber between the vena cava and the right atrium. Mammals have developed this chamber into a concentrated group of cells called the sino-atrial node (SA node), which is located at the entry of the superior vena cava. The heartbeat normally originates from the SA node because its signal is usually stronger than any other signals in the atria. Waves of excitation spread out from the SA node through the atrial muscle, resulting in the contraction of both atria. The contraction forces blood from the atria down through the atrioventricular valves (mitral and tricuspid) and into the ventricles.

Between the atria and the ventricles there is a fibrous septum which will not conduct the cardiac impulse because it does not contain cardiac muscle. Therefore the electrical activity fades away instead of spreading directly to the ventricles. There is only one pathway between the atria and the ventricles. This starts at the atrioventricular node (AV node), runs down the septum between the two ventricles as the atrioventricular bundle (bundle of His) and then travels to the right and left ventricles via the right and left bundle branches respectively. Within the ventricular muscle the contraction wave spreads rapidly via specialized tissue called Purkinje fibres. The end result is the normal action of the heart, i.e. atrial contraction, after which there is a short pause, followed by ventricular contraction. After the respective contractions both atria and ventricles relax before the next cycle. Atrial contraction is responsible for about 10–15% of ventricular filling. If this does not occur, e.g. in atrial fibrillation or nodal rhythm, the cardiac output may be significantly reduced, especially in patients whose cardiac function is already compromised.

When a cell is resting there is more potassium inside the cell and more sodium in the extracellular fluid. This inequality, which is maintained by the sodium pump, results in an electrical potential difference across the cell membrane. During electrical activity potassium moves out of and sodium moves into the cell (*depolarization*). Depolarization (as in the action potentials of nerve cells) is an 'all or nothing' event. It is not possible to depolarize only part of the atria or ventricles. The cardiac muscle cell then needs to 'recover' its ability to respond to electrical excitation by removing the excess sodium (*repolarization*). While this is happening the cell is said to be in a refractory state, i.e. it is unable to respond to further electrical stimulation.

If an extra impulse occurs after repolarization but before the next normal one, the heart will respond in the usual way. This means that the next normal beat will arrive during the refractory period and the muscle heart will not contract. There will therefore be a compensatory pause before the next normal contraction.

Heart muscle responds to an increase in tension by increasing the force of its contraction. Thus, if the volume of blood in the heart increases, so will the stroke volume (the volume of blood ejected from the heart with each contraction) until peak performance is achieved, when the heart will begin to fail and the stroke volume will fall. This is known as *Starling's Law*. Following the compensatory pause, therefore, more blood is present in the ventricle at the time of the next contraction and a greater volume of blood will leave the heart at the next contraction. This abnormality may be observed clinically by feeling the pulse: two quick pulses, followed by a prolonged pause and then a pulse of greater strength.

THE ELECTROCARDIOGRAPH (ECG)

The ECG (Fig. 6.3) is merely a recording of the electrical activity of the heart. It is a graphical representation of the action potentials generated in the myocardium during depolarization and repolarization of the cardiac muscle fibres. All ECG machines, whether an oscilloscope or paper readout, should run at a standard speed (2.5 cm/sec) and any paper used is printed with a standard grid, consisting of a series of large and small squares. Each large square is 0.2 seconds, so there are five large squares/sec or 300/min.

The height of the complexes both above and below the baseline depends on the lead used (see below) and the position of the electrodes.

Essentially, the ECG is a reading of the change in electrical charge (in mV) caused by the activity of the heart as viewed by a series of electrodes. When the depolarizing wave is moving toward the lead there will be an upward deflection of the reading and when the wave is travelling away from the lead the deflection is downwards. The depolarization wave moves in many different directions and the QRS complex (see below) shows the average direction of the spread of depolarization. Because the mass of ventricular muscle is greater than atrial muscle the deflection due to ventricular activity is usually greater than that representing the activity of the atria. Calibration is therefore important. A standard signal of 1mV should deflect the indicator (light or pen) vertically by 1 cm (two large squares), as indicated on all 12 lead ECG readings.

An ECG trace is obtained by placing electrodes on the limbs and chest and the picture varies depending on the site and grouping (lead) of the electrodes being used. The standard trace is known as the 12-lead ECG and consists of three bipolar limb leads, three unipolar limb leads and six chest leads. In the standard ECG the position of the limb leads is as follows:

Lead I	Right arm–left arm
Lead II	Right arm–left leg
Lead III	Left arm–left leg
aVR	Right arm lead
aVL	Left arm lead
aVF	Left leg lead
V_1–V_6	Chest leads

In all the leads the right leg is connected to earth. Each lead looks at the heart from a different position. For example, lead II is useful for changes in rhythm while chest lead V_5 will identify atrial activity and ischaemic changes. For routine anaesthetic monitoring of the heart, lead I is generally used. To expect a detailed knowledge of ECGs is unreasonable but the practitioner should have a general understanding of:

1. The electrical activity it represents.
2. How to calculate the heart rate from the ECG.
3. Identification of the normal cardiac rhythm.
4. Identification of changes in the reading and how to take the appropriate action.

ELECTRICAL ACTIVITY

The contraction of any muscle is associated with electrical changes and it is therefore important that the patient is fully relaxed when recording an ECG, because any extraneous muscle movement will affect the recording. In anaesthesia this is not normally a problem. Greasy skin and poor electrical contact may also lead to a poor-quality ECG.

The contraction of the atria causes the 'P' wave on the ECG while the 'QRS' complex represents ventricular contraction. Repolarization (the return of the ventricular mass to the resting electrical potential) is represented by the 'T' wave. The different parts of the 'QRS' complex are labelled as follows:

- If the first deflection is downwards, it is called a 'Q' wave.
- A deflection upwards is called a 'R' wave (whether or not it is preceded by a 'Q' wave).
- Any deflection below the baseline following an 'R' wave is called an 'S' wave.

HEART RATE

The ECG records the heart's electrical activity and this is not necessarily the same as the mechanical activity that produces the pulse rate. Heart rate can be calculated by reading the number of large squares between the 'R' peaks. Each large square represents 0.2 sec and so if the R–R interval is five large squares the rate is 60/min. Alternatively, there are 30 large squares in a minute and thus the number of complexes in 30 squares will give the rate.

RHYTHM

The use of squared paper allows one to study not only the heart rate but also the regularity and the timing of each wave and complex. For example, the conduction time taken for the impulse to spread from the atria to the ventricles (the P–R interval) should be less than 0.2 sec, while ventricular conduction (QRS) should be less than 0.9 sec. Normally the S–T segment should be isoelectric but long-standing cardiac ischaemia may cause S–T depression and acute ischaemia may show as S–T elevation.

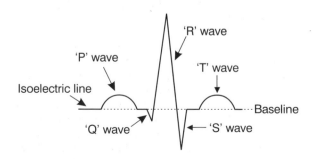

Figure 6.3   The electrocardiogram (not to scale).

An arrhythmia is an abnormal cardiac rhythm or rate. Arrhythmias may be the result of cardiac disease, drugs including anaesthesia, hypoxia and hypercarbia or electrolyte imbalance. The name of a cardiac arrhythmia consists of two parts: the first part indicates where the rhythm has come from and the second part indicates what the rhythm is doing. If each complex has one 'P' wave with each 'QRS' and the P–R interval is normal, it is known as a sinus rhythm. A rate of less than 60 beats/min is bradycardia while more than 100 beats/min is tachycardia in the adult.

A normal-looking 'QRS' complex indicates that the abnormality occurs before the ventricles. An abnormal atrial focus occurs in nodal rhythm (no visible or abnormal 'P' waves) and atrial fibrillation (no 'P' waves but rapid and totally uncoordinated atrial activity) while extra activity from the SA node results in atrial extrasystoles. Atrial flutter is a very rapid but regular arrhythmia, e.g. 250–300 beats/min. If conduction is impaired between the atria and the ventricles the condition is known as heart block. This varies from a slightly increased P–R interval to complete heart block where the ventricle beats at its own inherently slow rate due to the natural rhymicity of the muscle.

In ventricular extrasystoles the focus is somewhere in the ventricle and the 'QRS' complex looks abnormal. Ventricular tachycardia is due to a rapidly firing ventricular focus and requires urgent treatment. Ventricular fibrillation is totally disorganized activity that is universally fatal if untreated, because there is no effective mechanical pumping and hence no stroke volume.

Arrhythmias are most significant if they affect the cardiac output. This mainly occurs if the ventricle is unable to fill to its capacity (nodal rhythms, fibrillation and tachycardia). A useful indication of the severity of atrial fibrillation is the pulse deficit, i.e. the difference between the heart rate and the pulse rate. If this is large the patient needs treatment to slow the heart rate.

THE CONTROL OF CARDIAC OUTPUT

The cardiovascular system is the highway for the delivery of oxygen and nutrients to the tissues and for the removal of the products of metabolism. Although the body is adept at controlling blood pressure, by far the most important parameter in tissue oxygenation is perfusion. This in turn depends on the cardiac output, the maintenance of which is fundamental if the body is to survive. The level of the blood pressure is of secondary importance, provided the tissues are adequately perfused with blood and therefore in this chapter the control of cardiac output is stressed rather than the maintenance of blood pressure.

There are two basic formulae that determine cardiac output:

1. cardiac output (CO) = stroke volume (SV) x pulse rate;
2. cardiac output = blood pressure/peripheral resistance (PR).

Cardiac output may be defined as the volume of blood leaving the left ventricle each minute and is measured in litres/min.

STROKE VOLUME

Starling's Law (see above) states that the stroke volume varies with the stretching of the cardiac muscle fibres and this in turn must depend on the ventricle filling from the atrium. The effect of arrhythmias on ventricular performance has already been discussed and will not be mentioned further. As with all processes, what goes into the heart must match what comes out. The factors affecting cardiac output are summarized in Figure 6.4 but in view of the above, perhaps the most important is the venous return, i.e. the volume of blood returning to the heart from the great veins.

All blood vessels have smooth muscle that is able to respond to nervous stimuli from the brainstem and react to changes in the local environment. The heart

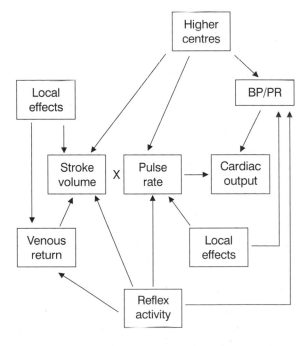

Figure 6.4   Factors affecting cardiac output.

and blood vessels are under the control of the autonomic nervous system, which consists of the adrenal glands and sympathetic and parasympathetic nerves. Sympathetic nerves produce sympathetic amines, including noradrenaline and adrenaline. These substances are known as neurotransmitters and, having been released from the nerve, react with receptors within the cardiac and vascular muscle to stimulate the cardiovascular system. Noradrenaline primarily increases vascular muscle tone while adrenaline increases cardiac output (the so-called fight or flight response). Acetylcholine is the parasympathetic neurotransmitter and tends to produce a slowing of the heart together with an increase in intestinal secretions. Although control of the autonomic nervous system is predominantly at reflex level, the higher centres of the brain also influence it and there is an increase in sympathetic activity resulting from pain and emotions, such as fear and anxiety. The overall 'tone' of the cardiovascular system is a balance between sympathetic and parasympathetic activity and it is not surprising therefore that those patients who are anxious or in pain have higher than normal blood pressures and tend to bleed more during surgery.

The venous system has a great deal of capacity and at any one time a significant proportion of blood is located within large veins known as capacitance vessels. When the muscle in these veins contracts, the volume of the venous system decreases and more blood is made available to return to the heart. Venous tone is under reflex control, mediated by receptors situated in the great veins and these respond to changes in the volume of these vessels.

An understanding of this physiology is useful in the positioning of patients for surgery. Venous and capillary bleeding generally account for the majority of blood loss, even though the rate of loss is greatest in arterial bleeding. If the patient is therefore positioned so that the operative site is above the level of the heart, the effect of gravity will decrease the venous return so that bleeding is reduced. Capillary bleeding may also be controlled by the use of local vasoconstriction. The local anaesthetic cocaine is a powerful vasoconstrictor and the addition of adrenaline to bupivacaine and lignocaine is widely used in ENT and plastic surgery. Coughing and straining, however, exacerbate bleeding by increasing the venous return and should therefore be avoided.

The affect of pathological changes, including local effects, on venous tone is discussed elsewhere but it must be stressed that acute changes may have a catastrophic effect on the ability of the body to maintain cardiac output. Arteries, however, have much thicker muscular walls and the arterial muscle tone plays a significant part in the maintenance of blood pressure.

PULSE RATE

The rate at which the heart beats (pulse rate) is under autonomic reflex control via the cardiac centre, situated in the hypothalamus, but it is also influenced by the higher centres of the brain, as described above. Thus, the inherent rhythmicity of the heart as controlled through the SA and AV nodes may be altered to maintain cardiac output. An increase in pulse rate will compensate for a fall in the stroke volume and in this way cardiac output may be maintained. Tachycardia may therefore be an early sign of a fall in stroke volume and hence cardiac output due to hypovolaemia or a failing heart.

Local factors, such as pyrexia and exogenous (added from outside the body) sympathetic amines, will increase the heart rate, while hypothermia and β-blocking agents that block the action of the sympathetic amines will slow the rate down. As previously stated, most bleeding is a result of blood loss from veins and capillaries. Blood flow through these vessels is more dependent on heart rate than blood pressure and thus controlling the pulse rate will reduce surgical bleeding. Managing patient anxiety and pain will minimize intraoperative tachycardia. This may be further enhanced by carefully positioning the patient and by judicious use of β-blocking agents. These methods are particularly useful for controlling the bleeding in superficial operations, such as the excision and skin/tissue flap repair of skin lesions, rhinoplasty and breast reduction.

THE CONTROL OF BLOOD PRESSURE

Equation 2 on page 59 relates cardiac output to blood pressure and peripheral resistance in exactly the same way that voltage overcomes electrical resistance to allow a current to flow. If the formula is rearranged BP = CO × PR. If blood pressure falls reflex vasoconstriction will, by decreasing the capacity of the veins, increase the venous return and tend to restore the blood pressure to normal. The reflex arc responds to pressure changes in receptors, situated for example in the aortic arch and the higher centres as previously described. Figure 6.5 illustrates the nervous pathways used in the maintenance of blood pressure and gives some examples of the factors influencing hypothalamic activity.

Unfortunately, the body attempts to maintain blood pressure at the expense of perfusion and, although this form of compensation may be acceptable in the early stages of hypovolaemic hypotension, increasing vasoconstriction will lead to local hypoxia. This is because vasoconstriction prevents adequate perfusion (blood flow) through the tissues and is of particular importance in the kidney. Severe hypotension and vasoconstriction may eventually lead to renal failure.

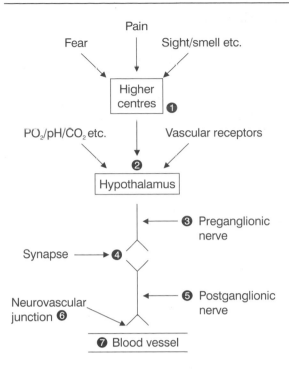

Figure 6.5   The nervous control of peripheral resistance.

The above refers to the situation in which blood pressure falls as a result of hypovolaemia but in severe systemic infection and anaphylaxis, the prime failure is the inability to maintain peripheral resistance. Although in both cases fluid replacement is essential, in this scenario sympathomimetic agents such as noradrenaline may be needed to restore the peripheral resistance to acceptable levels.

HYPOTENSIVE ANAESTHESIA

Bleeding may be reduced using methods previously described or, in peripheral operative sites, by applying a tourniquet but there are occasions when it is necessary to control bleeding by reducing the blood pressure. Examples include surgery for the middle ear, some neurosurgery and major head and neck surgery.

It has already been stated that the higher centres ❶ (see Fig 6.5) influence the nervous discharge of the hypothalamus ❷ and sympathetic nerves pass from this structure down the spinal cord as preganglionic nerves ❸. After synapsing ❹ in the cord postganglionic fibres ❺ leave the spinal cord and follow the vascular bundles to the site of action. At the neurovascular junction ❻ nerve endings release

sympathetic amines, which react with sympathetic receptors in the vascular muscle, leading to vasoconstriction. It is pharmacologically possible to influence blood pressure at all of these sites, as well as causing vasodilatation of the blood vessel by direct action on the muscular wall ❼. In practice only a few areas are used but the technique provides a good illustration of applied cardiovascular physiology.

By reducing anxiety (premedication) and pain (analgesia) and preventing awareness under anaesthesia, it is possible to reduce the influence of the higher centres. In a similar way, ensuring that the patient is well oxygenated with a low normal arterial partial pressure of carbon dioxide, may prevent reflex tachycardia and hypertension.

The pre- and postganglionic nerves synapse within the spinal cord and the neurotransmitter at this site is acetylcholine. It is possible to block the nerve impulse at this point but ganglion-blocking agents, e.g. trimetaphan, are not now in common use. Local anaesthetic agents administered during spinal and epidural analgesia prevent the transmission of neural impulses within the nerves leaving the spinal canal. Because all nerves entering and leaving the spinal canal are affected the nerve block obtained has analgesic (sensory nerves), muscle weakness (motor nerves) and hypotensive (sympathetic nerves) components. The degree to which each is affected depends on the dose, the height of the block and the speed of injection. Epidural blocks are most useful in controlling preeclamptic hypertension and are widely used in obstetric anaesthesia and for postoperative pain relief following major surgery.

Drugs that block neuromuscular transmission, e.g. to smooth muscle in blood vessels, are known as α-blocking drugs (as opposed to the β-blocking drugs that affect the adrenergic receptors in the heart). Because they affect vascular tone by directly altering the response of the effector organ (the organ which responds to a reflex action, in this case the blood vessel) to nervous stimulation, it is at this level that the most effective control of blood pressure is possible. Examples include sodium nitroprusside and glyceryl trinitrate. Both of these drugs are very short acting and are administered as an infusion. Unfortunately some patients respond to induced hypotension with reflex tachycardia. β-blocking agents such as atenolol are useful in controlling the heart rate if this occurs.

The volatile anaesthetic agents may also be used to control the blood pressure. This is partly as a result of the effect on the higher centres and the hypothalamus but these anaesthetic drugs also directly suppress myocardial activity.

If several of the hypotensive methods are used in combination, the overall effect is more than if they were used separately. For further information the reader should consult a standard textbook of anaesthesia.

THE MEASUREMENT OF BLOOD PRESSURE

This subject is dealt with in Chapter 10 but it is important to ensure that informed consent has been obtained if invasive monitoring is to be used.

RECOMMENDED READING

Guyton A.C., *Textbook of Medical Physiology* (7th ed). W B Saunders, 1986.

7

FUNDAMENTALS OF RESPIRATORY PHYSIOLOGY

E. C. Howard

LUNG MECHANICS

The lungs lie within the chest or thorax and are covered by the pulmonary pleura, which is a thin moist membrane. Over this lies a similar membrane, the parietal pleura, which lines the inner wall of the chest. Surface tension between these two layers helps to maintain lung inflation. The potential space between these two layers is called the parietal space and is filled with a thin layer of fluid. Entry of air into the pleural space produces a pneumothorax and results in the separation of the pleura and collapse of the lung.

On inspiration, the dome of the diaphragm contracts and moves downward while the ribs move upwards and increase the chest diameter. Inspiration therefore produces an increase in chest volume, which causes the internal pressure to fall with respect to atmospheric pressure and air is drawn in. During quiet respiration expiration is achieved entirely by the passive elastic recoil of the lung tissue. This results in the diaphragm being elevated and the chest wall being drawn inwards.

During quiet breathing inspiration is mainly achieved by diaphragmatic contraction which is innervated by the phrenic nerve from the third, fourth and fifth cervical nerve roots from the spinal cord. A network of muscles called the internal and external intercostal muscles attache the ribs to each other. The external intercostals run forwards and downwards and these aid inspiration by drawing up the anterior end of each rib, resulting in the increased chest width.

Larger strenuous inspirations need the assistance of the accessory muscles of inspiration such as the sternomastoid and scalene muscles of the head and neck to raise the sternum. Forceful expirations require the elastic recoil to be helped by muscle activity from the accessory muscles. Thus, at times of greater exertion abdominal and internal intercostal musculature actively contract. The internal intercostals extend diagonally upwards and forwards and therefore, as they contract, the ribs are forced downwards and the chest diameter decreases. At the same time the abdominal muscles contract and push the diaphragm upward into a dome, expelling gas from the lungs.

LUNG VOLUMES

Lung volumes are important in the assessment of respiratory function and combinations of lung volumes are called capacities (Fig 7.1).

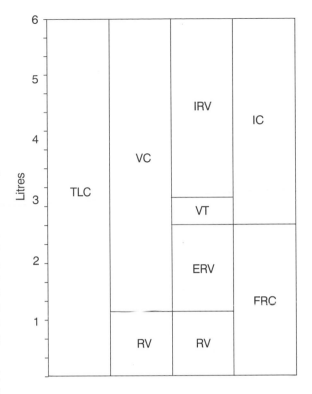

Figure 7.1 Lung volumes.

TIDAL VOLUME (V$_T$)

Volume of gas breathed in and out of the lungs. At rest this is about 500 ml.

TOTAL LUNG CAPACITY (TLC)

Volume of gas occupying the lungs at maximal inspiration (about 6 litres).

RESIDUAL VOLUME (RV)

Volume of gas remaining in the lungs after maximal expiration (about 1.2 litres).

EXPIRATORY RESERVE VOLUME (ERV)

Maximum volume that can be voluntarily exhaled after a normal expiration (about 1.3–1.5 litres).

INSPIRATORY RESERVE VOLUME (IRV)

Maximum extra volume that can be inhaled at the end of a normal inspiration (about 3 litres).

FUNCTIONAL RESIDUAL CAPACITY (FRC)

Volume remaining in the lungs at the end of a normal expiration. Therefore:

FRC = RV + ERV

VITAL CAPACITY (VC)

Volume of gas that can be shifted in and out of the lungs during maximal inspiration and expiration (about 5 litres). Therefore:

RV + VC = TLC

INSPIRATORY CAPACITY (IC)

Volume of gas that can be maximally inspired after normal expiration. Therefore:

IC = IRV + V_T

FEV$_1$

Volume of gas exhaled in one second from the start of a forced expiration.

SURFACE TENSION AND SURFACTANT

The small air sacs in the lungs are called alveoli and for adequate and efficient gas exchange to occur, these must be both ventilated and perfused. The laws of physics would lead us to expect that since the alveoli vary in size the larger ones would expand at the expense of the smaller. This is because of the expected differing wall tensions. Surfactant, a naturally occurring substance secreted by cells within the alveoli, considerably reduces the wall tension, particularly in the smaller alveoli, and therefore, the balance between the smaller and larger air sacs is maintained. Surfactant also improves alveolar function by inhibiting the accumulation of fluid filtered from lung capillaries. A deficiency in surfactant is frequently found in the underdeveloped lungs of the premature neonate. Artificially synthesised surfactant is now available and has done a great deal to improve the long-term outlook in these babies.

PHYSIOLOGY OF VENTILATION

COMPLIANCE

Compliance is a term that is used frequently with reference to lung function and is a measure of elasticity. The compliance of the lungs and thorax is defined as the change in volume per unit change in pressure, i.e. litres per centimetre of H_2O or, in SI units, L. Cm H_2O^{-1}. The higher the value, the better the lung function and the measurement specifically refers to static pressure/volume relationships. An understanding of lung compliance is important to us because of the following factors.

1. Pulmonary surfactant lowers surface tension and improves the overall compliance of the lungs.
2. Pulmonary oedema results in a decrease in compliance, as the lung fields become water-logged.
3. Ascites, pleural effusion, pericardial effusion and cardiomegaly all result in reduced compliance as a result of a reduction in FRC.
4. Conditions that destroy the elasticity of the lung walls will result in a reduction in compliance, e.g. fibrosing alveolitis.
5. Atelectasis (collapse of the lung) and pneumonia produce a reduction in FRC, surfactant and compliance.
6. Airway occlusion and bronchospasm result in a reduction in compliance secondary to a reduction in FRC.
7. Poliomyelitis and kyphoscoliosis also cause a reduction in FRC and thus also compliance.
8. General anaesthesia results in a fall in compliance as a result of reduced FRC.
9. Emphysema causes an increase in compliance due to the destruction of the elastic recoil of the lungs.
10. Spinal deformities, muscle diseases, abdominal disorders and marked obesity all result in reduced thoracic cage compliance.

A decrease in compliance results in an increase in the work of breathing.

AIRWAY RESISTANCE

Airway resistance is a measure of the driving pressure necessary to produce a given airflow. In SI units, it is measured in cm $H_2O.L^{-1}.s^{-1}$. Resistance is a result of friction between the molecules of flowing gas and the airway walls. This measurement refers to dynamic pressure/flow relationships.

Factors affecting airways resistance include the following.

1. Increased lung volume decreases airways resistance as the elastic tissues of the lungs expand the diameter of the airways.
2. Asthma results in an increased airways resistance as a result of bronchospasm and accumulated secretions.

3. Emphysema causes an increase in resistance as the airways collapse. There is further airway closure as these patients attempt forced expiration.
4. Airway resistance is increased by any cause of reduced airways diameter including, for example, infiltration by tumour, compression or fibrosis.
5. Iatrogenic causes of increased airway resistance include a narrow tracheostomy tube or a long narrow endotracheal tube.

Increased airway resistance prolongs the time required for exhalation. If the patient is being ventilated and the length of the expiratory phase is insufficient, there will be an increased FRC. Patients who are awake will have active exhalation, resulting in increased work. Increased airway resistance may cause respiratory distress, as in asthma. Commonly, patients with increased airway resistance will purse their lips in order to apply positive end-expiratory pressure (PEEP). This discourages airways collapse and is often used for this purpose in intermittent positive pressure ventilation.

RESISTANCE TO AIRFLOW

Resistance to airflow in and out of the lungs is largely due to airway problems rather than the lung tissue itself. The major sites are the upper respiratory tract and medium-sized bronchi. Airways without cartilage in their walls may collapse during forced expiration. Bronchoconstriction may occur as a result of parasympathetic stimulation, locally released chemicals, e.g. histamine, and inhaled substances. The accumulation of secretions as a result of a chest infection or reduced ability to cough will also result in an increased airway resistance.

Airway resistance is assessed in the pulmonary function laboratory by measuring the expiratory forced vital capacity, the volume expired in one second (FEV_1) and the peak flow rate.

ANATOMICAL AND PHYSIOLOGICAL DEAD SPACE

Dead space is the volume of gas not available for gas exchange and is made up of both anatomical and physiological components. Anatomical dead space is the volume of the conducting airways. There are parts of the alveoli which are not adequately perfused with blood, but in health the alveolar dead space is less than 5 ml. In lung disease, though, it may be considerably larger due to the mismatch of lung ventilation and perfusion. Physiological dead space is made up of anatomical and alveolar dead space.

GAS EXCHANGE

At rest the adult consumes about 250–300 ml of oxygen per minute (VO_2) and produces about 200–250 ml of carbon dioxide (VCO_2). The ratio of carbon dioxide produced and oxygen used ($VCO_2:VO_2$) is called the respiratory exchange ratio (for parts of the lung) or respiratory quotient (for the whole body) and is largely dependent upon the type of food we metabolise. If the substrate were entirely carbohydrate the quotient would be 1.0 but a mixed diet would be more likely to result in a value of around 0.8.

PROPERTIES OF GASES

The pressure exerted by one gas (the partial pressure of that gas) in a mixture of gases is equal to the total gas pressure in the mixture multiplied by the fraction of the total amount of gas it represents. This is Dalton's Law of Partial Pressure and applies to gases in a dry mixture and may be expressed as:

$Pgas = P_B \times F_{gas}$, where P_B is the barometric pressure and 'F_{gas}' is the fractional share. An alternative definition of Dalton's Law is that 'in a mixture of gases the pressure exerted in the system is the sum of the individual partial pressures of the constituent gases'. Therefore, $P = p_1 + p_2 + p_3 + p_4$ where P is the total gas pressure and p_1, p_2, p_3 and p_4 represent the partial pressures of the gases in the mixture.

When a gas enters the lungs it becomes saturated with water vapour. The saturated vapour pressure of water at 37°C is (6.25 kPa). This is always the same irrespective of barometric pressure. Thus, at body temperature:

$P_{gas} = F_{gas} (P_B - 6.25 \text{ kPa})$. This means that when the barometric pressure is low, e.g. at high altitude, there is less gas pressure available for the other gases in the mixture. Therefore, it is not always possible to use nitrous oxide at high altitude because the partial pressure available for the oxygen is too low to sustain adequate tissue oxygenation.

Expired gas is a mixture of that from the dead space (the same as the inspired air because it has not taken part in gaseous exchange) and that from the alveoli. The mean alveolar partial pressures of oxygen and carbon dioxide (PAO_2 and $PACO_2$) are usually 13.3 kPa and 5.3 kPa respectively. The composition of the inspired gas, the metabolic rate and the depth of ventilation will determine the actual values.

The Alveolar Gas Equation states the relationship between the partial pressures of oxygen and carbon dioxide in the alveoli as shown:

$$PAO_2 = PIO_2 - \frac{PACO_2}{R} + F$$

Where, PIO_2 = inspired partial pressure of oxygen, R = respiratory quotient and F = small correction factor.

Alveolar capillary oxygen and carbon dioxide equilibrate with the alveolar gases. If ventilation is perfectly matched to perfusion, blood leaving the lungs has a PO_2 of 13.3 kPa and a PCO_2 of 5.3 kPa. Venous blood returning from all over the body collects and enters the lungs as mixed venous blood with a PO_2 of 5.3 kPa and a PCO_2 of 6.1 kPa. Gas movement across the capillary walls is along a concentration gradient by diffusion. Successful gas transfer is dependent not only on alveolar ventilation but also on perfusion by blood and an effective diffusion process. The latter is a problem in some respiratory conditions where the alveolar membrane may be thickened.

SHUNTS

Any deoxygenated blood which is added to the left side (i.e. going to the tissues) of the circulation without passing through ventilated areas of the lungs is referred to as a 'right-to-left shunt'. In the normal lung there are two main sources of such a shunt: one from the blood supply of the heart and the other from the lungs themselves. This venous admixture results in a small reduction in the arterial partial pressure of oxygen leaving the left ventricle. Normally 1–2% of the cardiac output bypasses the alveoli and can be viewed as wasted perfusion.

PATHOLOGICAL SHUNTS

These may be divided into anatomical and physiological shunts. Anatomical shunts can result from cardiovascular disease, e.g. a patent ductus arteriosus, or arterial or ventricular septal defects. Physiological intrapulmonary shunts may be caused by airway blockage with secretions or alveolar collapse, provided, in both cases, the alveoli are still perfused.

A shunt-like picture may be seen if there is a reduction rather than a cessation of perfusion. The normal lung has less perfusion (Q_t) and ventilation (V) at the apices and more at the bases, but the ventilation:perfusion ratio (V:Q) increases down the lung. This is because perfusion increases faster than ventilation as the lung bases are approached. This mismatch of ventilation and perfusion adds a small amount to the venous admixture and results in a total reduction of the PAO_2 from 13.3 kPa to about 12.9 kPa. A true shunt can be distinguished from the above by administering 100% O_2 which, in the case of a true shunt, will not alter the final arterial PO_2.

By measuring the V:Q ratio, blood gases and the dead space, the effect of disease on respiratory function may be better assessed in terms of ventilation or perfusion problems.

CARRIAGE OF OXYGEN IN THE BLOOD

The transport of oxygen in the body is primarily carried out by haemoglobin in the red blood cells. In addition, a small amount is carried in the blood in solution. Each haemoglobin molecule binds four oxygen molecules (see also Chapter 21) to different degrees and a sigmoid curve can be plotted of the relationship between the partial pressures of oxygen (kPa) on the horizontal axis and the percentage saturation of haemoglobin on the vertical axis (Fig 7.2).

Several factors are involved in the affinity of haemoglobin for oxygen. If the affinity is decreased there is a shift of the curve to the right and an increase results in a shift to the left (Table 7.1). Shifts in either direction

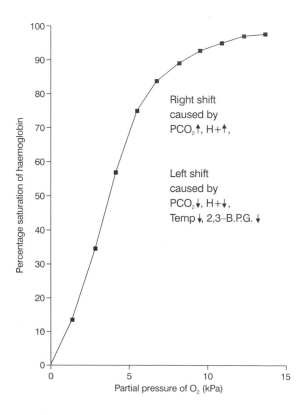

Figure 7.2   Haemoglobin dissociation curve.

Table 7.1 Affinity of haemoglobin for oxygen

Shift to left	Shift to right
O_2 affinity ↑	O_2 affinity ↓
P_{50} ↓	P_{50} ↑
As a result of	As a result of
PCO_2 ↓ , pH ↓	PCO_2 ↑ , pH ↑
Temperature ↓ , 2,3-BPG ↓	Temperature ↑ , 2,3-BPG ↑

are called the Bohr effect. A change in oxygen affinity is usually described by the P_{50}, which is the PO_2 at which the haemoglobin is 50% saturated.

2,3 Biphosphoglycerate (2,3-BPG), formerly known as 2,3 diphosphoglycerate, is very plentiful in red blood cells. It is a highly charged anion, which binds to the β chains of deoxygenated haemoglobin but not to those of oxyhaemoglobin. One molecule of deoxygenated haemoglobin binds one molecule of 2,3-BPG.

$$HbO_2 + 2,3 \text{-} BPG \leftrightarrow (Hb \text{-} 2,3\text{-}BPG) + O_2$$

In this equilibrium, an increase in the concentration of 2,3-BPG shifts the reaction to the right, causing more oxygen to be liberated.

In summary, therefore, as blood enters the lungs and carbon dioxide diffuses out of the blood into the alveoli, the reduction in blood PCO_2 and H^+ ions shifts the curve to the left. The affinity of haemoglobin for oxygen in the upper part of the curve increases at the site where oxygen is available for onloading. As blood enters the tissue capillaries and carbon dioxide is picked up, there is a reduction in the affinity of haemoglobin for oxygen at the site where oxygen needs to be released to the tissues. With exercise there is an increase in carbon dioxide production and temperature as well as an accumulation of H^+ ions as a result of lactic acid production. All of these metabolic changes will result in a shift to the right.

The actual amount of oxygen carried to the tissues is dependent upon the following.

1. The *cardiac output*. The more blood/unit time that is carried to the tissues, the more oxygen is available.
2. The *concentration of haemoglobin*. Haemoglobin is a viscous or sticky substance and, because of this, high concentrations may decrease the blood flow through the blood vessels. Thus, high levels of haemoglobin may have the potential for greater carriage of oxygen but in reality, the increased viscosity of the blood decreasing the cardiac output

to the tissues compromises this. It would appear, therefore, that a haemoglobin concentration of 10 g L^{-1} is the optimum for maximising the transport of oxygen.

3. The *percentage saturation of haemoglobin*. The higher the percentage saturation, the more oxygen is carried in each molecule of haemoglobin.
4. This in turn is dependent upon the *partial pressure of oxygen* in the blood. Typical values in arterial and venous blood are given in Table 7.2.

Thus, the amount of oxygen carried to the tissues can be calculated as follows:

Oxygen carriage (ml/min) = [Cardiac output × Hb% × Hb saturation × 1.34] + plasma oxygen

CYANOSIS

Cyanosis is a bluish-purple colour most evident in the mucous membranes, e.g. the lips, nailbeds and the skin. It is a result of a low O_2 saturation of haemoglobin in the arteriolar blood. The presence of cyanosis indicates a reduced oxygen content of the blood. In order to be clinically detectable, there must be at least 5 g L^{-1} of deoxyhaemoglobin (the reduced form of haemoglobin). It is therefore much more readily seen in polycythaemic patients who have an elevated haemoglobin level than in those who are anaemic.

CARRIAGE OF CARBON DIOXIDE IN THE BLOOD

The affinity of blood for carbon dioxide is decreased by oxygenation of the haem groups. This makes it more difficult for the globin to combine with the CO_2 molecules. Deoxygenated blood (venous blood) has a higher affinity for CO_2 and thus combines with it

Table 7.2 Typical values of the partial pressure of oxygen

Arterial blood	Typical value
PO_2	12.6 kPa
Hb concentration	150g.L^{-1}
Hb saturation	97%
O_2 content	195ml.L^{-1}
Venous blood	
PO_2	5.3 kPa
Hb saturation	70%
O_2 content	140ml.L^{-1}

better. The changes in CO_2 affinity caused by O_2 binding are called the Haldane effect.

Carbon dioxide is carried in the bloodstream as follows:

1. In the globin part of the haemoglobin molecule as a carbamino compound (approx. 30%).
2. In physical solution as carbon dioxide or carbonic acid (approx. 10%).
3. As bicarbonate (approx. 60%).

An enzyme is a protein that speeds up a reaction that is already taking place. The enzyme carbonic anhydrase is found in the red blood cell and causes the following reaction to increase in rate:

Water + carbon dioxide $\leftrightarrow$ carbonic acid $\leftrightarrow$ hydrogen ion + bicarbonate

This may be represented chemically as:

$$H_2O + CO_2 \leftrightarrow H_2CO_3 \leftrightarrow H^+ + HCO_3^-$$

The bicarbonate ion diffuses out of the cells and is replaced by chloride ions. The H^+ ions are buffered by globin. (A buffer is a substance that tends to absorb hydrogen ions without significant change in pH and therefore the pH of the blood is kept reasonably constant.) This process is known as the chloride shift (Table 7.3).

The pH of the plasma is dependent upon the ratio of HCO_3^- to PCO_2 so that the pH values of arterial and venous blood are 7.4 and 7.37 respectively. Whereas the PCO_2 is rapidly controlled by changes in lung ventilation the kidneys slowly excrete HCO_3^- to produce a longer term compensation.

The fate of carbon dioxide in the blood is summarised in Table 7.3.

CONTROL OF RESPIRATION

Breathing occurs rhythmically and without conscious effort. The regulation of respiration involves the coordinated interaction of central and peripheral chemoreceptors, medullary and pontine regulatory centres and the respiratory muscles.

The respiratory centres, which determine this rhythmicity, are found in the medulla oblongata and the pons areas of the brainstem. Mechanoreceptors in the lungs and chest wall provide feedback to the respiratory centres and determine the depth and frequency of the resting rhythm. Some stimuli, such as temperature and pain, affect breathing via the higher brain centres, e.g. the hypothalamus, which is part of the forebrain.

We have a degree of voluntary control over our breathing pattern which allows us, for example, to hold our breath or hyperventilate. This pathway involves the cerebral cortex and bypasses the respiratory centres. Protective reflexes such as coughing and sneezing are also superimposed on the normal pattern and irritants may initiate these.

The central chemoreceptors are located on the ventral surface of the medulla and respond to changes in the pH of brain extracellular fluid, which in turn is affected by the cerebrospinal fluid, local metabolism and blood flow. Peripheral chemoreceptors are found in the carotid and aortic bodies. Carotid bodies are located at the carotid bifurcation and respond to changes in the arterial blood while the aortic bodies are located near the arch of the aorta.

The role of the medulla and pons in the control of respiration is not as clearcut as was once thought. By itself, the medulla will produce a relatively normal pattern of rhythmic respiration but it is speculated that

Table 7.3 Carbon dioxide in the blood	
In plasma	*In red blood cells*
Dissolved as CO_2 or H_2CO_3	Dissolved as CO_2 or H_2CO_3
Formation of carbamino compounds with plasma protein	Formation of carbamino compounds with haemoglobin
Hydration in plasma to HCO_3^- and H^+ which is buffered	Hydration in red blood cells to HCO_3^- and H^+, which is buffered
70% of HCO_3^- diffused from red blood cells into plasma	70% of HCO_3^- diffuses into plasma
Cl^- shift from plasma into cells	Cl^- shift from plasma into cells

the pons is important in switching the respiratory phases of inspiration and expiration.

An elevation of $PaCO_2$ may be detected by both peripheral and central chemoreceptors, with the role of the latter being greater. The carotid body, however, appears to be mainly responsible for the increase in ventilation in conditions of hypoxia but the ventilatory response to hypoxia is accentuated by an elevation in $PaCO_2$. Thus, there is an interrelationship between chemoreceptors responding to hypoxia and hypercarbia. Ventilation is increased in response to reduced arterial pH and this is mediated by the peripheral chemoreceptors. Hypoxia and acidaemia also act synergistically at peripheral chemoreceptors to increase ventilation.

GENERAL ANAESTHESIA AND RESPIRATORY PHYSIOLOGY

AIRWAY OBSTRUCTION

Obstruction of the upper airways is the most common respiratory effect of anaesthesia. As anaesthesia deepens there is a loss of tone in the muscles of the soft palate; the tongue falls back into the oropharynx and the upper airways collapse. Because diaphragmatic movement is maintained better than that of the chest wall, the indrawing of the upper chest and an outpushing of the abdomen, due to strong diaphragmatic action, replace the natural heave of the chest and abdomen.

RESPIRATORY DEPRESSION

General anaesthesia causes changes in the control of respiration. Anaesthetic agents depress the sensitivity of chemoreceptors detecting hypoxia and hypercarbia and this is exacerbated by the opiate analgesics. The ventilatory response to hypoxia is depressed to a much greater degree than the response to hypercarbia. Volatile anaesthetic agents abolish the hypoxic ventilatory drive at about 1 MAC (MAC is the minimum alveolar concentration of a volatile agent that will prevent a response to surgical stimulation in 50% of patients) and significantly attenuate it at 0.1 MAC. This depression appears to be mainly sited at the peripheral chemoreceptors.

ANAESTHESIA, PATIENT POSITIONING AND LUNG FUNCTION

Ventilation and perfusion become mismatched and gas exchange deteriorates under general anaesthesia but in order to understand this process, we must define what is meant by closing volume and functional residual capacity.

Closing volume (CV) is the lung volume below which there is airways collapse, leading to a failure of ventilation, and functional residual capacity (FRC) is the volume of gas remaining in the lungs at the end of normal expiration.

The FRC is reduced by 20% under anaesthesia whether the patient is paralysed or breathing spontaneously. This fall is caused by a decrease in the thoracic volume because the diaphragm has reduced muscle tone and is displaced upwards. The FRC may fall below the closing volume although with general anaesthesia the CV also falls.

In the upright position lung gravity causes a variation in alveolar volume, compliance and ventilation. Intrapleural pressure is subatmospheric but to a greater degree at the apex than the base because the alveoli at the base of the lung are compressed and those at the apex are expanded. If a graph were plotted to show the change in alveoli volume in response to pressure, it would produce a curve which would show that dependent alveoli are better ventilated than alveoli in the upper part of the lungs. This can be applied to the lungs as a whole with the dependent lung being better ventilated than the non-dependent one.

The effect of patient position on ventilation is described below. In the supine position in an adult the FRC falls by about 0.5 L. The posterior aspects of each lung become the most dependent and are ventilated better than the anterior aspects.

Patients in the lateral decubitus position have the tidal ventilation distributed mainly to the upper lung, which is less well perfused. The dependent lung receives a greater proportion of the cardiac output but is well ventilated.

As the patient in the head-down position (Trendelenberg) is increasingly tipped, the intrapleural pressure gradient increases. This is the reverse of the upright position and the apical alveoli are decreased in volume, more compliant and better ventilated. The abdominal contents push against the diaphragm, resulting in less compliant lung bases. Both of these factors favour ventilation of the apices as compared to the bases.

The above is also exaggerated in gross obesity and to some extent in the later stages of pregnancy. This reduces the closing volume and increases the V:Q mismatch. The addition of PEEP and an increased FIO_2 will tend to correct this problem and as little head-down tilt as possible should be used.

PRINCIPLES OF THORACIC ANAESTHESIA

Thoracic surgery and anaesthesia illustrate many of the above points. During thoracic surgery, the anaesthetist usually employs the techniques of general anaesthesia, muscle relaxation, intubation and controlled ventilation. Obviously many of these patients already have poor respiratory function and reserve and must have a comprehensive 'work-up' before surgery. Patients with chronic lung conditions may well have a long history of smoking, which is also associated with ischaemic heart disease.

Thoracic surgery is associated with a high level of postoperative pain unless measures are taken to control it. This results in poor patient compliance with deep breathing exercises and chest physiotherapy, leading to an increased incidence of postoperative chest infection and pulmonary collapse. A thoracic epidural is therefore frequently used in these cases.

PREOPERATIVE PREPARATION

The purpose of the preoperative visit is to provide patient support and review the condition of the patient in relation to pre-existing disease and current medication. Frequently there is a history of chronic obstructive airways disease and investigation may reveal an obstructive picture with a low V:Q ratio and hypoxaemia. A reduction in pulmonary compliance peroperatively is a common finding in these patients. They may also lose the CO_2 drive to respiration, relying instead on hypoxia. Respiratory function postoperatively is affected by such factors as age, obesity, smoking and preoperative lung disease. Refraining from smoking for even just 12 hours preoperatively has been shown to have a beneficial effect on pulmonary ciliary function postoperatively. This will have a significant bearing on post-operative management, determining the need for controlled oxygen therapy.

The anaesthetic management of all patients should include determining their smoking habits in the preoperative visit. Information and advice regarding both their postoperative management and the long-term care of their respiratory system may produce benefits during their convalescence. It is also important to assess cardiac function and identify any cardiac strain or arrhythmias. Preoperative investigations should therefore include:

1. Electrocardiography.
2. Chest X-ray.
3. Pulmonary function tests (PFTs) including FVC and FEV_1.
4. Arterial blood gases.
5. Full blood count, together with blood urea and electrolytes.

Repeat readings of PFTs after bronchodilators are often carried out in order to ascertain how much of the bronchospasm is potentially reversible. The deterioration in postoperative lung function is related to the extent of lung tissue removed and lung resection is therefore contraindicated in patients whose FEV_1 is less than 0.8 L. In these cases great difficulty would be expected in re-establishing independent respiration at the end of the procedure.

The need for anxiolytic premedication is largely ablated by a careful and sympathetic preoperative visit. Antisialogogues may result in sputum retention and opiates should be avoided because of their respiratory depressant effects. Respiratory therapy, including bronchodilators and other drug treatment, should be continued up until the time of surgery.

PEROPERATIVE MANAGEMENT

Induction of anaesthesia should be smooth to minimise the risk of coughing and bronchospasm. Constant monitoring by pulse oximetry will help guard against hypoxia as a result of V:Q mismatch, loss of lung volume and reduction in pulmonary hypoxic vasoconstriction. This latter mechanism operates in poorly ventilated regions of the lung and diverts blood flow to areas with better ventilation. Unfortunately, many factors play a part in the effectiveness of this process and volatile anaesthetic agents seriously inhibit it. Intraarterial pressure monitoring is also advocated since repeated assessments of arterial blood gases may be needed and 'real-time' blood pressure monitoring is a major advantage, especially into the recovery period.

In many thoracic surgical procedures, one-lung ventilation is employed to:

1. Improve surgical access.
2. Reduce trauma to the lung tissue.
3. Limit soiling of the contralateral lung.

Once both ventilation and circulation to the operative site are stopped, the V:Q mismatch that results from collapsing that lung is minimised. In order that the procedure and recovery should progress smoothly, a double lumen tube must be sited so that ventilation of the lungs can be managed independently, thus allowing one lung to be collapsed. Any deflated lung remaining must be reinflated prior to closure of the wound.

During bilateral lung ventilation in a lateral thoracotomy position, the upper lung is ventilated preferentially while the lower lung is better perfused, resulting in a V:Q mismatch. This mismatch is reduced, as stated above, when ventilation is stopped to the upper lung but there is still circulation to this lung, leading to a shunt. A degree of hypoxic pulmonary vasoconstriction will to some extent reduce it. A number of factors complicate this scenario but one should remember that the disease process in the operative field might mean that perfusion is already compromised, thereby limiting this shunt.

In summary, therefore, to maintain adequate oxygenation during single-lung anaesthesia the anaesthetist should aim to:

1. Maintain the same tidal volume as was used when both lungs were ventilated. The limiting factor here may be the resultant airway pressures.
2. Use an inspired oxygen concentration of at least 50%.
3. Pass a catheter down to the unventilated lung and insufflate with oxygen.
4. Monitor pulse oximetry and arterial blood gases and guard against surgical compression of the dependent lung.

At the conclusion of the resection the residual lung tissue should be reinflated. Both the surgeon and the anaesthetist should check carefully that all areas appear re-expanded.

Postoperatively supplementary oxygen, chest drains, physiotherapy and adequate analgesia all require expert attention.

THE MANAGEMENT OF POSTOPERATIVE APNOEA

From time to time, the patient may fail to regain adequate respiration after a period of controlled ventilation. There may be one or more factors involved but certain problems are implicated more commonly than others and the anaesthetist needs to evolve a system for identifying the cause. A number of questions may be asked. Is the delayed recovery of respiration a direct result of the overenthusiastic use of certain drugs in the anaesthetic technique? Obvious examples are volatile agents, which maintain the patient deeply unconscious and depress respiration. The same clinical picture might also be seen with an overdose of narcotic analgesics, leading to pinpoint pupils and an absent or very infrequent breathing pattern. Usually narcotic depression causes a decrease in the frequency of respiration. The anaesthetist should consider ventilating with 100% O_2 with or without the use of naloxone, which is a specific antagonist to the opiate analgesics. It is important to note that naloxone has a shorter action than many of the opiates. This means that respiratory

depression may well recur and the patient should not be discharged from the recovery area until this possibility has been excluded.

Residual muscle relaxant alone may cause respiratory embarrassment but without the evidence of central nervous system depression. This may result from too large a dose of relaxant or because the patient was reversed too soon after the last increment of muscle relaxant. Rarely, an abnormality in the muscle endplates may be responsible for the failure of reversal. This condition is known as myasthenia gravis. Suxamethonium apnoea must also be excluded if suxamethonium has been administered. A true failure of reversal may only be diagnosed in the presence of normal blood gases and electrolytes and in the absence of respiratory depression due to volatile agents and/or analgesic drugs. Curtailing the administration of volatile agents and nitrous oxide runs the risk of the patient becoming aware but still being paralysed, a situation to be abhorred. A peripheral nerve stimulator is most useful in this situation.

Controlled ventilation resulting in hypocarbia deprives the respiratory centres of their most potent stimulus and the use of capnography should prevent this occurring.

The anaesthetist should also consider concurrent medical problems such as a head injury.

Medical problems occurring during anaesthesia including a stroke or embolism might, if suspected, require further investigation such as CT or MR scan and also transfer to the intensive care unit.

RESPIRATORY COMPLICATIONS POSTOPERATIVELY ON THE WARD

Hypoxaemia

The PaO_2 decreases after general anaesthesia even with apparently normal pulmonary function and all patients should receive added oxygen in the recovery ward.

Patients relying on a hypoxic drive should receive controlled oxygen therapy. Because they have lower than normal oxygen levels in the blood, any increase in inspired oxygen and hence PaO_2 will depress respiration. This results in an increase in carbon dioxide and the subsequent narcosis (a sleepy state induced in this case by carbon dioxide) will make the patient unrouseable. When the inspired oxygen is reduced the hypoxic drive returns, the carbon dioxide level falls and the patient wakes up again. In severe cases patients should not receive more than 24%–28% oxygen.

Sputum Retention

This is frequently the result of a reduction in respiratory effort, which may be due to inadequate pain relief, prolonged sedation or reduced ciliary action in the lungs affected by anaesthetic agents.

Humidification of inspired oxygen, adequate and efficient pain relief and physiotherapy are required to minimise this problem.

Atelectasis or Lung Collapse

Management of sputum retention will reduce the incidence of atelectasis. The treatment is the same, including considering an epidural for analgesia if not already instituted.

Pulmonary Aspiration

This may occur in the postoperative period if the laryngeal reflexes are still depressed and the patient not positioned safely. If associated with pregnancy the term Mendelson's Syndrome is used (see Chapter 26).

Pneumothorax

This is the introduction of air into the pleural space and is usually followed by some degree of lung collapse. The deflation of a lung may be caused by:

- Incomplete reinflation of the lung after thoracic surgery.
- Insertion of a CVP line.
- Rupture of an emphysematous bulla (an alveolus that has been weakened by disease) in the lung.
- Puncture of the pleura by the surgeon whilst performing a nephrectomy.
- Pleural damage during a cervical sympathectomy.

In all cases of suspected pneumothorax an urgent chest X-ray is required followed often by an underwater sealed drain to facilitate lung expansion.

RECOMMENDED READING

Atkinson RS. 1993 *Lee's Synopsis of Anaesthesia*, 11th edn Oxford: Butterworth Heinemann.

Bray JJ, Cragg PA, McKnight ADC *et al.* 1994 *Lecture Notes on Human Physiology*, 3rd Edn. Oxford:Blackwell

Faust RJ. 1994 *Anaesthesiology Review*, 2nd edn. New York:Churchill Livingstone

8

SCIENTIFIC PRINCIPLES IN RELATION TO THE ANAESTHETIC MACHINE

C.S. Ince, A.C. Skinner & E. Taft

WHAT IS AN ANAESTHETIC MACHINE?

All anaesthetics require the supply of respirable gases for the patient to breathe. In current UK practice this gas mixture is usually a major part of the maintenance phase of anaesthesia. Anaesthetic machines are the apparatus used for delivering to the patient this gas mixture in an accurate, controlled and safe manner. Early anaesthesia only made use of inhalational agents and as anaesthesia developed, so did the apparatus. Perhaps one of the earliest advances in this field was regulation of the concentration of anaesthetic vapours and in 1847 John Snow developed ether and chloroform inhalers. It was not until 1910 that E. I. McKesson introduced the first intermittent flow (demand) nitrous oxide and oxygen machine, which was able to determine the concentration of both gases in percentage terms given to the patient. In 1917 Edmund Boyle described a portable apparatus used for the delivery of oxygen and nitrous oxide. This was modified from an American design and was the forerunner of the modern Boyle's machine. Boyle is now a trademark of Ohmeda, formerly the anaesthetic division of the British Oxygen Company (BOC).

UNITS USED IN THE MEASUREMENT OF GAS PRESSURES

The SI unit of pressure is the Pascal (Pa). The CGS unit is the bar (b).

One atmosphere is

760 mmHg = 1b = 1000 mb = 100,000 Pa = 100 kPa = 15 lb/in^2 = 1000 cmH$_2$O where mb is short for millibar and kPa for kilopascal.

THE GAS LAWS

Gases obey physical laws, which determine how they must be supplied and used. In any container the molecules of a gas are evenly distributed throughout that container. As the molecules move about they will collide with each other and with the sides of the container and the speed with which the molecules move (and therefore the collision rate) increases with temperature. If more gas is added to the container or the size of the container is reduced, the rate of collision will also increase. The pressure the gas exerts on the container walls is a reflection of the collision rate of molecules with the container walls and with each other.

The volume (V), pressure (P) and absolute temperature (T) for any fixed amount of a gas are therefore dependent on each other so that the pressure multiplied by volume is proportional to absolute temperature. Symbolically this becomes PV ∝ T. A more useful relationship is PV = RT and this is called the *universal gas equation*.

R is a known physical constant and is the same for all gases. Thus, for a given amount of gas, compressing it to half the original volume will require doubling its pressure. A 10% increase in absolute temperature, about 30 K (°Celsius) at normal temperature, will increase pressure by 10% unless the volume is allowed to expand.

The relationships of volume, pressure and temperature were all described independently by physicists in the past, so for a fixed amount of gas:

1. At a constant temperature the pressure of a gas is inversely proportional to its volume (Boyle's law), i.e. P ∝ 1/V.
2. At a constant pressure the volume of a gas is directly proportional to its absolute temperature (Charles' law), i.e. V ∝ T.
3. At a constant volume the pressure of a gas is directly proportional to its absolute temperature (Gay-Lussac's law), i.e. P ∝ T.

A gas that obeys the gas equation is known as an ideal gas but no gas is a true ideal gas. The gas equation makes no allowance for intermolecular forces and molecular volume, but in practice it describes the behaviour of most gases well enough. It is well known that applying pressure increases the boiling temperature of liquids, for example in pressure cookers or steam autoclaves. Similarly applying pressure increases the temperature at which it is possible to liquefy any gas. There is, however, a temperature above which it is impossible to liquefy a gas by pressure alone. This is the critical temperature and is different for each gas.

The critical temperature is defined as the temperature above which no application of pressure alone will liquefy the gas. This temperature determines whether a gas will exist in the liquid or gaseous state when compressed in cylinders.

Oxygen, Entonox™ and air have critical temperatures well below normal temperatures and so exist in gaseous form in cylinders. Because of this they behave according to the gas equation and the pressure in the cylinder is roughly proportional to the contents. Nitrous oxide, carbon dioxide and other gases like butane and propane fuels, have critical temperatures above normal temperatures and so exist as liquids (with gas in the free space above the liquid) in compressed gas cylinders. This means that pressure is no guide to contents until all the liquid is used up and the cylinder is virtually empty. The gas pressure in these cylinders is a product of the specific gases' physical properties and the temperature. This pressure is known as the saturated vapour pressure, which rises with the temperature and differs for each gas. Thus, the temperature of the liquid nitrous oxide in effect solely determines the pressure in nitrous oxide cylinders.

The change from liquid to gaseous state needs energy in the form of heat (as in boiling a kettle). This energy is known as latent heat of vaporization (see Chapter 19). Thus as liquid oxygen (at low temperatures) or nitrous oxide (in cylinders) is used, the liquid is cooled. If a nitrous oxide cylinder is used for a long period it is not uncommon to see frost on the outside of the cylinder as a result of this cooling. Because of this cooling the pressure in a nitrous oxide cylinder will fall with use, but this is due to the cooling and is not an accurate guide to the volume remaining in the cylinder.

THE ANAESTHETIC GAS SUPPLY

It should be self-evident that incorrect delivery of any of the gases used risks either inadequate oxygen supply to the patient, with perhaps death or serious injury, or inadequate anaesthesia, risking painful recall of surgery.

The anaesthetic gases are delivered to the patient from two main sources: via pipelines or from cylinders directly attached to the anaesthetic machine. Oxygen, air and nitrous oxide are generally used from a pipeline. Carbon dioxide (when available) is only supplied in cylinders while Entonox™ is supplied for analgesia either via a pipeline or cylinders, though the latter is more common as the apparatus is essentially portable. Almost all anaesthetic machines have reserve cylinders of oxygen and usually nitrous oxide attached in case of pipeline failure.

CYLINDERS

Modern gas cylinders are made of molybdenum steel and because of its strength, the walls are now thinner and lighter than older cylinders constructed from carbon steel. Cylinders are visually checked at each filling and every five years a cylinder undergoes hydraulic testing, to pressures that are well in excess of maximum working pressures.

IDENTIFICATION OF MEDICAL GAS CYLINDERS

Each gas cylinder carries its own specific mark and history in order that it may be uniquely identified. In the UK this is in the form of a plastic disc, the shape and colour of which identify the year when it was last examined. Cylinders are produced in a variety of sizes (Fig. 8.1), each denoted by a capital letter (A through to J in ascending order of size). Sizes A and H are not produced for medical gases. J-sized cylinders are about four feet tall and need careful handling.

Medical gas cylinders are colour coded by gas contents. The UK and ISO standards are the same, but the USA and Germany use different colourings (Table 8.1). Cylinders consist of a valve and a body, with the curved upper part of the body below the valve called the shoulder.

The valve is a separate unit, secured to the cylinder by a screw thread. The valve that connects a cylinder to the anaesthetic machine is known as a pin-index valve. Each valve block has one or two locating holes drilled into the valve face. The cylinder yoke, where the cylinder fits onto the anaesthetic machine, contains locating pins that correspond to the holes on the valve. Each gas has a different pin arrangement (Table 8.1) so only the correct gas cylinder can be attached to each yoke.

Larger cylinders (used to supply some pipelines and for some portable uses) use 'bull-nose' valves and

Table 8.1 Identification of the most common gas cylinders			
Gas	Cylinder colour	Shoulder colour	Pin index holes
Oxygen	Black	White	2 & 5
Nitrous oxide	Blue	Blue	3 & 5
Entonox™	Blue	Blue & White	Central
Carbon dioxide	Grey	Grey	1 & 6
Compressed air	Grey	Black & white	1 & 5

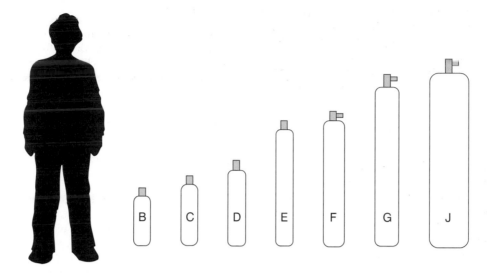

Figure 8.1   Cylinder sizes in relation to a 6 foot man

occasionally "hand wheel" valves. These use screw-in connectors to attach to apparatus. Some gas cylinders have different threads to prevent cross connection, but the uniqueness of the pin-index system makes this impossible. Bull-nose and pin-index cylinders need a key to open the valves but hand-wheel cylinders do not.

PIPED GAS SUPPLY

Piped nitrous oxide and Entonox™ (and oxygen for small users) come from separate banks of J-sized cylinders arranged in a group with pressure-reducing valves and control gear, called a manifold. The manifold usually has two banks of cylinders to allow changeover without interruption. Each bank usually consists of 4–6 interconnected cylinders and, within the bank in use (known as the running bank), all the cylinders empty simultaneously. When the available gas in the running bank is nearing exhaustion the supply is transferred to the second (reserve) bank. This is changed automatically by a pressure-sensitive control device, linking both banks. The control unit is connected to a display panel that gives both an audible and a visual alarm to the theatre staff, who then should arrange for replacement of the empty cylinders (Fig. 8.2). The replaced cylinder bank then becomes the new reserve bank.

Piped oxygen (except for low-volume users) originates from a liquid oxygen supply. Liquid oxygen is stored in large vessels that work in the same way as a vacuum flask and are known as vacuum insulated evaporators (VIE). These are double-walled vessels with the inner vessel holding the liquid oxygen. A vacuum is main-

tained between the inner and the outer skins and this insulation helps to maintain the temperature of the stored oxygen at about -180°C. (constant evaporation of oxygen gas for use, from the liquid, cools the contents.) The size of the evaporator depends on the hospital demand and the plant is rented from a supply company (usually BOC), who installs and maintains it. The vessel is usually filled from a liquid oxygen tanker about once each week. Due to the risk of fire liquid oxygen must be sited in a locked compound in the open air.

The VIE is maintained at pressures higher than atmospheric since this allows the oxygen to remain liquid at higher temperatures. The pressure in the VIE will vary with the temperature of the liquid, which in turn depends on oxygen usage. Higher usage cools the liquid because of the heat energy needed to evaporate the liquid oxygen. The initial pressure in the VIE is 1000 kPa, which is reduced to pipeline pressure (400 kPa) through a series of regulators. If the demand is high liquid oxygen is automatically withdrawn from the bottom of the VIE and passed through an evaporator (a length of copper tubing with fins to absorb heat from the surrounding air) into the main system. All the gas is passed through a superheater (further copper piping) to warm it to ambient temperature before the final pressure reduction. A conventional cylinder manifold backs up this main supply.

In addition to the medical gases, there is usually a central compressed air and suction supply. Compressed air is supplied from a compressor on site. Air is supplied at two pressures, 420 kPa (for respi-

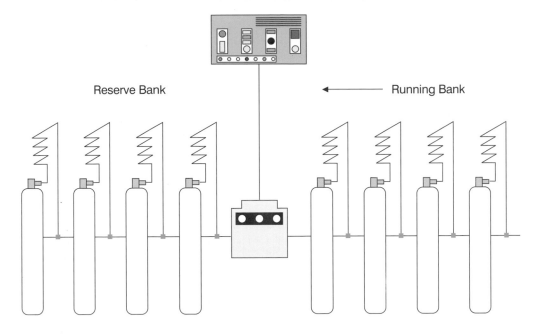

Figure 8.2   Manifold and alarm panel, which is displayed in operating department, to alert staff to arrange replacement of empty bank.

ratory use, the standard pipeline pressure) and 700 kPa to drive power tools in theatre. Pipeline installations treat these as if they were two separate gases. Pipeline pressure is the same for all gases except the high-pressure air supply.

Piped gases in theatre

Piped gas outlets are strategically placed in the theatre suite. Oxygen, nitrous oxide, compressed air and suction outlets are grouped together. Cross connection is prevented by colour coding and couplings specific to each gas or suction. These couplings are known as Schraeder valves and contain a valve to ensure that the gas flow is shut off when there is no probe *in situ*. The fitting on the anaesthetic machine is also unique to each gas. The pipelines themselves are colour coded: oxygen – white; nitrous oxide:–blue; compressed air – black; and suction–yellow.

In order to prevent incorrect reassembly the flexible hoses must never be repaired on site. Before any gas supply is handed over to the user (either after installation or following maintenance or modification) pressure tests and anti-confusion tests are carried out to make absolutely certain that the central supply is delivering the correct gas to each outlet. Both the manufacturer and a representative of the user sign a document to this effect.

THE USE AND STORAGE OF OXYGEN CYLINDERS

Because the critical temperature of oxygen is -116°C it cannot exist as a liquid at room temperatures and therefore an oxygen cylinder only contains gas. Oxygen cylinders are designed to withstand pressures of 20,000 kPa (about 3000lb/in^{-2}) but are only commercially filled until the pressure reaches 13,700 kPa, which is 2000lb/ in^{-2}. Although the cylinder pressure increases proportionately with an increase in temperature this rise is not significant within the temperature range found in the British Isles.

When oxygen is removed from the cylinder the gas pressure falls roughly in proportion to its use (Fig. 8.3), so that when a third of the gas has been used the cylinder pressure will also have fallen by about 33%. Thus this pressure accurately reflects the amount of gas remaining in the cylinder.

THE USE AND STORAGE OF NITROUS OXIDE CYLINDERS

The critical temperature of nitrous oxide is 36.5°C and because the cylinders are filled under pressure, at temperatures below 36.5°c they will contain both liquid and gaseous nitrous oxide. Until all the liquid is used up a cylinder of nitrous oxide, at a

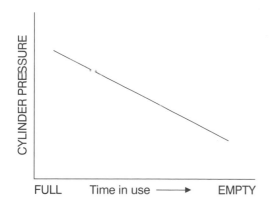

Figure 8.3   Pressure changes in an oxygen cylinder.

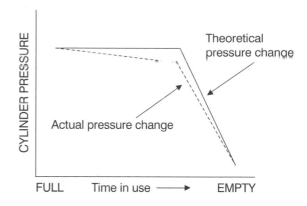

Figure 8.4   Diagrammatic representation of the pressure changes within a nitrous oxide cylinder.

temperature of 20°c, has an internal pressure of 5100 kPa (750lb/in⁻²).

If a nitrous oxide cylinder is left in the sun or is stored in a hot climate the critical temperature may easily be exceeded and all the liquid nitrous oxide becomes a gas. The pressure exerted by a gas depends on the number of molecules existing in the gaseous phase and, therefore, if the critical temperature is exceeded there will be a massive increase in the cylinder pressure. At 65°C a full cylinder will have an internal pressure of some 17,500 kPa. It is for this reason that nitrous oxide cylinders are subjected to the same pressure tests as cylinders containing oxygen and are not filled to capacity but to a safe level. This is usually expressed as the 'filling ratio', defined as the mass of contents placed in the cylinder divided by the mass of water that would completely fill the cylinder. A filling ratio of 0.67 is used for commercially filled cylinders destined for both the UK and tropical countries.

When nitrous oxide gas is withdrawn from a cylinder the number of gaseous molecules decrease. As a result molecules pass from the liquid to the gaseous phase until equilibrium is reestablished. The saturated vapour pressure does not change unless the temperature falls. It is only when all the liquid has been converted into gas that the pressure begins to fall in a similar manner to an oxygen cylinder. The continuous line in Figure 8.4 illustrates this concept but the actual change is represented by the dotted line. Energy (as heat) is needed to convert liquid nitrous oxide to a gas (latent heat of vaporization). This heat energy is taken from the cylinder and from the contents, thus cooling both of these. Because the saturated vapour pressure of nitrous oxide decreases with temperature, the pressure in the cylinder falls even though there is still liquid

remaining in the cylinder. (If the cylinder is turned off the temperature gradually returns to room temperature and the cylinder pressure increases again.)

As the temperature of the cylinder falls, the air around it is cooled. Chapter 9 describes how a fall in air temperature results in an increase in relative humidity, reflecting the fact that the air cannot hold as much water vapour. When the relative humidity reaches 100% any further decrease in temperature means that the air is unable to hold all the water it is carrying and the excess will condense onto the cold surface. It appears firstly as condensation and then as the temperature continues to fall, frost appears on the surface of the cylinder.

THE USE AND STORAGE OF ENTONOX CYLINDERS

Entonox™ is a mixture of 50% oxygen and 50% nitrous oxide and is used as an analgesic. It is described elsewhere but is mentioned in this chapter because it behaves differently from either oxygen or nitrous oxide. Just as sugar may be dissolved in water, so liquid nitrous oxide is effectively dissolved in oxygen. This is achieved by bubbling oxygen through liquid nitrous oxide in a cylinder. The resulting mixture behaves as if it were a single gas providing the temperature is maintained above −7°C.

Below −7°C liquid nitrous oxide separates out and above this liquid is a mixture of oxygen and some nitrous oxide gas. When the cylinder is used the initial gas has a high percentage of oxygen and less nitrous oxide. As the oxygen is used up the percentage of nitrous oxide increases in the mixture and eventually a hypoxic mixture can result. It is therefore important that Entonox™ is not used if the cylinder has been subjected to temperatures below 0°C unless steps have been taken to reconstitute the mixture after re-warming. This does not necessarily occur merely when the temperature rises and ideally Entonox™ cylinders should be kept rigorously frost-free. Therefore:

1. Entonox™ cylinders should be stored for at least 24 hours before use at a temperature above 10°C.
2. Cylinders should be stored on their side to allow the maximum surface area for reconstitution.
3. Before use portable cylinders should be inverted repeatedly to ensure mixing.

CHANGING A GAS CYLINDER

Because of the prevalence of piped gas supplies this is a task that is not often performed within the theatre area. It is, however, important to be familiar with the procedure because the need may well occur when least expected, e.g. a pipeline failure. The method is described below.

1. Select a new cylinder of the correct type and make sure it has a plastic sheath around the valve. This protects the valve from dust but also indicates that it is likely to be an unused cylinder.
2. Close the empty cylinder and remove it from the yoke.
3. Check the Bodok seal situated between the cylinder and the valve block to make sure it is in good condition.
4. Remove the plastic sheath from the new cylinder and briefly open the valve with a key to blow out any dust ('snifting').
5. Close the valve, replace the cylinder in the yoke and tighten the screw to fix it securely in position. Most authorities recommend that oxygen cylinders be left hissing slightly during fitting to prevent dirt entering the valve after snifting.
6. Open the cylinder to check that there is no leak and to ensure the cylinder is not empty. Bear in mind that gauge pressure does not indicate the contents of a nitrous oxygen cylinder.
7. If there is a leak check the Bodok seal, gland nut and securing screw. Discard the cylinder and fit a new one if problems persist.
8. Replace the used cylinder in the store.
9. Label the new cylinder as 'full' and the previous spare as 'in use'.

PRESSURE-REDUCING VALVES

There are three main reasons why anaesthetic machines are fitted with reducing valves:

1. To maintain a safe, easily managed working pressure in the anaesthetic machine. The working pressure is, like pipeline pressure, about 400 kPa, which is considerably less than cylinder pressures.
2. To maintain a more or less constant flow rate. If a cylinder is used without a reducing valve the flow rate would vary with the pressure within the cylinder. Thus as the gas was used up the flow rate would decrease and the needle valve would need constant adjustment to maintain a steady flow.
3. To facilitate the adjustment of the flow rate. In a high-pressure system a small change in the needle valve produces a large fluctuation in flow rate and makes adjustment of flows difficult. Adjusting the flow rate is therefore easier to manage if there is a lower pressure within the system.

HOW A PRESSURE REDUCING VALVE WORKS

Within the pressure-reducing valve (Fig. 8.5) high-pressure gas enters the bottom of the regulator or reducing valve. Pressure reduction takes place immediately where the gas enters the valve, with the valve needle, acting against the valve seat, regulating the entry of gas into the main valve chamber. The gas outlet is from the main chamber of the valve and the

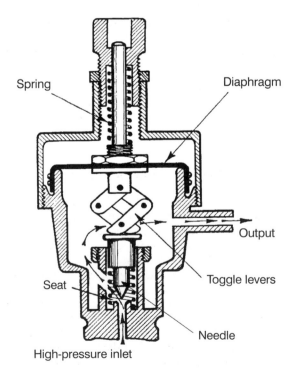

Figure 8.5   Pressure reducing valve

main chamber pressure is regulated to the desired outlet pressure. If the pressure in the main chamber is higher than the set pressure, the diaphragm is displaced upwards against the spring. The toggle levers turn this upward movement of the diaphragm into a downward movement of the needle into the seat. This closes the high-pressure inlet so the main chamber pressure falls.

Conversely, if the pressure in the main chamber is lower than the set pressure the diaphragm is displaced downwards by the tension in the spring. The toggle levers turn this downward movement of the diaphragm into an upward movement of the needle into the seat. This opens the high-pressure inlet so the main chamber pressure rises as more high-pressure gas is allowed in.

The force exerted by the gas in the main chamber, pushing the diaphragm upwards, is the regulated gas pressure multiplied by the area of the diaphragm (force = pressure × area). The valve is therefore in equilibrium when this force is equal to the tension in the spring.

Changing the tension on the spring sets the regulated (reduced) pressure. Most anaesthetic machine regulators are preset but some devices, such as tourniquets and air cylinders used to drive power tools, still use variable regulators. The input pressure will slightly affect output pressure since the high-pressure gas will tend to lift the needle slightly. As the cross-sectional area of this needle is small this is only a modest effect and two-stage reduction is sometimes used to reduce this.

Reducing valves are cooled by the expansion of gas within them and older valves had heating fins cast into their bodies to prevent freezing. As medical gases are now effectively dry, icing is no longer a problem.

GAS FLOWS – ROTAMETERS™

In most current anaesthetic machines the flow of gases is adjusted by needle valves and a Rotameter™ - is used to measure this flow rate. Rotameters™ are tapered glass tubes (the tube is wider at the top than bottom) through which gas flows from bottom to top. Within this tube is a bobbin float, the height of which is a balance between gravity (pulling the bobbin down) and the force of the gas flow (pushing the bobbin up the tube). Thus the greater the gas flow, the further up the tube the float rises. The flow rate is read from the top of the bobbin against the calibrations on the glass tube. Oblique grooves cut in the bobbin cause it to rotate (Fig. 8.6), showing it is not stuck but is floating freely. Sticking is more likely to occur at low-flow rates

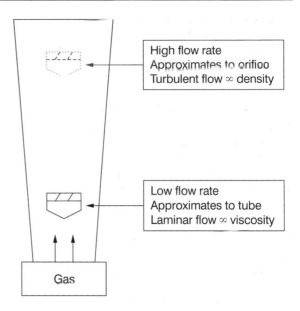

High flow rate
Approximates to orifice
Turbulent flow ∞ density

Low flow rate
Approximates to tube
Laminar flow ∞ viscosity

Gas

Figure 8.6   The Rotameter™

and is due to the build-up of electrostatic charge, which is minimized by treating the wall of the tube with a conductive coating, but dirt can also cause sticking. Rotameters™ must always be vertical or the float will tend to stick badly.

At low gas flows near the base of the tube the gap between the bobbin and the wall of the Rotameter™ is long and narrow (Fig.8.6). This means the gas flow is mainly laminar and the flow rate is determined mainly by the viscosity of the gas. At high flow rates near the top of the Rotameter™ the gap between the bobbin and the wall approximates to an orifice, its width being larger in relation to its length. Flow through an orifice is turbulent in nature and varies mainly with the density of the gas. Thus the Rotameter™ is a variable orifice device within which there is a mixture of laminar and turbulent flow.

Medical gases all have different densities and viscosities and therefore each Rotameter™ tube must be calibrated for a specific gas and not used for any other. Some Rotameters™ use two tubes in series (cascade), one of which is calibrated for the accurate delivery of low flow rates. Although this is useful in low flow anaesthesia, it is by no means essential.

Leaks in Rotameter™ banks can cause selective loss of different gases. Modern flow meter banks place the oxygen flow meter downstream to protect against selective loss of oxygen and consequent hypoxic gas mixtures. Modern anaesthetic machines also interlock the nitrous oxide and oxygen controls to prevent the delivery of hypoxic gas mixtures.

The combined output from the flow meters is passed to the 'backbar', a common gas conduit to which the vaporizers and other devices are fixed.

Ball float flow meters are used in less critical applications such as on wards. They are not as accurate as Rotameters™ and the flow rate is read from the equator of the ball.

VAPORIZERS

Nitrous oxide alone is not an effective anaesthetic. Additional inhalational drugs are usually added to the gas flow to ensure unconsciousness. Most modern inhalational agents are liquids at room temperature and pressure (so-called volatile agents). They must therefore be vaporized into the gas flow for administration to the patient. Vaporization of a liquid depends on:

1. The physical properties of the liquid.
2. The temperature of the liquid.
3. The surface area available for vaporization.

Early administration of volatile agents was carried out by placing gamgee placed over the mouth and nose with the volatile agent administered from a dropper bottle. In an attempt to make administration more predictable, anaesthetic vaporizers were designed early in the development of anaesthetics. Typical examples, which survived into the modern era, were the Boyle's bottle and the Goldman vaporizer. In these a control valve passes part of the gas flow through the chamber containing the volatile agent and the rest flows through a bypass. Various devices could be used to increase the output of these primitive vaporizers, such as home-made wicks or a plunger which would direct the gas flow close to or through the liquid agent. Although the principle of a variable bypass is still used to control most modern vaporizers, many improvements have been made to make output highly predictable.

MODERN VAPORIZERS

All volatile agents have different physical properties and therefore vaporizers are designed and calibrated for use only with a specific agent. There are many different patterns in use and being developed. The purpose of this section is to give an overview rather than describe particular types.

Almost all modern vaporizers work by dividing the gas flow (often called the carrier gas) into two streams. The larger part passes through a bypass channel and is unal-tered. The smaller passes through a carefully designed vaporizing chamber with a large surface area (usually increased by means of wicks), which saturates the gas with the volatile agent. Since at any particular temperature the saturated vapour pressure of the volatile agent is known, the composition of the gas leaving the vaporizing chamber is also known. The controls of the vaporizer accurately split the gas flow between the bypass and the vaporizing chamber and it is changing this 'splitting ratio' that controls the output of the vaporizer.

Energy (as heat) is needed to evaporate the volatile agent and this causes the system to cool. The saturated vapour pressure of the agent decreases with the fall in temperature and reduces the output of the vaporizer. To reduce the cooling, the vaporizer is made from metal of high thermal conductivity acting as a heat sink, readily giving up heat to the anaesthetic agent and helping to maintain the temperature. Modern vaporizers also have a temperature-compensating device, commonly utilizing a bimetallic strip. When metals become hot they expand and if two dissimilar metals are fixed together as a strip they will expand at different rates, resulting in the bending of the strip. This property is used to control the splitting ratio. If the temperature of the vaporizer falls more gas flows through the vaporizing chamber and vice versa if there is an increase in temperature. Vaporizers that have the facility of compensating for change in temperature are known as temperature compensated vaporizers. The name 'TEC', used by Ohmeda for their vaporizers, is a contraction of temperature compensated.

Desflurane boils at about room temperature. For this reason a variable bypass vaporizer is unsuitable. The desflurane vaporizer is a 'vapour generator'. Liquid desflurane is heated to generate pure desflurane vapour, small volumes of which are added to the gas flow that never enters the vaporizing chamber. The desflurane vaporizer is electrically heated and controlled by electronics. In use it seems like the other temperature compensated vaporizers. Older designs of vaporizer for diethyl ether were vapour generators, for example the Oxford Vaporizer and others, so the principle is not new.

Older ventilators exert an intermittent back pressure on the backbar components, including vaporizers. This so-called 'pumping effect' can affect vaporizer output, causing the concentration of volatile agent to increase. Modern vaporizers are designed to prevent this occurring.

In early vaporizers, either the vaporizer jar was simply unscrewed and filled or, a funnel shaped filling port sealed by a screw stopper was used. In the late 1970s, however, both systems were criticized because neither eliminated the potential for filling the vaporizer with the wrong volatile agent. Agent-specific, colour-coded filling devices (the Fraser Swetman pin safety system) were introduced by Cyprane (now Ohmeda) in the early 1980s for use in filling and draining vaporizers. One end of the filler is keyed to fit a specific vaporizer and the other fits a collar on the neck of the bottles for the correct agent. This system minimizes filling errors but also prevents the overfilling of vaporizers and reduces atmospheric pollution during the filling process.

'Draw-over' vaporizers are used in applications where the patient's respiratory efforts drive gas through the vaporizer, rather than supply gas pressure. They are used in field (usually military) apparatus, as portable analgesia apparatus (now uncommon) and in some circle systems (see below). They are not usually used on anaesthetic machines as the low resistance to gas flow needed is often at the cost of less accurate output.

Vaporizers are sited on the backbar of the anaesthetic machine and are usually removable by a quick-release mechanism such as the Selectatec™. This allows rapid changes of anaesthetic agents on the machine and rapid replacement if the vaporizer becomes empty or malfunctions during use. The system does, however, have a number of potential hazards and it is important to observe the following safety precautions.

1. Do not carry the vaporizer by the control dial.
2. Check that the mounting port 'O' rings on the Selectatec™ manifold are intact and undamaged and that the mating surfaces are clean.
3. Make sure that the vaporizer control knob is in the 'off' position and that the locking lever is in the 'unlock' position.
4. Lower the vaporizer onto the manifold and move the locking lever to the 'lock' position.
5. Make sure that the vaporizer is properly seated.
6. Leak test the system with the vaporizer off and then turned on. A leak can be catastrophic for the patient.

OXYGEN FAILURE ALARMS, PRESSURE RELIEF VALVES AND OXYGEN FLUSH

These components are the final parts of the anaesthetic machine before the gas mixture passes to the common gas outlet. The hazard of an unobserved failure of oxygen supply should be obvious. Almost all machines in current use will have a combination of oxygen failure warning devices that may include:

- A whistle sounded by oxygen pressure alone as the oxygen pressure fails: the dying oxygen alarm. This should sound for at least seven seconds and the remaining gas flow must be cut off and vented harmlessly. Machines without this type of alarm are potentially lethal and it is difficult to justify their continued use.
- A second alarm driven by this vented gas or high-pressure nitrous oxide.

Some devices cut off the nitrous oxide before the Rotameters™. A visual indicator was common in the past. Finally, of course, oxygen concentration in the breathing system should be monitored.

Sometimes it may be useful to bypass the conventional gas supply in order to deliver pure oxygen at high flows (about 35 l/min). Every anaesthetic machine has a clearly marked emergency oxygen button for this purpose. It may be used to:

- Flush out anaesthetic gases from the circuit prior to preoxygenation.
- Increase gas flow to facilitate ventilation despite leaks.
- Deliver a high oxygen concentration in an emergency.

It should be used with care, however, because it is easy to subject the patient to potential barotrauma from the high-pressure gas. In addition, in some older machines it is possible to lock the oxygen flush on, leading to inadequate anaesthesia.

The final component on the machine is a pressure relief valve and non-return valve. These are to protect the vaporizers from the pumping effect and the machine from occlusion of the common gas outlet. The pressure setting (about 30 kPa, 300 cmH$_2$O) is far in excess of that which would protect the patient from barotrauma.

BREATHING SYSTEMS

Anaesthetic gases leave the anaesthetic machine via the common gas outlet, usually a Cardiff swivel. Breathing systems transport the anaesthetic gases from the anaesthetic machine to the patient. There are many different circuit designs but the ideal features of a breathing system are:

- Efficient elimination of expired carbon dioxide.
- Low resistance to gas flow.
- Safety and robustness.
- Low dead space.
- Light and easy to use.

Their design and function can affect the final composition of the gas that reaches the patient and are also used in classifying breathing systems.

PARTS OF A CIRCUIT

Corrugated rubber (so-called 'elephant') or plastic tubing is used to carry the gases to the patient. Ideally it should be light in weight, flexible without kinking and with a low resistance.

The reservoir or rebreathing bag is included in the circuit to match the varying inspiratory flow, which the patient demands, to the constant flow produced by the anaesthetic machine. It may also be used as a means of manual ventilation. Adult reservoir bags are 2 litres in capacity but paediatric bags may be 1 litre or 500 ml in size. The use of a bag within a circuit acts as a very effective pressure-limiting device, as pressures in excess of safe pressures are relieved by the bag distending, thus limiting the rise in pressure.

Expiratory valves allow the escape of expired gases without the ingress of air. Commonly, they are called Heidbrink valves and allow the opening pressure to be varied by means of a spring controlled by a screw top. Modern valves include a pressure relief valve (commonly set at 60 cm H_2O) and a cowling that conducts the waste gases to the scavenging system. Strictly, the name Heidbrink should only be applied to the obsolete, non-scavenged pattern of valves.

CLASSIFICATION OF CIRCUITS BY FUNCTION

There are many classifications of anaesthetic circuits but different classifications may contrast or contradict. Often, they complicate rather than elucidate.

OPEN OR SEMIOPEN ADMINISTRATION

Holding a delivery tube before a child's face for induction is an example of this. The gases are essentially unconstrained. It is wasteful and little used nowadays.

NON-REBREATHING SYSTEMS

This is a conventional system fitted with a special valve (a non-rebreathing valve, for example Reubens or Ambu valve) that discards all exhaled gas and ensures each inhalation is entirely fresh gas. Because it is a wasteful and often awkward system to use it is only seen commonly nowadays in resuscitation equipment. Minute volume dividing ventilators are non rebreathing systems.

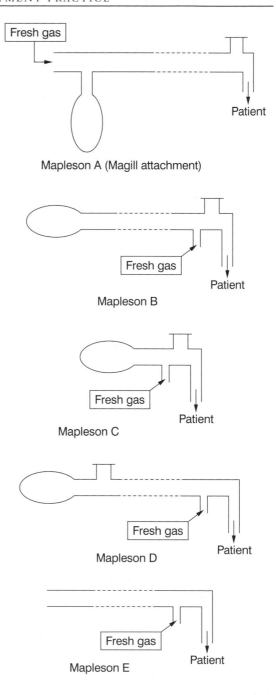

Figure 8.7   Mapleson's classification of rebreathing systems.

REBREATHING SYSTEMS

Most systems in use today allow limited rebreathing of expired gas. The design of these systems (classified A–E by Mapleson and illustrated in Figures 8.7, 8.8) determines how much gas flow is needed to prevent

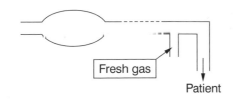

Jackson-Rees modification of Ayre's T-piece
(functionally D/E)

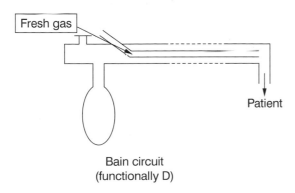

Bain circuit
(functionally D)

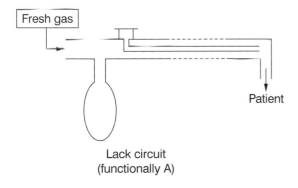

Lack circuit
(functionally A)

Figure 8.8   Types of non-rebreathing circuits

carbon dioxide accumulation with either spontaneous or controlled ventilation (Table 8.2). In practice, the best division of these systems is into afferent reservoir, junctional reservoir and efferent reservoir systems. Rebreathing systems without carbon dioxide absorption need fresh gas flows equal to at least the patient's alveolar ventilation if well chosen for the intended use, often much more if badly chosen. The Mapleson A (afferent reservoir) systems eliminate carbon dioxide very efficiently with spontaneous ventilation and although ventilators can be made to function similarly, ordinary afferent reservoir systems need high gas flows for controlled ventilation. Conversely, the Mapleson D and E efferent reservoir

systems (in practice, the D and E are functionally the same) work well with controlled ventilation but need high gas flows with spontaneous ventilation. Mapleson B systems are not used in practice and the Mapleson C system should only be for short-term use. Both need high gas flows for either spontaneous or controlled ventilation, as they are junctional reservoir systems. Systems that are switchable between A and D/E modes are available.

CARBON DIOXIDE ABSORPTION

Chemical absorption of carbon dioxide offers the possibility of satisfactory elimination at flows much lower than are possible even with the most efficient rebreathing system. Both soda lime and barium lime are used as carbon dioxide absorbents but in the UK only soda lime is commonly used.

Soda lime is composed of 90% calcium hydroxide, 5% sodium hydroxide, (1% potassium hydroxide), silicate and a Ph-sensitive indicator. It has moisture content of between 14% and 19% but soda lime is hygroscopic (it absorbs water from the atmosphere). Soda lime is made by fusing its components together and allowing them to cool into sheets. These sheets are then broken up into granules. Carbon dioxide absorption is most efficient if the granules are very small because they have a large surface area-to-volume ratio. However, small granules have little gas space between them and thus would cause a considerable resistance to breathing. Granule size is therefore a compromise. Granules are measured using mesh size, as illustrated in Figure 8.9, which shows an 8-mesh size screen. This means that there are eight holes per inch and each hole is therefore one-eighth of an inch square. Thus there are 16 in each square inch. Similarly, 4-mesh is quarter inch square size. Soda lime has a mesh size of between four and eight.

It is important that the granules do not break up in use, producing dust. Hardness is assessed by means of a hardness number. Soda lime granules are agitated for 30 minutes in a pan with 12 steel balls of fixed diameter. They are then placed on a 40-mesh grid and shaken for a further three minutes. At the end of this period at least 75% should remain above the grid and this is known as the hardness number.

CHEMISTRY OF SODA LIME

Carbon dioxide gas dissolves in the water contained in the soda lime, producing bicarbonate (HCO_3^-) ions and hydrogen (H^+) ions. These in turn react with the sodium hydroxide to produce sodium carbonate, water and heat.

Table 8.2 Approximate gas flows to ensure adequate CO_2 elimination in non-rebreathing systems

Circuit	Spontaneous respiration	Controlled ventilation
Mapleson A (Magill)/Lack	0.7–1.0 times MV	2–3 times MV
Mapleson B	2.0 times MV	2.0 times MV
Mapleson C	2–3 times MV	2.0 times MV
Mapleson D/Bain Jackson Rees circuit	1.5–2.0 times MV	1.0 times MV
Mapleson E/Ayre T-piece	1.5–2.0 times MV	2–3 times MV
Humphrey ADE circuit	>50 ml/min/kg	>70 ml/min/kg

MV = minute volume

$$H_2O + CO_2 \leftrightarrow HCO_3^- + H^+$$

$$2NaOH + HCO_3^- + H^+ \leftrightarrow Na_2CO_3 + 2H_2O + heat$$

The sodium hydroxide is reformed as a product of the reaction between sodium carbonate and calcium hydroxide forming insoluble calcium carbonate.

$$Na_2CO_3 + Ca(OH)_2 \rightarrow CaCO_3 + 2NaOH$$

It is for this reason that soda lime is capable of some regeneration after it has been used. In addition, the calcium hydroxide is neutralized by the acid to produce calcium carbonate.

$$Ca(OH)_2 + HCO_3^- + H^+ \rightarrow CaCO_3 + 2H_2O + heat$$

The pH-sensitive indicators are dyes that change colour as the alkaline absorbents are used up and the acidic gas carbon dioxide determines the pH of the absorbent. Thus exhausted soda lime can be made to change colour by addition of indicators. It is important to know which indicator is in use because the fresh (unused) colour of one may be the same as the exhausted colour of another (Table 8.3). These substances are only indicators and often the efficiency of absorption will fall before the colour changes. An increasing inspired carbon dioxide concentration is the only truly reliable method of assessing when the soda lime is exhausted. Efficient absorption also depends on the even packing of absorbent.

CHEMISTRY OF BARIUM LIME

Barium lime consists of 80% calcium hydroxide, 20% barium hydroxide and a pH-sensitive indicator. Its moisture content is between 11% and 14%. Barium lime is much harder than soda lime and therefore no silica is needed to maintain its integrity but the chemical reactions are of a similar nature.

$$H_2O + CO_2 \rightarrow HCO_3^- + H^+$$

$$Ba(OH)_2 + HCO_3^- + H^+ \rightarrow BaCO_3 + 2H_2O + heat$$

$$Ca(OH)_2 + HCO_3^- + H^+ \rightarrow CaCO_3 + 2H_2O + heat$$

Unlike sodium carbonate, barium carbonate is insoluble and thus there is no potential for regeneration. Barium lime is therefore less efficient than soda lime.

Many anaesthetic agents have the potential to break down in contact with soda lime or barium lime. Mostly with modern agents, any breakdown products are harmless in clinical practice.

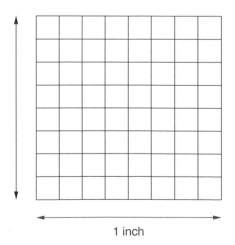

1 inch

Figure 8.9   An 8-mesh screen

Table 8.3 Colour changes in pH-sensitive indicators

Indicator	Fresh	Exhausted
Clayton yellow	Pink	Yellow
Ethyl violet	Colourless	Purple
Methyl orange	Orange	Yellow
Phenolphthalein	Colourless	Pink

However, in a report from the USA three patients were described who were subjected to unacceptably high levels of carbon monoxide (>30% carboxyhaemoglobin). Investigation of this revealed that isoflurane, enflurane and desflurane all produce carbon monoxide in reaction with the alkaline absorbents. The effect is more marked with barium lime than soda lime and is seen most with desflurane. Drying of the absorbent appears necessary to promote the reaction. The US cases were desflurane anaesthetics using barium lime as the absorbent. They occurred early on Monday mornings after the absorbent had dried out over the weekend. The following recommendations are therefore suggested.

- Turn off gas flow between cases as this can dry out the absorbent.
- Change the absorbent regularly, if it might have dried out or after a period of non-use.

- Avoid high gas flows when using carbon dioxide absorbents.
- Avoid barium lime, especially with desflurane.

LOW-FLOW ANAESTHESIA

Dr Peter Horsey defines low-flow anaesthesia as 'methods which make use of fresh gas flows of one to one and a half litres per minute'. It has regained its previous popularity because of economic and (largely misplaced) environmental concerns. The theory supporting low-flow anaesthesia is the key to its management and allows the theatre practitioner to guide individuals, including anaesthetists, into the areas of best practice.

DELIVERY OF LOW-FLOW ANAESTHESIA

The delivery of low-flow anaesthesia is facilitated by double-tube (cascade) Rotameters™ but these are by no means essential. Low-flow anaesthesia is only really practical using a modern circle system. Although the Waters' system has been used it is obsolete and will not be discussed further. The circle system comprises an absorber canister, inspiratory and expiratory tubing, inspiratory and expiratory unidirectional valves and a reservoir bag, which is often replaced by a lung ventilator (Fig. 8.10). Fresh gas is fed into the system and is moved around the system in a circular path by the

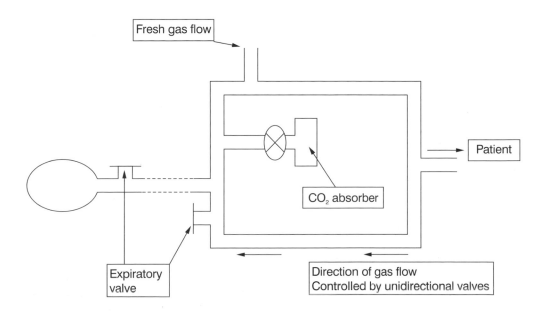

Figure 8.10   The Circle System

patient's lung ventilation. The exact arrangement of these components is important under some circumstances, but is outside the scope of this book. All body tissues eventually equilibrate with the gas breathed. Normally this will be the nitrogen-oxygen mixture of air. When the gas breathed is changed to an anaesthetic gas mixture, nitrogen is given up by the body and anaesthetic gases are taken up. Nitrogen leaves the body rapidly at first and the vast bulk of it is given up in the first 10–20 minutes of anaesthesia. Nitrous oxide uptake is rapid for about the first 10 minutes but goes on at a few hundred ml per minute (gradually declining) for the first two hours of anaesthesia. Volatile agent uptake is similarly rapid at first but goes on for many hours because of the higher solubility in blood and fat of these drugs compared to nitrous oxide.

Uptake of oxygen is constant at about 250 ml/min for an anaesthetized adult, as is excretion of carbon dioxide at about 200 ml/min.

Patient uptake and excretion of gases are not easily seen in high-flow anaesthesia, since the constant inflow of gas keeps the circuit gas mixture very close in composition to the gas delivered by the anaesthetic machine. As flows decrease the uptake and excretion of gases by the patient become much more significant.

For the first five minutes or so of anaesthesia, a high-flow (say 6 l/min) will speed equilibration of the circuit gas volume with the desired gas mixture. After this an intermediate flow (say 3 l/min) can be used until the rapid uptake of agents and excretion of nitrogen has slowed. Many anaesthetists will maintain an intermediate flow until the inspired and expired nitrous oxide concentrations are similar, signifying that the most rapid changes seen early in anaesthesia have slowed. Others reduce the flows to their target level earlier in the anaesthetic, accepting that frequent readjustment will be needed for the next 20 minutes or so.

In practice little economy is gained by using flows lower than 1 l/min. This flow is high enough to mask most of the effects of uptake of gases by the patient and the problem of small circuit leaks. Flows of about 300 ml/min of oxygen and 200 ml/min of nitrous oxide plus a volatile agent will work well in an adult after the rapid equilibration phase, but the final circuit gas mixture will be very different to the gas leaving the machine. Most importantly, the volatile drug concentration is about halved by patient uptake at these flows. An oxygen concentration of between 40% and 50% is necessary to produce an inspired concentration approximating to 30%. These changes are due to the fact that the small volume of fresh gas entering the circle is diluted by the much larger volume of expired gas.

Dependence on monitoring therefore increases as flows decrease below 1 l/min. High-quality monitoring is vital in low-flow anaesthesia to ensure that hypoxia, hypercapnia and inadequate anaesthesia are prevented. The following modalities are suggested:

- Oximetry.
- Tidal volume and respiratory rate.
- Airway pressure.
- Oxygen concentration leaving the anaesthetic machine, though this will not accurately reflect the circuit concentration at low-flows.
- Inspired and end-tidal concentrations of oxygen, carbon dioxide and nitrous oxide and volatile agent measured as close to the patient as possible.

There are a number of advantages in using low-flow anaesthesia. Clinically, the most important is the conservation of heat and moisture. It has been shown that fresh gas flows in excess of 3 l/min negate this advantage but below 1.5 l/min the heat and moisture content within the circuit gradually increase. A fresh gas flow of 600 ml/min will maintain a temperature above 30°C with adequate water content. This is particularly advantageous during prolonged anaesthesia.

The potential decrease in pollution in theatre is important but efficient scavenging has made this less of an advantage. Environmental pollution by anaesthetic drugs is probably unimportant. By far the bulk of atmospheric nitrous oxide (a 'greenhouse' gas) comes from the gut of ruminant animals and the volatile agents are too short lived in the atmosphere to take part in the ozone destroying reactions that chloro-fluro carbons cause.

The most important non-clinical advantage must be the cost savings that are achieved, equating to approximately 90% of the fresh gas flow and about 75% of the volatile agent. If the technique is used effectively the cost of the low-flow system and the necessary monitoring equipment will be paid for within about 2–3 years in a typical UK hospital.

Low-flow anaesthesia however also has some disadvantages:

- High-flows are needed early in the anaesthetic, so savings for short cases are limited.
- The presence of leaks within the circuit becomes more significant when low flows are used and will be obvious if the leak is equal to or greater than the fresh gas flow. The exact effect of leaks depends to some extent on the circuit set up and on the type of ventilator used and unexplained changes in gas monitor readings should make the user suspicious. Most current ventilators for circle systems are of the

rising bellows type and with these a leak is obvious. Although a hole in the circuit tubing or any loose connection may be the cause, leaks from the carbon dioxide absorber are by far the most common. Soda lime granules remaining on the rubber seals often cause such a leak and the seals should always be cleaned before replacing the canister. The gas analyser removes in excess of 300 ml of gas each minute from the circuit and this should be returned to the system, ideally into the expired gas before the carbon dioxide absorber.

- A thorough check for leaks must always be performed prior to using an anaesthetic machine, particularly if low flows are contemplated.

- Because only small volumes of gas are added to the circuit each minute, rapid changes of gas or volatile agent concentration cannot be achieved at low-flow rates. If rapid change is needed it is imperative to increase the fresh gas flow until the effect has been achieved, after which low flows may be reinstated. Similarly, if rapid lightening of the anaesthetic is indicated the flows must be increased to wash the anaesthetic drugs out of the circuit.

VAPORIZERS AND THE CIRCLE SYSTEM

Vaporizers may be used as vaporizer outside circle (VOC) or inside circle (VIC). VOC is common, since it uses the vaporizer already fitted to the machine backbar. However, at very low flows it can be difficult to deliver enough volatile agent into the circle to maintain the desired concentration. At low flows the concentration of volatile agent in the circle may be reduced by 50% to 80% of the dial setting on the backbar vaporizer. Since there is little advantage to flows below 1 l/min. VOC is usually satisfactory and is, in effect, the only commonly used technique.

VIC (vaporizer in circle) is limited nowadays in the UK to eccentrics and enthusiasts. The vaporizer, which must be a 'draw-over' type, is placed in the inspiratory limb of the circle. The lower the fresh gas flow, the more times the gas will pass through the vaporizer before being lost to the exhaust, so as the fresh gas flow decreases the concentration of the volatile agent in the circle rises above the concentration the vaporizer could deliver in non-rebreathing systems. The concentration can easily reach 500% of the set concentration and can do this especially rapidly when controlled ventilation is used. Unlike VOC, even at low-flows anaesthesia can be deepened with frightening speed using VIC. Although VIC offers the prospect of truly basal flow anaesthesia (250 ml/min of

oxygen alone), this potentially catastrophic spiral of increasing concentration requires very close monitoring and the technique has no place in day-to-day practice. Occasional demonstrations of the technique might aid understanding of the behaviour of the circle at low flows but little else can be said to commend VIC in modern hospitals.

SCAVENGING SYSTEMS

It used to be common for anaesthetists to complain of headaches and feelings of listlessness after a busy day in theatre. With the introduction of scavenging systems many anaesthetists believe that these complaints are less frequent, though attempts to prove this consistently fail. Health and safety issues are very important in the modern NHS and acceptable exposure levels for all anaesthetic gases have been set. The monitoring of anaesthetic pollution is now easy with hand-held analysers. It should be emphasized that, at the time of writing, there are no proven health hazards from anaesthetic gas pollution of the working environment.

Pollution may be minimized by low-flow anaesthesia but in any case waste gases should be removed from the theatre environment. This may be achieved by passive or active means. All UK anaesthetic equipment now uses expiratory ports with 30 mm antipollution fittings. These cannot be cross connected with the standard 22 mm fittings used in the 'live' parts of the circuit.

The first widespread attempt to reduce theatre pollution was the use of canisters filled with activated charcoal (the Cardiff Aldasorber). These absorbed volatile agents but not nitrous oxide. After a fixed usage time or weight increase they were discarded. They are no longer used, since nitrous oxide pollution is unchanged.

Passive systems rely on the activity of the patient to force the waste gases through a series of pipes to a point where they may be discharged to the atmosphere, generally via a hole drilled directly in the theatre wall. Unfortunately, there is a real danger that the outflow may become obstructed, causing the pressure within the circuit to rise to dangerous levels or that change in wind direction could force the gases back into the system. Pressure relief valves can be fitted but obstruction of the scavenging hose between the patient and any such valve will still cause overpressure.

Active systems rely on low-pressure suction to remove the anaesthetic gases. Although apparently more efficient, it is important to ensure that pressure-relieving devices (air breaks) are present to prevent the development of very low pressures within the anaesthetic circuit. These also protect against obstruction of the system but again obstruction of the scavenging hose between the patient and any such unit will still cause overpressure. The medical suction should not be used for scavenging. Volatile drugs can damage some pumps, the suction is high pressure but low-flow, whereas low pressure, high-flow is needed and the safety systems are lacking.

The design and installation of active scavenging is complex and outside the scope of this book, other than to say that the commonest cause of failure, is failure to connect the pipes or to switch on the pump.

SUPPLEMENTARY ANAESTHETIC EQUIPMENT

This equipment is usually left ready for use on the anaesthetic machine. It includes such items as:

- Oral and nasopharyngeal airways.
- Facemasks.
- Laryngeal masks.
- Laryngoscopes.
- Catheter mounts.
- Endotracheal tubes.
- Syringes.
- Artery forceps.
- Magill's forceps.
- Gum elastic bougies and stilettes.
- Tape and ribbon gauze for fixing airway devices.
- Local anaesthetic spray.
- Mouth packs.
- Eye ointment.
- Suction devices.

SIMPLE AIRWAY MANAGEMENT

The anaesthetic circuit is finally connected to the patient's airway. This might be by means of a facemask with or without an additional airway, a laryngeal mask or a tracheal tube. Selecting and using these various airway devices is the single most important and skilled part of anaesthetic practice.

The simplest way of ensuring airway patency is to place the patient's head in the 'sniffing' position and lift the mandible forward. Oropharyngeal (Guedel) or nasopharyngeal airways may be used to improve the airway by separating the tongue from the hard palate and by holding the base of the tongue forward. Anaesthetic gases can then be administered by means of a close-fitting facemask. There are several different types of facemask and selection depends partly on the patient but mainly on the preference of the anaesthetist.

Laryngeal mask airways are anatomically formed airways, mounted on a tube not unlike an endotracheal tube, that fit over the opening of the larynx. Newer developments include a flexible, reinforced laryngeal mask and a laryngeal mask designed as an aid to tracheal intubation. These devices have greatly reduced the use of tracheal intubation and are useful as an alternative to difficult intubation. Laryngeal masks appear to protect the airway from debris above the mask but do not protect against aspiration of gastric contents. They are easy to insert and might become the airway of choice in resuscitation if there is no-one present who can pass a tracheal tube. Their role in management of failed intubation is still unclear.

TRACHEAL INTUBATION

Tracheal intubation offers the most secure airway. Intubation is indicated to secure the airway for prolonged surgery, head and neck surgery and for controlled ventilation. The laryngeal mask has partly taken over for some of these indications but intubation also protects the airway from contamination by surgical debris or gastric contents and is absolutely indicated when these are a hazard.

INTUBATION EQUIPMENT

Endotracheal tubes placed directly into the trachea through the larynx, provide continuity with the anaesthetic circuit. An inflatable cuff seals the tube to the tracheal wall. Paediatric endotracheal tubes are often uncuffed but this subject is discussed elsewhere. Modern endotracheal tubes are hypoallergenic and may be left *in situ* for some time before there is a need for tracheostomy. Intubation can be either orotracheal or nasotracheal. Oral intubation is the norm; nasal intubation is only common for intraoral surgery.

The first tracheal intubations were for resuscitation, the tube being guided blindly into the larynx using the fingers, but use of a laryngoscope soon became common in anaesthetic practice. Laryngoscopes allow visualization of the vocal cords and hence the introduction of the endotracheal tube under direct vision.

When the endotracheal tube is in place it is connected to the anaesthetic circuit. The cuff is inflated, using a 20 ml syringe, via a pilot tube with just enough air to prevent a gas leak (slight overinflation probably protects better against aspiration of gastric contents if this is thought a hazard). The pilot tube usually has a non-return valve or is closed with an artery forceps. The endotracheal tube is then secured either by tying or using sticky tape.

The Magill laryngoscope was based on that of Chevalier Jackson, an ENT surgeon, and had a straight blade. The Mackintosh laryngoscope has a curved blade and is regarded by most as easier to use. It is the most commonly used laryngoscope in the UK. The light source is a small light bulb situated near the tip of the blade or, in more modern laryngoscopes, a fibre-optic light guide from a bulb in the handle. Power is from two 1.5-volt batteries that are housed in the handle. Fibreoptics and a prefocused lamp produce better and more reliable illumination. The blade is attached to the handle either by the American 'hook on' fitting or by the Longworth fitting which uses a small screw to hold the blade in place. The Mackintosh laryngoscope is introduced through the mouth until the tip lies between the base of the tongue and the larynx (the vallecula fossa). It is then lifted along the axis of the handle. Operators should not use the teeth as a fulcrum because the leverage will almost certainly damage or dislodge one or more of the teeth.

The McCoy laryngoscope is a modification of the Mackintosh laryngoscope. It has a hinged tip. As the operating lever is depressed the hinged tip is flexed and this may make the larynx easier to visualize in some patients.

In patients who are grossly obese or in women with very large breasts, the use of the standard laryngoscope may be difficult. The polio blade is set at an angle of approximately 120° to the handle and makes introduction of the blade much easier (it was designed to intubate patients in 'iron lungs', hence 'polio'). Obtuse blades, left-handed blades and larger blades (#4, instead of the usual #3) all have their place in difficult intubation.

Straight blades (like that of Magill) are used to intubate infants and occasionally adults who are difficult to intubate using a Mackintosh laryngoscope. Instead of sitting in the vallecula the tip of the straight blade passes posteriorly over the epiglottis in order to lift it directly and expose the vocal cords. (Infants have a large leafy epiglottis, which favours the use of a straight blade.) The Miller blade is probably the most widely used straight blade, being slightly better shaped than the Magill.

The gum elastic bougie, which is threaded through the endotracheal tube, is a device for aiding difficult intubation and is passed through the vocal cords either under partial vision or blindly. Bougies enter into the trachea more easily than a tube because of their small diameter and malleability. The tube is then introduced over the bougie, which is then carefully removed, leaving the endotracheal tube in place. Although described many years ago, the technique has only recently been rediscovered. It has been described as 'quietly revolutionising anaesthesia'.

Fibreoptic laryngoscopy is used in cases of difficult intubation and the patient may be awake, when it is performed under local anaesthesia of the airway, or anaesthetized. A thin flexible endoscope is passed through a tracheal tube and is then introduced into the trachea by visualizing the larynx through the endoscope and manipulating the steering controls of the endoscope. The tube is then introduced into the trachea and the fibreoptic laryngoscope is carefully removed. This technique is difficult and inexperienced operators are unlikely to succeed and may damage the laryngoscope.

TRACHEOSTOMY

Tracheostomy tubes are endotracheal tubes that are inserted into the trachea through a surgical opening below the level of the larynx. In practice, they are used after surgical removal or trauma to the larynx, to secure the airway if intubation is impossible or unduly hazardous or if there is a need for prolonged intubation, since this can damage the larynx. The exact safe duration of intubation before a tracheostomy is needed is a hotly debated subject but several days intubation seems safe, possibly much longer.

SUCTION MACHINES

It is imperative that the anaesthetist always has access to suction equipment. Suction is needed to remove secretions to aid visualization of the larynx and to remove blood, secretions or gastric contents from the pharynx to prevent contamination of the lungs. Clearly this might arise as an emergency and the formerly common practice of 'sharing' suction with the surgeon is no longer acceptable, except perhaps during intraoral surgery.

Suction may be generated from a central supply, an electrical or mechanical sucker or from a gas-driven Venturi. The latter uses high-pressure oxygen from the anaesthetic machine to generate a vacuum using the Venturi effect. Before piped suction was common, many machines used Venturi suction and it is still commonly seen on patient trolleys.

CHECKING THE ANAESTHETIC MACHINE

The Association of Anaesthetists of Great Britain and Ireland has produced guidelines for the preoperative

ANAESTHETIC MACHINE AND EQUIPMENT ODA/ODP PRESESSIONAL CHECK

ANAESTHETIC MACHINE
CHECK CONDITION OF SODA LIME
CYLINDERS ON MACHINE CHECKED AND TESTED
PIPELINE GASES CHECKED AND TESTED
VAPORIZERS CHECKED, FILLED, TESTED (INC O RINGS)
FLOW METERS FUNCTIONING, CHECK % O_2 WITH CAPNOGRAPH
O_2 FLUSH, POS+ PRESSURE RELIEF VALVE TESTED
ANAESTHETIC MACHINE CLEANED, NEW PAPER AFTER CHECK

MON	TUES	WED	THUR	FRI	SAT	SUN

AIRWAY MAINTENANCE
MAGILL CIRCUITS CHECKED AND TESTED
RESERVOIR BAGS AND VALVES CHECKED AND TESTED
FACEMASKS – AVAILABLE SIZES 1-5
ALL LARYNGOSCOPES CHECKED AND TESTED
CATHETER MOUNT, SPENCER WELLS, 20ML SYRINGE
MAGILL FORCEPS, GUM ELASTIC STILETTE, INTRODUCER
FERGUSON MOUTH GAG
ET TUBES- APPROPRIATE SIZES, CUFFS, LUMENS CHECKED

MON	TUES	WED	THUR	FRI	SAT	SUN

SUCTION
SUCTION AVAILABLE AND WORKING
SUCTION CATHETERS AVAILABLE

MON	TUES	WED	THUR	FRI	SAT	SUN

MONITORING: ALL EQUIPMENT TESTED, CHECKED, CLEANED AND FUNCTIONING
STETHOSCOPE ON BOTH ANAESTHETIC MACHINES
BP MONITORING
ECG MONITOR
GAS MONITORING
PULSE OXIMETER
IV DRIPS LEFT OUT (IF PREPARED, DATE AND SIGN)

MON	TUES	WED	THUR	FRI	SAT	SUN

VENTILATOR
LEAK TEST WITH CO_2 ABSORBER ON AND OFF
WATER TRAPS EMPTIED IF NECESSARY
CLEANED, CHECKED AND FUNCTIONING

MON	TUES	WED	THUR	FRI	SAT	SUN

SUNDRIES AVAILABLE
EYE OINTMENT
KY JELLY ON BOTH MACHINES
TAPE INCL $\frac{1}{2}$ INCH ZINC OXIDE AND 1 INCH MICROPORE
VENFLON TAPE CUT AND AVAILABLE
SWABS – STERILE PACKETS AVAILABLE
STERETS AVAILABLE/ STERILE GALLIPOTS CHANGED DAILY
ALL THEATRES STOCKED PROPERLY BEFORE/AFTER OP LIST

MON	TUES	WED	THUR	FRI	SAT	SUN

MONDAY CHECKS
CHANGE ALL CIRCUITS, CHANGE SODA LIME, CALIBRATE GAS MONITORS [   ]

	A.M DATE	SIGNATURE	P.M DATE	SIGNATURE
MONDAY				
TUESDAY				
WEDNESDAY				
THURSDAY				
FRIDAY				
SATURDAY				
SUNDAY				

THEATRE. . . . . . .

Figure 8.11   Anaesthetic and equipment checklist.

checking of anaesthetic machines. Although the assistant to the anaesthetist often performs these routine tests, it is the final responsibility of the anaesthetist to ensure that the anaesthetic machine is safe. This is where the 'buck' really stops! Particular care should be taken when commissioning machines on delivery or after service. Most hospitals have adapted these recommendations for local use and the one used at St Helens and Knowsley Hospitals Trust is illustrated in Figure 8.11.

RECOMMENDED READING

Moyle, JTB, Davey A, Ward C 1992 *Ward's Anaesthetic Equipment*: London, W B Saunders Co. Ltd

Baum J.A. 1996 *Low-flow Anaesthesia*: Oxford, Butterworth Heinmann

9

FUNDAMENTALS OF ARTIFICIAL VENTILATION OF THE LUNG

R. R. Macmillan

HISTORY OF ARTIFICIAL VENTILATION

Artificial ventilation of the lungs can be performed without any equipment at all. Early descriptions of resuscitation include the use of expired air ventilation, which was used in victims of drowning. This involved manipulation of the arms to expand the thorax and draw air into the lungs but has been superseded by 'the kiss of life' with ventilation using expired air. However, as long ago as 1788, Kite of Gravesend described oral and nasal intubation for the resuscitation of the apparently drowned patient. In 1871 Trendelenberg anaesthetized a patient through a tracheostomy wound and occluded the trachea with an inflatable cuff but it was Langton Hewer who, in 1939, reintroduced the concept of the pilot tube.

In 1934 Guedel and Treweek introduced artificial ventilation of the lungs into anaesthesia and in 1936 Waters first used the term 'controlled respiration'. Guedel and Treweek controlled breathing using deep ether anaesthesia to raise the threshold of the respiratory centre. Controlled ventilation was greatly facilitated by the development of muscle relaxants. Much of this work in the UK was done by Gray and Rees in Liverpool and resulted in the so-called 'Liverpool Technique' of anaesthesia.

During the 1950s in Sweden there was a major epidemic of poliomyelitis. Medical students were paid to help with the ventilation of these patients and this event helped to speed up the development of mechanical ventilators.

USES OF ARTIFICIAL VENTILATION

Artificial ventilation of the lungs is used on a daily basis across the world, predominantly as part of an anaesthetic technique associated with muscular paralysis. Assisted ventilation is mainly used within intensive care units as a means of life support whilst recovery from disease or injury is awaited. Cardiopulmonary resuscitation also relies upon artificial ventilation until spontaneous respiration is restored. An infrequent but important use of artificial lung ventilation is for patients who have problems from which they are unlikely to recover and for whom artificial ventilation is a lifelong necessity.

This variety of need has led to the production of a wide range of devices that can be used to provide artificial ventilation. The vast majority of techniques provide an intermittent supply of gas at a positive pressure when compared to the ambient atmospheric pressure in the trachea. This is usually delivered via an endotracheal tube or similar device, which protects the airway from soiling. The term intermittent positive pressure ventilation (IPPV) describes this process. This chapter describes the general aspects of IPPV, the effect this has on the patient and how harmful effects of the process may be minimized. The indications of other techniques of artificial ventilation are also discussed.

VENTILATION EQUIPMENT

The range of ventilators available is enormous and many are multifunctional. Classifications using pressure, volume or time as the cycling trigger have previously been used but are of little value because many machines can be set to function in different ways according to clinical need. The most reliable information relating to the characteristics of any particular device is best obtained from evaluations specific to that ventilator. Because of the continuous development of ventilators manufacturers are often the best able to fully describe the functional capabilities of their products. Objective comparison between ventilators is more difficult as such tests are often out of date as newer ventilators are produced.

As previously stated, originally artificial ventilation was performed without any specialized equipment. A variety of devices are now available that permit ventilation using either a facemask with a valve to prevent rebreathing or a self-inflating bag, again with a one way-valve and mask to enable ventilation. The self-inflating bag may also be attached to an endotracheal tube via the non-rebreathing valve and ventilation maintained in this way. Such manual methods are only suitable for brief periods but remain an important application of artificial ventilation. A number of small portable ventilators exist that are powered by compressed oxygen and they are most often used for patient transfer within hospital or out of hospital by the emergency services. They all utilize a non-rebreathing valve and are of varying degrees of sophistication.

Because they consume large volumes of oxygen, adequate amounts of compressed oxygen are essential when using such devices for patient transport, as the following example illustrates. Transporting a patient with 100% oxygen, a tidal volume of 700 ml and rate of 10 breaths per minute will consume 420 litres per hour (700 × 10 × 60 ml.), assuming there are no leaks. Many portable transport ventilators permit the use of air entrainment, thus reducing the inspired oxygen concentration and the amount of oxygen consumed.

INTERMITTENT POSITIVE PRESSURE VENTILATION (IPPV) IN THE OPERATING THEATRE AND INTENSIVE CARE UNIT

IPPV requires a ventilator capable of providing a tidal volume at an appropriate pressure via a circuit connected to an endotracheal tube sited in the major airways. The placement of an endotracheal tube into the trachea is not a physiological process and exposes the airway and trachea to the risk of traumatic injury. This risk extends to all areas traversed by the laryngoscope and endo/nasotracheal tube, from the lips or anterior nares to the larynx. Strategies to minimize these potentially harmful consequences are therefore necessary.

DESIGN AND SELECTION OF ENDOTRACHEAL TUBES

Originally mass manufactured from red rubber, endotracheal tubes are now produced from biologically inert substances such as silicone rubber and plastic. Tubes are available with or without a cuff, the inflation of which is by means of a pilot tube. This cuff has an important role in maintaining a gaseous seal to prevent leaks but it also protects the bronchial tree from the aspiration of oral secretions and blood. The circular nature of the cricoid cartilage at the commencement of a child's trachea, together with the fact that this is the narrowest part, means that an uncuffed circular tube will often achieve an acceptable seal in paediatric patients. However, the adult trachea, with its horseshoe shape in cross-section, needs a cuff to give an adequate seal. Many studies have shown however, that an inflated cuff cannot be assumed to provide an absolute barrier to the aspiration of orogastric secretions. Cuff design is such that high-volume, low-pressure (HVLP) cuffs with a substantial surface area in contact with the tracheal mucosa have superseded cuffs with a small, high-pressure contact area. This development is to reduce the pressure injury that the mucosa will suffer if the cuff pressure exceeds the perfusion pressure to the mucosa.

The volume and pressure of gas within a cuff may alter during anaesthesia because nitrous oxide diffuses into the cuff, as it does into any of the other cavities within the body. This may be avoided by inflating the cuff with saline, a method also necessary if air transport or the use of a hyperbaric chamber is envisaged. Monitoring of cuff pressure, though seldom undertaken in practice, is useful to reduce the likelihood of mucosal damage that excessive pressure can induce and is particularly relevant during prolonged operations.

The individual needs of the patient and the increasing range of surgical techniques have influenced the development and design of endotracheal tubes but both the diameter and length of the tube must be appropriate to the patient. Some of the specialized endotracheal tubes are listed below.

- Preformed tubes are useful for improving access for surgical procedures about the face and head.
- Reinforced tubes are resistant to kinking and are used when the patient is placed in the prone position.
- Very small diameter tubes with large cuffs allow visualization of the vocal cords.
- Tubes suitable for use with lasers.
- Tubes permitting differential lung ventilation (double lumen tubes) allow one lung to be collapsed to facilitate thoracic and high abdominal surgery.

Movement of the tube in the trachea is another cause of mucosal damage and fixation devices are used in intensive care where patient movement is more commonplace than in anaesthetic practice.

CHOICE OF ORAL, NASAL AND TRACHEOSTOMY TUBE PLACEMENT

Endotracheal tubes may be placed orally, via the nose or directly into the trachea using a tracheostomy. Each method has advantages and disadvantages but the choice depends on the surgical procedure or reason for intubation and the length of time that the tube will be in situ.

Oral intubation is by far the most common technique in use. The tube is usually introduced under direct vision using a rigid laryngoscope blade but if intubation is difficult a flexible or rigid fibreoptic laryngoscope may be used. The oral route permits the rapid and in most patients, easy placement of a short wide-bore endotracheal tube. An oral endotracheal tube is poorly tolerated, particularly in young, fit patients, and considerable gagging and retching may occur if the level of anaesthesia or sedation is inadequate. Oropharyngeal trauma during placement is possible and fixation can be troublesome. The tube may migrate or be malpositioned into one of the major bronchi, usually the right main bronchus, and only partial ventilation of both lungs will then be possible.

Nasotracheal intubation, though less common than oral intubation, is nevertheless a popular technique and absence of the tube from the mouth may be a surgical advantage in operative procedures where oral access is required. In addition, it is easier to introduce a tube by this route if there is a problem with intubation and totally blind nasal intubation is a most useful skill in spite of the development of fibreoptic laryngoscopy. Nasal tubes are longer and rather narrower than oral ones but substantial trauma to the soft tissues of the nasopharynx is common, with bleeding and occasionally submucosal placement of the tube. Breathing may be easier through one of the nostrils and if the better side is used the trauma may be minimized. Some anaesthetists also spray the mucosal lining of the nose with a vasoconstrictor in order to reduce the bulk of the mucosa. Patients with large adenoids or chronic nasal obstruction are particularly liable to postintubation bleeding. The nasal tube is also better tolerated than an oral one and with good fixation, the tube is generally more stable but malposition can still occur.

The surgical placement of a tube directly into the trachea is unusual outside intensive care but tracheostomy may be part of a surgical procedure such as laryngectomy. Compared with other endotracheal tubes, the awake patient with a tracheostomy tolerates it extremely well and does not need sedation. Fixation is straightforward though misplacement into the subcutaneous tissues can occur. The risk of this is greatest at the time of insertion and in the first few days thereafter if exchange of the tube is attempted. Bedside tracheostomy is possible using dilatational techniques and is popular in intensive care. The confirmation of intratracheal placement of the dilators using a fibreoptic bronchoscope or similar device is a sensible precaution and a recently described technique involving dilatation from within using a translaryngotracheal approach is being evaluated at present.

APPLIED PHYSIOLOGY

The introduction of an endotracheal tube bypasses a number of important physiological processes undertaken by the upper airways and the naso-oropharynx. The processes disturbed are:

1. Humidification and particle filtration.
2. Glottic closure (an essential part of the physiological cough and protection of the bronchial tree).
3. Speech and swallowing (including drainage of the sinuses).

HUMIDIFICATION AND FILTRATION

The nasopharynx is a very effective heat and moisture exchanger with filtration properties resulting from the nasal hairs. Each change in the direction of the gas flow also causes particulate matter to fall out of the airstream onto the moist mucosal surface. However, endotracheal tubes are capable of delivering dry unwarmed gases directly into the major conducting airways, thus resulting in loss of heat and moisture (latent heat of vaporization) together with the drying of pulmonary secretions. The increased viscosity causes disturbance of the normal ciliary function and ultimately the loss of effective clearance of the pulmonary secretions. Inspired gases are physiologically fully saturated (44 mg of water in 1000 ml of gas) and the ideal is to match this by artificial means. The presence of water within breathing circuits may, however, predispose to corrosion and to the malfunction (sticking) of valves designed to maintain a one-way flow of gases.

METHODS OF HUMIDIFICATION OF INSPIRED GAS

Active humidification utilizing a heating device relies upon the generation of sterile water vapour in a manner similar to a kettle boiling water. Though apparently straightforward it introduces the risk of thermal injury and near patient monitoring of the inspired gas temperature and a negative feedback loop is necessary for patient protection. A potential culture medium of warm water is provided and cross-infection associated with contamination in hot water and cold water humidifiers and nebulizing systems is well documented.

The use of small volumes of water heated to high temperatures has become the preferred system. It is the temperature sensor near the patient that determines the time for heating and because of the small volume of water used, this time is short and the system is more responsive. The danger of overheating is reduced because there is no large reservoir of heated water and the high temperature reduces the risk of bacterial growth in the humidifier.

A number of cold water nebulization systems may be used to atomize sterile water. They work by entraining water droplets into a stream of gas using the Venturi effect and then causing them to be broken into many much smaller droplets by hitting an anvil. Ultrasound has also been used to generate droplets. Some devices are disposable, containing reservoirs of sterile water, and once the reservoir is empty the device is replaced with a new system. These are suitable for the non-intubated patient in need of extra humidification as well as the intubated and ventilated individual. Sterile water is hypotonic and has been implicated in inducing bronchospasm in some patients. Fluid overload due to absorption of water has also been described, particularly in paediatric practice.

The conservation of heat and water using heat and moisture exchangers is often combined with a filtration capability sufficient to act as a bacterial or even viral barrier, thus protecting patients from cross infection. They mimic the physiological process whereby during exhalation the water content of the expired gas condenses on a surface only to be vaporized with the inhalation of the next breath. These devices are less efficient as tidal volume increases and their effectiveness as a biological filter is compromised if they become wet. They are, however, disposable items. To work well all gas flow must pass through them so that they are only effective for intubated patients and they need to be positioned within the breathing system as near to the patient as possible. Because the exchangers form part of the dead space of the circuit and this may be significant in children, small volume devices are available for paediatric use. Their presence increases the number of junctions within a breathing system, thus increasing the likelihood of a circuit disconnection.

The use of low-flow circuitry recycles the moisture present in expired gas. In addition heat and water are generated by the soda lime as it is used to absorb the carbon dioxide. This technique has again become popular in anaesthetic practice and the main reason for its resurgence relates to the economy of gas and volatile agent consumption resulting from the low fresh gas flows. Thus, there are both financial and environmental benefits in addition to the conservation of heat and water.

In general, active humidification is used for prolonged artificial ventilation in intensive care settings, low-flows in anaesthesia and heat moisture exchangers in both areas. The use of bacterial/viral filters has become commonplace as a means of reducing contamination of ventilator circuitry and minimizing the risk of crossinfection. Heat moisture conservation is an added benefit with the use of such devices. The need for humidification in brief anaesthetic procedures is slight but for long procedures, particularly in patients with pulmonary disease and copious secretions, it is beneficial. Humidification is essential for patients receiving long-term ventilation in the intensive care setting.

THE MEASUREMENT OF HUMIDITY

It is unusual to measure the extent of humidification of respired gases in clinical practice but avoiding extremes of environmental humidity is important for the comfort and safety of those working in theatre. If the theatre environment is too wet there is an increased risk of spreading infection and in the extreme situation water may even run down the walls of the operating theatre. If the atmosphere is too dry there may be problems with static electricity.

There are two different ways of recording humidity and an appreciation of the two will lead to a better understanding of the whole concept of humidity and its measurement. Humidity may be defined as absolute or relative humidity.

Absolute humidity is the actual amount of water present in a gas expressed in terms such as the volume of water vapour present in a standard volume of gas or the weight of water present in a given gas volume. No matter how the temperature of the gas varies, the amount of water vapour present will be the same – hence the term absolute humidity.

Relative humidity compares the amount of water that is actually present in a gas with the maximum amount of water that the gas is able to hold at a particular temperature. Thus, if the maximum amount of water that a gas could hold at 35°C is Y, the relative humidity at 35 °C would be:

$$\frac{\text{Absolute humidity (X)} \times 100\%}{Y}$$

It can therefore be seen that the relative humidity is a percentage of the total water that can be held by the gas at that temperature. How then does the relative humidity vary with a change in temperature if the water content of the gas remains the same? As the temperature of a gas increases it can hold more water vapour in any given volume of that gas but because the absolute humidity is the same, the relative humidity falls (Y increases in the above formula but X stays the same). Similarly, as the gas cools, it can hold less water vapour and the relative humidity increases. By definition the relative humidity cannot be greater than 100% at any given temperature (X and Y are the same) and at this temperature the gas is completely saturated with water vapour. Because the gas is unable to hold any more water, further cooling will mean that water vapour has to be deposited in the form of water droplets on a surface. This is exactly what occurs when clouds give up water as rain and this process is also responsible for the frosting on the outside of nitrous oxide cylinders during prolonged use.

The humidity of environmental air may be measured by means of Regnault's Hygrometer, the wet and dry bulb thermometer or by the horsehair hygrometer. Regnault's Hygrometer relies upon the observation of water vapour condensing on a cold surface. Air is bubbled through ether in a silvered tube. The temperature of the ether falls during evaporation and this is recorded by means of a thermometer situated within the ether. The clouding of the silver finish marks the start of condensation, which occurs when the air is fully saturated. This is known as the Dew Point and the temperature of the Dew Point is recorded from the thermometer placed in the ether. The water content of air that is saturated with water vapour at that temperature, i.e. the Dew Point, can be calculated from a graph. Because the actual (absolute) amount of water present in the air has not changed but only the temperature, the water content recorded is actually the same as the absolute humidity (see definition above) at the original or air temperature. By again referring to the graph, we can read off the maximum amount of water that air can hold at the original or air temperature. This corresponds to Y in the above equation and thus we now know both X and Y and can calculate the relative humidity of the air using the formula.

The Wet and Dry Bulb Thermometer works on the principle that when water evaporates it cools the surface with which it is in contact (latent heat of vaporization) and the rate of evaporation is dependent upon the humidity and the ambient temperature of the air. Thus, the lower the humidity, the greater will be the rate of evaporation and the greater will be the cooling and hence the fall of temperature. Similarly, the higher the ambient air temperature, the lower will be the relative humidity (see above) and the greater will be the cooling and hence the fall of temperature. The equipment has two thermometers, one dry and one with its bulbous reservoir surrounded by damp muslin; the latter thermometer cools in response to evaporation and the magnitude of the difference is dependent upon the relative humidity prevalent at the time the temperatures are measured.

To calculate the relative humidity, the dry bulb and the wet bulb temperatures are recorded. Using a graph, the dry bulb temperature is measured against the temperature difference between the two thermometers in order to obtain a direct reading of the relative humidity.

The Horsehair Hygrometer relies upon the increasing elasticity of horsehair with increasing humidity. Within the hygrometer is a horsehair spring which coils or uncoils with changes in humidity and is attached to a recording mechanism. It is commonly used in devices such as barometers that directly measure humidity.

GLOTTIC CLOSURE AND SPEECH

The intubated patient is unable to speak or close the vocal cords but in the case of individuals having an anaesthetic the endotracheal tube is removed at the time of recovery. For a brief period the voice may be affected and rarely granulomas of the vocal cords can follow what is only a relatively short period of intubation. In those undergoing more prolonged periods of ventilatory support within an intensive care unit, the loss of communication can be a major issue for all involved. Tracheal injury and stenosis are much more common if prolonged endotracheal intubation is undertaken and this includes tracheostomy. Laryngeal damage with cord granulomas, stenosis and adhesions can also occur.

The normal cough sequence is the most effective means for clearing the lungs of secretions and maintaining patency of the smaller airways. It consists of inspiration, glottic closure and a rise in intrathoracic pressure caused by muscular contraction followed by a sudden opening of the glottis. This produces a very rapid outflow of gas, which carries the secretions with it. Intubation of the trachea and artificial ventilation interfere with all these processes and contribute to the high incidence of pneumonia in patients who undergo prolonged ventilation. Rapid recovery and extubation with return of full muscle power are clearly beneficial postoperatively for patients who only undergo transient artificial ventilation.

SWALLOWING AND PULMONARY ASPIRATION

The disturbance in swallowing and glottic closure resulting from airway instrumentation, combined with abnormal upper airway reflexes for a period following extubation, all increase the incidence of aspiration into the bronchopulmonary tree and this is probably a contributory factor in the development of postoperative chest infections. Local pressure has been suggested as inducing nerve damage within the larynx, thus disturbing its function. Fixation of the larynx by the endotracheal tube prevents its normal rise towards the head with swallowing. This mechanism is part of the process involved in closure of the larynx, which directs material towards the oesophagus and minimizes aspiration of secretions.

THE PHYSIOLOGY OF NORMAL VENTILATION

Although the physiology of normal respiration is fully discussed in Chapter 7 it is summarized here in order to achieve a better understanding of the problems associated with artificial ventilation of the lungs. Normal spontaneous ventilation is controlled centrally and relies upon an intact spinal cord with neuromuscular transmission causing the muscles of respiration to act on the chest wall. The expansion produced by muscle activity lowers the intrathoracic pressure, drawing respirable gases into the lungs. It is possible to voluntarily suspend respiration for a brief period but it continues during sleep in an involuntary manner. Adequate ventilation is necessary to provide sufficient oxygen to meet metabolic demand and to excrete the carbon dioxide produced by the body as a result of the metabolism of the cells.

Normal ventilation depends upon the following:

- An intact central nervous system to sense and drive respiration.
- Intact neural pathways.
- Normal neuromuscular transmission.
- Normal muscular contraction and relaxation.
- An intact chest wall.

These constitute the 'pump' that has to overcome the resistance offered by the airways and to expand the lung tissue and chest wall. The total work of breathing is variable, depending upon the metabolic needs of the body and the following factors:

- Airway resistance.
- Pulmonary compliance or elasticity.
- Chest wall compliance.

The negative intrathoracic pressure of spontaneous ventilation has important effects upon the cardiovascular system. Venous return to the right atrium is enhanced by the fall in intrathoracic pressure and the corresponding increase in atrial filling contributes to maintaining the cardiac output. This maintenance of right atrial filling is disturbed by the change from a negative to a positive intrathoracic pressure, as occurs in positive pressure ventilation.

PHYSIOLOGICAL DISTURBANCES RESULTING FROM IPPV

RESPIRATORY

Positive pressure applied to the bronchial tree will result in distension of the most easily expanded areas of the lung, i.e. those with the greatest local compliance. Spontaneous respiration is a consequence of local muscle contraction so diaphragmatic contraction has an expansive effect on the lower lobes that is lost with IPPV. It is these areas of the lung that have the greatest perfusion of blood and thus there is a ventilation:perfusion (V:Q) mismatch, because the lower lobes are less compliant than those areas that are underperfused and better ventilated, situated higher in the lung. As a result the association of blood in the alveolar capillaries with gas in the alveolus is lost, with some alveoli being ventilated but not perfused and others being perfused but not ventilated. This mismatching within the lungs may lead to varying degrees of hypoxaemia but in most cases it can be effectively managed by increasing the inspired oxygen concentration although this does not resolve the underlying problem.

Expiration remains passive and is dependent upon the elastic recoil of the lungs. Prolonged expiration secondary, for example, to bronchospasm may mean that inspiration occurs before full exhalation has taken place. This may be exacerbated by a rapid respiratory rate with the relative times permitted for inspiration and expiration (the I:E ratio) less than 1:2. If expiration is incomplete then air trapping will occur with hyperinflation of the lungs and a rise in the intrathoracic pressure. Potentially this can produce a tension pneumothorax and this is most likely to occur if bullae become overdistended to the point of rupture. Patients with preexisting lung disease are at the greatest risk but any failure of equipment that exposes the lungs to excessive pressures can produce this devastating complication of IPPV. Pressure relief valves and monitors of airway pressures within ventilator circuits are mandatory for this reason.

CARDIOVASCULAR

The major effect of IPPV on the cardiovascular system, which has already been referred to, is the reduction in cardiac output secondary to the fall in venous return. This may present as a fall in pulse volume or blood pressure with the inspiratory cycle and the effect is increased if the patient is hypovolaemic prior to the induction of IPPV or if there is limited cardiac reserve, e.g. in the elderly and patients with valvular heart disease. The use of cardiac depressant drugs in association with anaesthesia and ventilation aggravates the situation and may be sufficient to reduce cardiac output to the point of myocardial ischaemia or a cardiac arrest. Regional changes in blood flow inevitably follow even modest falls in cardiac output and the splanchnic blood flow is reduced.

The increased intrathoracic pressure means that the forces involved in producing stretch of the atria walls in the heart are reduced. As a result atrial natriuretic hormone (sodium-excreting hormone) is no longer produced and there is retention of salt and water. This manifests itself as a reduction in urine flow, responding to loop diuretics such as frusemide, and normally is self-correcting on cessation of IPPV. Salt and water retention can, however, be significant in patients who are ventilated for prolonged periods.

CENTRAL NERVOUS SYSTEM

Artificial ventilation can produce states of hypocapnia, hypercapnia or normocapnia. End-tidal CO_2 monitoring now permits the maintenance of normocapnia regardless of changes in gas flow and the characteristics of the ventilator breathing system. The changes in cerebral blood flow resulting from these states, together with acute changes in pH from the production of respiratory alkalosis (hypocapnia) or respiratory acidosis (hypercapnia), may induce a wide variety of effects ranging from epileptiform seizures to narcosis. Normocapnia is desirable in almost every circumstance and the restoration of spontaneous ventilation may be affected by induced hypocapnia with lack of respiratory drive though the effect of this is often overstated. Induction of hypocapnia will reduce intracerebral (intracranial) pressure by reducing cerebral blood flow. Cerebral perfusion pressure (arterial pressure minus jugular venous pressure) may be reduced by IPPV, which produces a fall in blood pressure and a rise in the venous pressure. Intraocular pressure follows intracerebral pressure and can be reduced by the induction of hypocapnia.

MODES OF VENTILATION AND VENTILATOR JARGON

There are many different modes of ventilation described, the majority relating to intensive care medicine. Some are applicable only to intensive care because patients who are anaesthetized for surgery are pharmacologically paralysed and therefore have no spontaneous respiratory activity. There is little convincing evidence that one mode is better at achieving oxygenation than another or that weaning is simplified. The main factors remain airway and intrathoracic pressure, lung volume and the presence of positive end-expiratory pressure (PEEP). Ventilators are now under development which will achieve a variety of goals, as set by the attending physician. The combination of oximetry, carbon dioxide, oxygen and pressure monitoring with feedback loops permits the ventilator to modify itself to achieve a number of preset functions.

CONTROLLED MECHANICAL VENTILATION (CMV)

CMV describes the total control of breathing by the ventilator in which no spontaneous activity occurs and

disconnection will render the patient apnoeic. This is the usual state of affairs associated with anaesthesia. The volumes, I:E ratio and all other ventilatory variables are the responsibility of the anaesthetist and overdosage of volatile agents is possible. Patient awareness is a potential risk if paralysis and ventilation are continued without adequate anaesthesia being administered.

POSITIVE END-EXPIRATORY PRESSURE

PEEP is not a ventilatory mode but can be added to almost any mode. If added to patients breathing spontaneously, it is conventionally referred to as Continuous Positive Airway Pressure (CPAP). PEEP is achieved using a low-resistance threshold resistor, which produces a predictable positive pressure with different flow rates having little effect on that pressure. The early technique of immersing the expiratory limb of the circuit in water to a depth of 10 cm in order to produce 10 cm of PEEP demonstrates the principle. PEEP can improve oxygenation in many patients and probably does so by recruiting lung units previously not ventilated. It also increases intrathoracic pressures and therefore can reduce cardiac output. Intrinsic PEEP describes the situation when at the end of expiration the intrathoracic pressure has not fallen to zero and the lung remains inflated above the FRC. This may occur in airway obstruction with a prolonged expiratory phase or may be induced by manoeuvres such as reversing the I:E ventilation ratio. PEEP has yet to be demonstrated conclusively to alter outcome in conditions such as Adult Respiratory Distress Syndrome (ARDS) though most clinicians believe its benefit to be greater than its risk if it is maintained at levels of 5–15 cm H_2O.

PRESSURE-REGULATED VOLUME-CONTROLLED VENTILATION

This recently introduced mode guarantees a volume and manipulates the pattern of inspiration to produce the lowest inflation pressures achievable for the given tidal volume and rate. The rationale is to minimize the adverse effects of high airway pressures.

INVERSE I:E RATIO VENTILATION

The normal ratio of 1:2 (inspiration to expiration) may be unsatisfactory in lungs with regional disease processes. By convention, if the I:E ratio is greater than 1:1 then inverse ratio ventilation is present. The shortened expiratory period will increase the intrathoracic volume and recruits alveoli in a manner similar to applied PEEP. Locally altered compliance may make some alveoli less easily distended and increasing the period for inspiration may thus improve regional distribution of ventilation.

PRESSURE RELIEF VENTILATION

The application of a positive pressure to a preset limit with the tidal volume being dependent on this is another approach to reducing the effect of excessive airway pressure. Changes in pulmonary mechanics will alter the delivered tidal volume.

INDEPENDENT LUNG VENTILATION

This infrequently used technique relies upon the independent intubation of the left and right lungs using a dual-lumen endotracheal tube. Each lung is then ventilated with a separate ventilator or one lung may be collapsed to permit surgical procedures to be undertaken. Independent lung ventilation may have a role where there is unilateral lung pathology and it does not appear to be necessary for the ventilators to be synchronized in any way.

WEANING MODES

These are ventilatory modes that permit the support of ventilation by mechanical means whilst permitting the patient to breathe for themselves to a greater or lesser extent. These modes are appropriate in managing the transition from full mechanical ventilation to sustained spontaneous ventilation in the intensive care unit. Many ventilators will allow spontaneous ventilation to take place in any mode. They are designed to minimize the swings in intrathoracic pressure that would occur if respiration were attempted against closed valves in the ventilator circuit. A great deal of effort has been directed towards achieving the sensitive detection and rapid response to any inspiratory activity on the part of the patient. The use of flow or pressure detectors is the usual means of achieving this.

SYNCHRONIZED INTERMITTENT MANDATORY VENTILATION (SIMV)

Originally developed as unsynchronized intermittent mandatory ventilation (IMV), this mode permits the patient to breathe whilst the ventilator guarantees a preset (mandatory) number of breaths of a given tidal volume. The synchronization refers to the detection by the ventilator of the patient's respiratory cycle so that machine inspiration does not occur whilst patient expiration is taking place.

MANDATORY MINUTE VOLUME

This mode ensures that the patient achieves a predetermined minute volume of ventilation. The minute volume may be entirely mechanical or entirely spontaneous with any intermediate combination and the mode is designed so that a very high frequency of small tidal volumes will not be considered as acceptable.

SPECIALIZED VENTILATORS

HIGH FREQUENCY JET VENTILATION (HFJV)

This mode of ventilation uses frequencies in the range of 60–200 breaths per minute and specific ventilators to generate this high frequency of ventilation have been developed. The 'breaths' are delivered via a fine catheter that is either introduced as a separate cannula into an endotracheal tube or uses a special endotracheal tube with extra lumina in the wall of the tube for jet insufflation and distal pressure monitoring. HFJV causes the entrainment of gases along with the jet stream and measurement of the combined (jet plus entrained) flow is not possible. The frequent measurement of blood gases is therefore necessary to determine if adequate ventilation is taking place.

As yet, the indications for jet ventilation remain unclear. There is a lower intrathoracic pressure with HFJV and this is a benefit, particularly in patients with a bronchopleural fistula. It has been used in patients with a multitude of pulmonary pathologies, including ARDS, but its benefit remains unproven.

NON-INVASIVE VENTILATION AND VENTILATORY ASSIST DEVICES

This refers to techniques of ventilation that are possible without intubation of the airway. They are of particular value in the management of patients with severe chronic diseases. Typical examples of such conditions are paralytic diseases or injury affecting the muscles of respiration in which the loss of muscle power may be complete or partial. The problem may be muscular, as in the muscular dystrophies, neural, such as occurs with spinal cord lesions, or central with loss of the central control of ventilation. The combination of gross musculoskeletal deformity or the loss of lung parenchyma associated with chronic lung disease can also contribute to the need for ventilatory support. Ventilatory support may be necessary for the entire 24 hours or only for part of the time, most frequently at night. Rare disorders that affect the normal maintenance of respiration during sleep, such as Ondine's Curse, cause the patient to become hypercapnoeic and hypoxic. Sleep apnoea that occurs in the Pickwickian Syndrome, which is associated with gross obesity and daytime somnolence, will also cause periods of hypoxia.

Non-invasive ventilation has been used in the management of all these conditions and has become popular of late for the management of patients with chronic pulmonary disease in an attempt to prevent deterioration to the point of needing conventional invasive ventilation.

NASAL VENTILATION

Nasal ventilation can provide assistance to patients with sleep apnoea or severe chronic airways disease. The application to the conscious cooperative patient of a tight-fitting nasal mask, connected to a high flow of gas above atmospheric pressure, provides assistance to inspiration. This is nasal continuous positive airway pressure (nasal CPAP). Combining this with a cyclical increase and decrease in the pressure constitutes nasal ventilation and exhalation can occur via the mouth or against the relief pressure of the system. The use of non-invasive nasal ventilation can avoid the need for intubation in a proportion of patients who become hypercapnic and would otherwise need conventional IPPV. The risks of ventilator-associated pneumonia are correspondingly reduced. The patient with little in the way of secretions appears to be the most likely to benefit.

THE IRON LUNG

The iron lung was developed as a means of ventilatory support for victims of poliomyelitis and heralded the use of artificial ventilation for extended periods of time. It was as a consequence of the polio outbreaks in the 1950s that long-term mechanical ventilator support was realized. The body was encased in a container with the head outside and cyclical reductions of the pressure in the container drew air into the lungs. Access to the patient was greatly limited but, nevertheless, it enabled patients to survive who would not have done so otherwise.

CUIRASS VENTILATION

A plate shaped like a tortoise shell is placed over the thorax and upper abdomen. Negative pressure is cyclically produced causing the thoracic volume to increase and gas to enter the lungs. Expiration is passive though the most recently produced cuirass ventilator has a positive phase enhancing expiration and a very wide range of frequencies available. This device (Hayek Ventilator) has resurrected interest in cuirass ventilation amongst enthusiasts of non-invasive ventilation.

POSTURAL VENTILATION

Tilting of the supine patient can offer some modest enhancement of tidal volume and has been used as an assist device for patients without sufficient muscular activity to permit spontaneous ventilation, particularly during the night.

THE IDEAL VENTILATOR

To meet the varying needs of patients an ideal ventilator would have to fulfil many criteria because the needs for intensive care and theatre ventilators are different. The ability to use the same ventilator for all patients is appealing but would lead to a complexity that is not justified for routine theatre use. All anaesthetic ventilators need to be safe with current and future volatile agents, capable of withstanding corrosion from the anaesthetic gases and due to water condensing from the expired gases. The ability to function with low fresh gas flows is essential for anaesthetic ventilators but inappropriate for intensive care. 'Bag in a bottle' ventilators that circulate the gases around a circle system are characteristic of many theatre ventilators and the use of low fresh gas flows together with carbon dioxide absorption is commonplace. Such ventilators separate the respired gases from those involved in driving the ventilator. Also used extensively are minute volume dividers that permit the division of the total fresh gas flow into a number of equal, preset volumes (tidal volume) and sometimes frequencies. These have the benefit of only functioning when gas flow is present but are unsuitable for use with low fresh gas flows.

RELIABLE

Reliability is an essential prerequisite of any device that is intended to provide life support. The ventilator must be able to function with minimal maintenance for prolonged periods of time and all components should be readily accessible for maintenance and inspection. Robust design and simplicity are desirable, yet inevitably at odds with the need for close accurate monitoring and measurement of the many variables associated with artificial ventilation.

INEXPENSIVE

The market for ventilators is limited and the development costs are high. The life expectancy for most ventilators is in the range of 10–15 years and although initial costs can be high, the cost per year is more modest. When considering the cost per patient treated, the expense is probably comparable to the costs associated with surgical consumables. Running costs such as filters, specific disposable items and maintenance need to be considered when trying to compare the true cost of any particular ventilator with another.

EASY TO STERILIZE

Crossinfection is an ever-present risk to patients and rapid turnover of patients in the operating environment makes infection control a more difficult issue to manage. The use of bacterial/viral filters has resolved the problem to a great extent even though the efficacy of such filters can be compromised by humidity within the filter and the pressure across the filtration membrane. In addition, the introduction of such filters increases the number of potential leaks in any ventilator circuit.

SIMPLE TO USE

Ergonomic design has an important role in the construction of ventilators. The separation of alarm settings from those that determine the tidal volume, rate and other parameters will help to make the machine safer to use.

MONITORING AND ALARMS

Integral monitoring is usual for intensive care ventilators and is commonplace in many of the more recent anaesthetic ventilators. The use of separate monitoring devices in anaesthesia remains very common and there are arguments in favour of both the totally integrated system and one with free-standing options.

Parameters that are monitored include the follwing.

Inspired and expired oxygen

This identifies the use of a hypoxic mixture and can give some indication of oxygen consumption. With suitable volume measurements metabolic rate may also be determined. The use of oxygen cells to continu-ously measure oxygen can be expensive because their life is shortened when working in a high oxygen environment.

Tidal volume, minute volume and respiratory rate

Measurements of tidal volume and rate are the most basic parameters of ventilation. Comparison of inspired and expired tidal volume may reveal any leaks within the breathing system but may also be due to the expansion under pressure of the ventilator circuitry. This apparent loss of volume is known as the internal compliance of the ventilator. Measurement of the expired gas volume and composition is made more complex by the presence of moisture because the condensation of water may interfere with a transducer's ability to measure flow and volume.

Airway Pressure

The cyclical change in airway pressure is often the basis of a disconnection alarm device. Pressure monitors are useful to detect changes in airway resistance, pulmonary and chest wall compliance but excessive airway pressure may reflect other problems such as a tension pneumothorax or endobronchial intubation. The ability to provide and measure PEEP is a helpful option on anaesthetic ventilators for the small number of critically ill patients who may require surgery.

VERSATILITY

Ventilators should ideally be suitable for anaesthesia and intensive care but although this may be an advantage, the reality is that most patients undergoing anaesthesia have normal pulmonary function whereas those on intensive care units do not. The provision of a variety of ventilatory modes is of benefit in intensive care medicine. It is for these and similar reasons that the development of two families of ventilators has evolved though small numbers have been designed for use in both anaesthesia and intensive care.

RECOMMENDED READING

1997 *Handbook of Mechanical Ventilatory Support*, 2nd edn. Baltimore: Williams and Wilkins.

10

SCIENTIFIC PRINCIPLES IN RELATION TO MONITORING EQUIPMENT

C. S. Ince & A. C. Skinner

This chapter is intended to provide an understanding of the physical principles of anaesthetic monitoring devices and reference will only be made to individual monitors in order to further this understanding. Alternative texts will provide detailed descriptions of specific devices if required. The measurement of temperature and humidity has been discussed elsewhere.

PHYSICAL PRINCIPLES

The waveform is a good way of describing how many types of energy are transmitted. This is represented as a 'sine' wave, which is a repetitive, cyclical waveform moving about a horizontal axis (Fig. 10.1). The distance between repeating parts of the cycle is called the *wavelength*, measured in metre (m), and the distance between the horizontal and the maximum deflection is called the *amplitude*. *Frequency* is the number of cycles each second, measured in Hertz (Hz). *Velocity*, the product of frequency and wavelength, is dependent on the medium through which the wave is moving, being reduced in denser media. Sound waves are correctly thought of as a form of (mechanical) energy propagated as a wave.

Electromagnetic radiation (visible light, X-rays, gamma rays, radiowaves, microwaves, infrared [heat] radiation and ultraviolet light) shows many properties of being propagated as a waveform. Unlike sound, however, this is not a complete description of its behaviour because some of the properties of electromagnetic radiation are more like a stream of particles than a waveform. These various types of energy make up the so-called *electromagnetic spectrum* (see Fig. 11.1). Within the spectrum there is a great variation in wavelength. Radiowaves may have a wavelength of up to 3 km, with a frequency from less than 10^5 Hz to 10^9 Hz, but microwaves have shorter wavelengths and higher frequencies. Infrared radiation has a shorter wavelength than microwaves and that of visible light is even shorter, with the wavelength of red light longer than that of violet light. Beyond this is ultraviolet light, with an even shorter wavelength, then X-rays followed by gamma radiation. All electromagnetic radiation propagates in a vacuum at the same speed (of light), about 3×10^8/ms, and thus the product of wavelength and frequency for any electromagnetic radiation is constant.

Just as numbers may be added together or subtracted, so two or more waveforms may interact with each other. If the waves are synchronized (*in phase*), their amplitudes will add together but if they are out of phase, the effects will cancel out and the amplitude will decrease.

By combining waves of different amplitudes and frequencies, complex wave patterns may be produced. The electrocardiogram, for example, can be thought of as a mixture of many sine waves between 0.5 Hz and 80 Hz. Therefore, in order to display the ECG satisfactorily without distortion, the apparatus must have a frequency response that exceeds these limits. Similar analysis of any repetitive waveform can be used to estimate the apparatus' frequency response needed to handle it satisfactorily.

Electrons are the negatively charged particles that surround the positively charged nucleus of an atom. (Atoms may obtain an excess of electrons by means of a chemical reaction, a magnetic field or by developing a static charge.) An *electric current* is a flow of electrons along a conductor. The force driving the current flow round the circuit is known as the electromotive force, potential difference or voltage and is measured in volt (V). Electrons flow easily through conductors but not through insulators. Resistance within the circuit will impede (slow down) the flow of electrons and increases with an increase of temperature in normal conductors. This principle is used in some temperature-measuring devices (see Ch. 19).

If the current flow regularly changes direction it is known as an *alternating current* (AC), being again expressed graphically as a sine wave. Current which flows in one direction only is known as a *direct current* (DC).

SI UNITS OF ELECTRICITY

Current flow (abbreviated to I) is measured in amperes (A), the potential difference (V) in volts (V) and the resistance (R) in ohms (Ω). Their relationship (described in Ohm's Law) is expressed in the following formula:

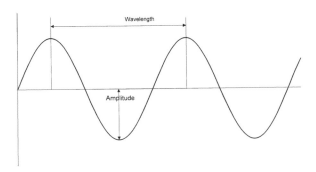

Figure 10.1   A sine wave

$I=V/R$ (which transposes to $V=IR$ or $R=V/I$).

Expressed as words, this means an increase in resistance will cause a decrease in current if the voltage is unchanged.

The power (P) dissipated by an electrical system is measured in watts (W). A power of 1 watt represents 1 joule of work being done per second. In an electrical system, power = current × voltage, that is, 1 watt is 1 ampere volt. Thus, a domestic 13 A supply at 230 V has a maximum power of 2990 W or 2.99 kW. (Energy used by an electrical installation is generally metered in kW hour, not the SI unit joule. One kW hour is therefore equal to

1000 × 60 [minutes in 1 hour] × 60 (seconds in 1minute] = 3 600 000 joule.)

The unit of electrical charge is the coulomb (C) and is the amount of electrical charge passed when a current of 1 ampere flows for 1 second. (It is the charge carried by approximately 6.25×10^{18} electrons.) One joule of energy is needed to raise the potential of a charge of 1 coulomb by 1 volt.

INTRODUCTION TO MONITORING EQUIPMENT

Monitoring equipment may be thought of as devices for sensing and interpreting signals received from patients. The process includes some or all of the following steps:

Patient → Sensor → Transducer →
Amplifier → Display → Recorder.

THE SENSOR

Sensors receive signals from the patient in many different ways, e.g. heat energy causing a liquid to expand (temperature measurement with a mercury in glass thermometer), variation in pressure (blood pressure monitor) and electrical energy from biological potentials (electrocardiograph). They may be placed within the substance of the body (invasive), such as balloons for measuring intracranial pressure, or on its surface (non-invasive), such as an ECG or blood pressure cuff. Monitoring devices introduced into the gastrointestinal tract are generally thought of as non-invasive because they still remain outside the substance of the body.

TRANSDUCERS

A transducer is a device for changing one form of energy into another, usually mechanical energy into an electrical impulse. Almost the only time in routine clinical practice when transducers are used is in invasive blood pressure measurement or temperature measurement. There are several techniques of transduction, some of which are described below.

Strain Gauge Transducer

Stretching a wire will cause its diameter to decrease and length to increase, thus increasing the *resistance* of the wire. The strain gauge pressure transducer responds to changes in resistance caused by stretching and relaxing an electrical wire attached to a diaphragm, which moves in response to pressure changes within the transducer.

Heating a wire will also increase its resistance and this principle is utilized in the resistance wire thermometer, used to measure gas temperatures in industry, although this device is only useful for high temperatures, not those found in clinical practice.

Transducers that utilize changes in resistance are usually connected to a *Wheatstone Bridge*. This circuit is illustrated in Figure 10.2 and consists of four resistances arranged as shown, one of which, e.g. R4, is the transducer. When R1/R2 = R3/R4 no current flows through the galvanometer (G), but when R4 changes the bridge becomes unbalanced and the resulting flow of electric current is proportional to the change in resistance. It is this current that is used as the transducer output.

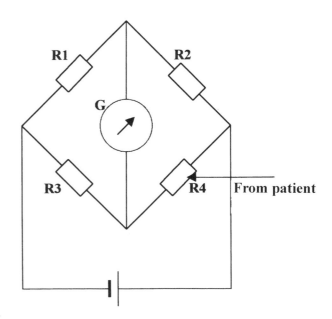

Figure 10.2   The Wheatstone Bridge

Inductance Transducer

If a coil of wire that can conduct electricity is moved in and out of an electrical field, a potential difference will be generated in proportion to the speed of movement. This is the principle of *inductance* used in the inductance coil pressure transducer and the electromagnetic flow meter, the latter being used to measure blood through a vessel.

Unfortunately, magnetic fields generated by apparatus can induce electrical currents in neighbouring equipment with resulting interference.

Capacitance Transducers

If a circuit is broken by a small gap between two electrodes (a capacitor, as illustrated in Fig. 10.3) a direct current will be unable to flow and a charge will build up on the plates when a DC voltage is applied. However, if the capacity of the capacitor is large enough, an alternating current will pass as the charge on the plates is repeatedly reversed. Capacity of a capacitor is measured in farad (Fd). A capacitor of 1 farad will store 1 coulomb of charge when a potential of 1 volt is applied. (A 1 Fd capacitor actually reflects huge capacity and capacities of 10^{-10} Fd are more normal in electronic devices.) The capacity depends on the area of the plates and their separation; thus increased plate area or decreased separation increases the capacity of the capacitor. If a capacitor is charged from a DC source through a high resistance, the voltage across the capacitor can be used to measure the separation of the plates, since this affects capacity, the amount of charge being constant. This principle is used in capacitance pressure transducers, in which the diaphragm is attached to one of the plates, the other being fixed. The commonest device that uses this principle is the capacitor microphone.

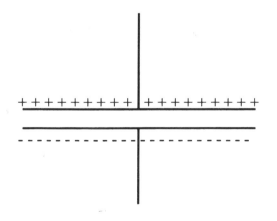

Figure 10.3   A capacitor

Zeroing Pressure Transducers

Modern transducers have very reliable calibration, i.e. a given change in the input (usually pressure) will reliably produce the same change in output signal. Manufacturers of transducers supply calibration data for each pattern or occasionally for each batch of transducers. How these are programmed into the monitor varies with each type of monitor, but will usually not need to be done for each usage. However, the output of the transducer for zero pressure (or other signal) is not reproducible and may even 'drift' with time. Because of this, transducers need to be 'zeroed', which simply means exposing the transducer to zero signal (for pressure transducers open to atmosphere) and telling the monitor to use this signal to 'zero'. The exact technique varies with each pattern of monitor but it is usually a very simple operation. It is important to bear in mind that changes in the level of the transducer relative to the patient will render the zero point useless and the transducer will need to be relevelled.

Since physiological pressure signals can range in value from a few mmHg to up to 300 mmHg, monitors provide different selectable pressure ranges. Like the ECG, an appropriate frequency response of the whole system is needed to realistically reproduce the pressure waveform. Using extension sets not designed for the pressure measurement system, defects in the set (commonly kinking or partial obstruction of the cannula) or air bubbles in the correct system can affect frequency response and produce incorrect readings or waveforms.

Thermistors

Some types of semiconductors are capable of conducting electricity but this ability is increased with heat (thermistors). The alterations in resistance in these devices can be used to measure temperature (see Ch. 19). Thermistors are commonly used in clinical temperature probes.

Thermocouples

A circuit that comprises a conductor of one metal with conductors of a second metal at either end will generate a very small potential difference if the temperature of the two metal junctions is different. This will not measure temperature absolutely but the difference between the unknown temperature and the other junction at a known temperature, the so-called *reference junction* (see Ch. 19).

AMPLIFICATION, DISPLAY AND RECORDING OF ELECTRONIC MONITORING

Amplifiers

Most of the devices above produce only very small signals and the signal must be amplified before it can be displayed. The way that amplifiers work is unimportant for practising theatre staff, considerations such as frequency response and compatibility being the concern of the manufacturers. Each amplifier is usually within the monitoring device and therefore incapable of being improperly connected by the end user. Devices like this, where end users need not be concerned with the details of their function, are often referred to as 'black boxes'.

Display

Display modes are used according to the parameter being displayed. Parameters that change slowly will usually be displayed numerically, for example body temperature. If the parameter changes rapidly a faster response time is needed and a graphical display is often used, usually with a numerical display, which is updated several times each minute.

Display technology is rapidly evolving but at the time of writing both cathode ray tubes and liquid crystal displays are in widespread use.

Recorders

There are many ways of generating a printout of monitored parameters. Some institutions use printouts widely, others hardly at all. ECG monitors are the devices most commonly supporting direct printout, usually using thermal techniques. (In order to help interpretation some printouts, such as ECGs, use recording paper marked with gridlines). Modern inkjet and laser printing technologies, together with the ability to connect monitors to an institution-wide computer network, are likely to revolutionize record keeping over the next few years.

MEASUREMENT OF BLOOD PRESSURE

Pressure is force/area and is therefore recorded as Newtons/square metre, with the SI unit being the Pascal. However, because of the small size of the Pascal, pressure is usually measured in Kilopascals. Units other than SI units are still used to record pressure, i.e. Bar and mm of mercury (mmHg). One bar is approximately equal to atmospheric pressure at sea level but the relationship of these three units is shown below:

$$760 \text{ mmHg} = 1.01 \text{ bar} = 101 \text{ kPa}.$$

Central venous pressure manometers are graduated in cms of water but transducers are calibrated in mmHg or kPa. Because of this, errors in interpretation may arise. Mercury is 13.6 times heavier than water and thus a 13.6 cm column of water is equivalent to a 1 cm column of mercury or, similarly, a 1.36 mm column of water is equivalent to a 1 mm column of mercury.

Pressure gauges may measure pressure including or excluding atmospheric pressure. For example, the pressure inside an empty nitrous oxide cylinder is recorded on the pressure gauge as zero but the true pressure is atmospheric. This is explained because atmospheric pressure + gauge pressure = total pressure (absolute pressure). Pressure gauges may therefore be calibrated to read either absolute (total) pressure or gauge pressure.

The Bourdon gauge (aneroid gauge) consists of a coiled tube connected to a pointer. As the pressure increases, the coil is inflated and straightened and the pointer moves around the dial until the force tending to expand the coil is equal to the opposing force. The Bourdon Gauge is used to measure cylinder pressures.

An alternative way to measure pressure is by use of a narrow manometer tube filled with liquid, usually mercury or water (Fig. 10.4). The pressure supporting the column of liquid is equal and opposite to the pressure to be measured and is usually read off a graduated scale on the manometer. When the device is used to measure atmospheric pressure the tube is sealed, e.g. the barometer, and this creates a vacuum above the liquid. If it is used for the measurement of blood pressure it is open to the atmosphere and may be connected to the circulation (invasive monitoring) or to a blood pressure cuff (non-invasive monitoring).

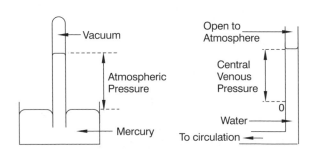

Figure 10.4   Measurement of atmospheric and central venous pressure

SETTING UP INVASIVE MONITORING

All equipment should be checked and prepared in advance. It is important that informed consent is obtained for any invasive procedure. Ideally, for arterial cannulation, a peripheral artery should be selected so that the whole limb is not threatened should a blood clot or haematoma form. Although some physicians use the brachial artery, the radial artery is usually preferred but if this is not possible the dorsalis pedis or posterior tibial arteries may be cannulated.

Before arterial cannulation the viability of a collateral circulation must be established. This is achieved by performing an Allen's test. First, the patient is asked to clench their fist and the radial and ulnar arteries are occluded. Following this, the patient is requested to open their hand, the ulnar artery is released and the palmar skin observed; flushing should occur within 5 seconds. If flushing does not occur or is delayed, poor ulnar circulation is present and another limb should be used. If possible, it is preferable to use the non-dominant hand.

A 20 or 22 gauge Teflon cannula is ideal for arterial pressure monitoring and it may be introduced over a needle or using a guidewire. Local anaesthetic should be infiltrated prior to cannulation if the patient is conscious.

Veins most commonly used for venous pressure monitoring are the internal jugular, subclavian, femoral and cephalic. The catheter should be inserted using a full sterile technique and the number of lumens within it will depend on its clinical use. Because veins are part of a low-pressure system, it is very easy to entrain air into a vein during insertion of the catheter. For this reason, subclavian and internal jugular lines should be introduced in the head-down position. It is also important to make sure that there is a free flow of fluid within the monitoring system.

PROBLEMS WITH INVASIVE MONITORING

Damping

Zero, scale and display

Zero in the case of central venous or arterial blood pressure measurement should be set at the level of the sternal angle or the mid-axillary line. The manometer tube should always read in the vertical plane and readings are taken from the bottom of the meniscus in the case of water and from the top of the meniscus if mercury is used.

Although the system may have been properly opened to air and calibrated, errors may still arise, from changes in the position of either the patient or the transducer. If the transducer is relatively higher than the level at which zero was set, the apparent pressure reading will be lower than the actual level and if it is lower, the reverse will be true. Although digital values will be recorded on the screen, a waveform will not be displayed if the recorded pressure is outside the range of the selected scale.

Overshoot

If the sensitivity of the system is too great, an overshoot will appear on the trace and the pressure will be recorded as higher than it is in reality.

COMPLICATIONS OF INVASIVE MONITORING

Bleeding

It is very important to ensure that the cannula or catheter is firmly fixed in place and that all connections are tight. Patients may easily exsanguinate if arterial bleeding is unnoticed.

Infection

Infection commonly arises from the tip of a central venous catheter, especially if it has been in position for several days. If infection is suspected the catheter should be changed and the removed tip placed in a sterile container and sent to the laboratory for culture and sensitivity.

Pneumothorax

Pneumothorax may occur if the pleural lining is punctured during the procedure. It is important therefore to check the position of the central line by performing a chest X-ray. This complication is most likely following insertion using the subclavian route. Nitrous oxide diffusing into an existing pneumothorax may make it bigger and IPPV may lead to the formation of a tension pneumothorax. It is therefore prudent not to give a general anaesthetic to a patient who has had a subclavian catheter inserted unless an X-ray of the chest has excluded a pneumothorax. If a patient with a pneumothorax requires a general anaesthetic, chest drains must be introduced before the start of the procedure.

Haemopneumothorax may result from the operative procedure or as a result of subsequent trauma by the catheter.

MONITORING EQUIPMENT

As previously mentioned, blood pressure may be measured by connecting the graduated column of mercury to an inflatable cuff situated around a limb. This apparatus is known as a *sphygmomanometer*. The cuff, which should be 20% wider than the diameter of the limb, is sited over an artery and inflated until the palpable pulse (e.g. radial) disappears. Systolic blood pressure is approximately the pressure at which the pulse reappears. If a stethoscope is placed over the artery, sounds known as *Korotkoff sounds* may be heard, the significance of which is given in Figure. 10.5.

An obsolete device, the Von Recklinghausen oscillotonometer, detected these oscillations as a means of estimating the blood pressure without auscultation or palpation of a distal pulse. Although sufficiently accurate for routine use, it was unreliable in hypotensive and hypovolaemic patients.

It has now been entirely replaced by modern non-invasive blood pressure (NIBP) monitors that detect the pressure changes by means of an electronic transducer. These modern automated oscillotonometers are the basis of almost all current automatic blood pressure devices.

FLOW PROBES

The Doppler effect, the drop in pitch of a note when a rapidly moving source of sound (say a police siren) passes the observer, is well known. Sound reflected from moving objects has its frequency altered in the same way. This effect is used to detect flow in blood vessels, so-called Doppler probes, the sound being reflected from moving blood cells. The Doppler effect is widely used in non-invasive cardiac ultrasound investigations.

1st phase	Sound first appears	Systolic blood pressure
2nd phase	Slight muffling of sound	
3rd phase	Increase in volume	
4th phase	Abrupt fall in sound	Sometimes used as diastolic pressure
5th phase	Disappearance of sound	Usually used as diastolic blood pressure

Figure 10.5   The Korotkoff sounds

MEASUREMENT OF VOLUME

The theatre practitioner may be required to measure the volumes of both gases and liquids. Although both are fluids, they behave in very different ways. Unlike liquids, gases are compressible and therefore changes in the pressure and temperature of a gas may have a significantly greater effect on the volume that is actually recorded.

MEASUREMENT OF GAS VOLUME

There are two main principles involved in the measurement of gas volume. The flow of gas may either change the volume of a bellows, which is attached through an arrangement of levers to a recording device, or rotate a series of vanes attached via a system of gears to a dial that is calibrated to record volume. Examples of the former are the Benedict Roth Spirometer, the vitalograph (a more portable version of the Spirometer) and the dry gas meter, which is used to measure larger volumes, e.g. recording the volume of gas used in the home. The Wright respirometer is an example of the latter and it has been specifically calibrated for the intermittent measurement of tidal and minute volumes. It is not accurate if used for continuous measurement.

MEASUREMENT OF LIQUID VOLUME

The simplest way of measuring the volume of a liquid is using a graduated measuring device, which in theatre is usually a suction bottle, although syringes are used for determining the doses of liquid drugs. An assessment of blood and body fluid loss plays a major part in the anaesthetic management of the patient and is discussed in Chapter 20. This chapter is only concerned with the principles involved.

Blood loss may also be estimated by weighing swabs. If the weight of a dry swab is known, the amount of blood on the swab may be calculated as follows:

Weight of blood loss = weight of used swab –
weight of dry swab

For practical purposes, 1 ml of blood weighs approximately 1 g and therefore the weight in grams may be expressed as millilitres of blood loss. The swabs should not be allowed to dry out but should be weighed immediately. Even so, the result is always an underestimate because it takes no account of the blood on the drapes and elsewhere in and around the patient.

Dilution techniques are more accurate and are especially useful for the measurement of small volumes of blood, e.g. in paediatric surgery. All the swabs, towels and drapes are put into a washing/agitating device and the blood is extracted into a large, known volume of diluent. Water, to which is often added some detergent and ammonia, is usually used as the diluting fluid. The detergent ensures disruption of the red blood cells, thus releasing the haemoglobin, while the ammonia converts the haemoglobin to methaemoglobin, the concentration of which may be measured using a *colorimeter*. Light absorption by the haemoglobin solution is directly proportional to the amount of haemoglobin present. The colorimeter includes two small glass containers, one filled with the diluting solution and the other with the solution containing haemoglobin. When viewed together, the haemoglobin solution appears darker because the haemoglobin pigment has absorbed more light. The intensity of the light passing through the test solution is increased (by decreasing the resistance of the circuit) until both containers appear the same intensity. This is achieved by rotating a graduated wheel, which in turn alters the resistance of the circuit.

Prior to its first use the colorimeter must be calibrated with a series of readings for different blood volumes, taking into account the haemoglobin concentration of the sample. If the same volume of diluting fluid is used each time, estimates of blood loss may be obtained from the graph so obtained. The result must then be corrected for the patient's haemoglobin. (If the patient's haemoglobin concentration is higher than normal more haemoglobin will be present for each unit volume of blood and the apparent blood loss will be greater than it is in reality. The reverse will happen if the patient is anaemic.)

There is now equipment available that will produce an electronic result from a reading of the haemoglobin. The method only works if the volume of blood is small compared to the volume of diluting fluid and thus the accuracy of the method decreases as the volume of blood loss increases. It is not applicable if a large amount of non-body fluid, e.g. Hibitane or Betadine, is present on the swabs. The more sophisticated methods of estimating blood volume and blood loss such as the radio tagging of red blood cells and albumin are beyond the scope of this book.

MEASUREMENT OF FLOW

Flow is defined as volume/unit time and may be measured by integrating volume with time. Alternatively, any of the parameters that affect the flow of a fluid may be used to measure flow indirectly. It is therefore necessary to be aware of these factors. Flow may be laminar or turbulent. In *laminar flow*, the particles of fluid move along in lines parallel to the sides of the tube. Flow in the centre of the tube is greater than that next to the tube wall and laminar flow is more likely to occur at low flow rates. The flow rate varies directly with the pressure difference across the length of the tube and the fourth power of its radius and inversely with the length of the tube and the viscosity of the fluid, as shown below in the Hegan-Poiseuille Formula:

$$\text{Flow rate} = \frac{\pi \times (\rho_1 - \rho_2) \times r^4}{8 \times l \times \eta}$$

where π = 3.142
$\rho_1 - \rho_2$ = pressure difference across the tube
r = radius of tube
l = length of tube
η = viscosity of fluid

On the other hand, the movement of particles in *turbulent flow* is haphazard and occurs in eddies and swirls. It takes place at the junctions and bends of circuits and if the flow rate reaches a critical level, laminar flow is converted into turbulent flow. Under turbulent conditions the flow rate varies directly with the square root of the pressure difference and the square of the radius and inversely with the length of the tube and the density of the fluid.

If the radius and length of the tube were constant and the same fluid were used (thus eliminating any variation of flow with viscosity and density) the pressure difference across the tube would vary with the flow. The *pneumotachograph* works on this principle (Fig. 10.6). It consists of a series of parallel tubes or a perforated gauze disc with a pressure-measuring facility on either side of the disc or tubes as shown. Pressure transducers record the pressure difference $(p_1 - p_2)$ across the device. The pressure difference is calibrated in respect of known flow rates and this is then integrated with time and displayed as volume. Because it is used to record tidal flows, expired water vapour may condense within the tubes, thereby impeding its performance. This is prevented by electrically heating the tubes. The pneumotachograph should be calibrated for each different gas used, so as to compensate for the variation in density and viscosity.

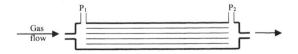

Figure 10.6   The Pneumotachograph

If gas passes through a constriction the pressure distal to the narrowing falls. This is known as the *Venturi effect* and is utilized in some humidifiers and oxygen masks. The pressure drop varies approximately with the square of the flow rate and this is the basis of the Venturi Flowmeter.

Anaesthetic gas flow meters all work on the principle of balancing increasing gas flows against gravitational forces. They may have a variable or a fixed orifice and have been described in detail in Chapter 8. Doppler flow meters measure blood flow in specific blood vessels and have been described above.

MEASUREMENT OF CARDIAC OUTPUT

Cardiac output is measured using a dilution technique that involves the injection of a dye or the injection of a cold liquid. If the blood volume is known (or calculated) the cardiac output can be worked out from the rate of the serial dilution of the dye (or a drop in the temperature, as the cold fluid is diluted by the warmer blood). Once the patient parameters have been programmed into the computer, the cardiac output is calculated very rapidly.

MEASUREMENT OF CARBON DIOXIDE AND ANAESTHETIC GASES IN GAS MIXTURES

Carbon dioxide can be measured by direct analysis of arterial blood. However, this is unsuitable for the monitoring of ventilation in the operating room. Routine monitoring of carbon dioxide is achieved by measuring the carbon dioxide levels in exhaled end-tidal (alveolar) gas. Since the alveolar gas has been equilibrated with arterial blood in the lung, measuring carbon dioxide in end-tidal gas effectively measures carbon dioxide in the blood.

The volatile anaesthetic agents equilibrate in the lungs with the blood in a similar way to carbon dioxide. Measuring each in end-tidal gas gives a fairly accurate idea of the levels in the patient's blood.

All the anaesthetic gases and volatile agents except oxygen and nitrogen absorb infrared light. Each substance can be measured in exhaled gases by using the absorbance of infrared light, either in a cell that is part of the breathing circuit (mainstream measurement) or via a continuous sample pumped from the circuit into the analyser (sidestream measurement). Because each anaesthetic agent has a different infrared absorption spectrum, different wavelengths of infrared light are measured for each gas. Usually mainstream analysers measure only carbon dioxide and sidestream analysers measure a wider range of anaesthetic gases.

MEASUREMENT OF GASEOUS OXYGEN

Oxygen, like carbon dioxide, can be measured by direct arterial sampling but this is unsuitable for routine use. End-tidal oxygen concentration gives a good idea of the oxygen delivered to the lung, while the difference between inspired oxygen and end-tidal oxygen gives a measure of uptake of oxygen by the patient. Oxygen in anaesthetic gas mixtures can be measured using the following methods.

A FUEL CELL

This is in effect a battery, the voltage of which varies with the oxygen concentration to which it is exposed. Fuel cells have a slow response time and need regular replacement. In addition, not all fuel cells are suitable for use in nitrous oxide-containing gas mixtures.

A PARAMAGNETIC ANALYSER

Oxygen is the only common paramagnetic gas. (A paramagnetic gas moves weakly in a strong magnetic field.) This property is used in most modern gas monitors and results in a rapidly reacting oxygen analyser.

A POLAROGRAPHIC CELL

(as in blood gas analysers)

MEASUREMENT OF HAEMOGLOBIN SATURATION

Unfortunately, the efficiency of oxygen transfer in the lung is much more variable than that of carbon dioxide and for this reason end-tidal oxygen measurement does not accurately reflect the level of oxygen in the patient's blood. To overcome this problem, pulse oximetry is used.

PULSE OXIMETRY

The pulse oximeter detects changes in the oxygen saturation of haemoglobin. Prior to its development, pulse meters were used but they only measured changes in the volume of an extremity, such as a finger, ear lobe or nose, during and after systole. Near infrared electromagnetic waves are able to pass through the body tissue and are detected by a sensor suitable for that particular wavelength. As the volume of the tissue expands with an influx of blood, more light is absorbed and less light passes through the tissue to the sensor. These changes are displayed as a 'pulse wave' on an oscilloscope. The method is known as *pulse plethysmography* and the principle is also used to produce the trace in modern pulse oximeters.

Oxygenated haemoglobin (HbO_2) is redder than deoxygenated haemoglobin (Hb), which is somewhat bluer, and the colour difference between arterial and venous blood is usually obvious. The electromagnetic absorption spectra for HbO_2 and Hb are different, except at a frequency of 660 nm where they are the same. A pulse oximeter placed on a finger, toe, ear lobe or nose transmits alternate beams of infrared light (with wavelengths of 660 nm and 940 nm respectively, the cycle time of which is about 1 kHz) through the tissue. The tissues, including the blood vessels, absorb some of this light energy and a semiconductor sensor detects the remainder as it emerges from the body. Because the absorption spectrum for HbO_2 and Hb is the same at 660 nm, this frequency may be used as a reference point, representing background tissue absorption.

Thus, by comparing the absorption at this frequency with that at 940 nm, electronically eliminating the background activity and incorporating a complex algorithm, the oximeter is able to detect changes in the colour of the pulsatile element of the tissue due to the variation in haemoglobin oxygen saturation. The results are averaged out over a few seconds.

There are, however, problems associated with the use of oximeters. Pulse oximeters are accurate to about ± 2% but sometimes there is a delay between a change in the saturation and its detection. This is usually because of alterations in blood volume or cardiac rhythm. It is important to remember that desaturation is the final common path of many hypoxic disasters. Pulse oximetry is not an acceptable early warning tool and cannot replace the monitoring of anaesthetic gases. In addition, under- and overreading may occur in small infants and specially designed paediatric probes should be used for these patients. Excessive light or electrical interference may also make these devices inaccurate.

Because the display is based on the normal haemoglobin curve, oximeters are unable to detect abnormal haemoglobins. The most important of these is carboxyhaemoglobin (HbCO) and for every 1% of HbCO present the oximeter will overread by about 1%. The use of oximeters in patients who may have been exposed to carbon monoxide is negligent practice. Co-oximeters that sample several different absorption spectra should be used in these patients. Some dyes used in diagnostic procedures, including indocyanine green and methylene blue, have a short but dramatic effect on the accuracy of oximeters. Coloured nail polishes have also been reported to interfere with pulse oximetry.

Oximeters cannot distinguish between pulsatile veins and arteries and may therefore underread in patients with tricuspid incompetence. Poor positioning of the probe and excessive movement are common causes of malfunction but because pulse oximetry relies on a good pulse wave, artefacts may also occur in patients who are hypotensive or who have a poor peripheral circulation.

Patients undergoing magnetic resonance imaging and nuclear magnetic spectroscopy are at risk because all metal objects must be removed from the operative field. Special apparatus using optical fibres to transmit the electrical information has been designed to overcome this problem.

RESPIRATION, HYDROGEN ION CONCENTRATION AND RESPIRATORY GASES

Animals need a constant supply of oxygen for cellular metabolism and enzymes involved in metabolism only function within a very narrow range of hydrogen ion concentration (pH). Because pH is intimately related to carbon dioxide levels, the partial pressure of carbon dioxide (PCO_2) in the blood must also be strictly controlled. This is regulated by changes in the depth and rate of breathing. Anaesthesia, surgery and acute illness all potentially change respiratory gas exchange and acid–base balance and for this reason, in recent years companies have invested large amounts of money in the development of blood gas monitors.

REGULATION OF BODY HYDROGEN ION CONCENTRATION

For convenience, hydrogen ion concentration, unlike other ions, is usually expressed on a logarithmic scale. This is known as pH and is defined as the negative logarithm of the hydrogen ion concentration. This arrangement serves to make the very small values involved into more convenient numbers. Thus, 10^{-6} M (10^{-6} mole/litre) becomes a pH of 6, 10^{-7} M becomes a pH of 7 and 10^{-8} M becomes a pH of 8.

Acids in solution in water dissociate and yield hydrogen ions:

$$acid \leftrightarrow base + H^+$$

For example, hydrochloric acid (HCl) dissociates into hydrogen ions and chloride ions thus:

$$HCl \leftrightarrow H^+ + Cl^-$$

The free hydrogen ion concentration in any acid solution is determined according to the following formula:

$$pH = pKa + \log (base/acid)$$

Where pKa is a measure of the 'acidity' of that particular acid–base pair.

The main acid–base system in the body is the carbon dioxide/bicarbonate system. Acid carbon dioxide reacts with water to produce carbonic acid and this dissociates reversibly into hydrogen and bicarbonate ions thus:

$$CO_2 + H_2O \leftrightarrow H_2CO_3 \leftrightarrow HCO_3^- + H^+$$

So the formula for body pH becomes:

$$pH = pKa + \log (HCO_3^-/k \star CO_2),$$

where k is a constant, the value of which depends on the units used.

The pH of the body is therefore controlled both by respiratory factors (the level of carbon dioxide) and by metabolic factors (the body's production and the kidney's excretion of acidic and basic molecules, which effectively determine the HCO_3 ion concentration). Acid–base disturbances are referred to as metabolic or respiratory according to the original cause and acidosis or alkalosis according to the direction of the disturbance. The body attempts to correct metabolic disturbances by respiratory changes and vice versa. For example, a patient with diabetic acidosis (a metabolic problem) will hyperventilate to decrease the partial pressure of carbon dioxide in the blood in order to compensate for the acidosis. Similarly, the kidneys of a patient with chronic lung disease (who persistently hypoventilates, resulting in a respiratory acidosis) will retain bicarbonate (HCO_3^-) ions to produce a compensatory metabolic alkalosis. Therefore, a knowledge of both the pH and carbon dioxide level of the blood is necessary to interpret the body's acid–base status.

MEASUREMENT OF pH, CO_2 AND O_2 IN BLOOD

Usually pH, $PaCO_2$ and PaO_2 are all determined from a single arterial blood sample using an automated blood gas analyser. The analysis is usually performed by an end user as the machines are pretty 'foolproof' and the results are often needed with minimal delay. Modern blood gas machines often include the ability to measure blood electrolytes, such as sodium, potassium, calcium and magnesium.

An ion-specific electrode (in effect a small cell, similar to those found in alkaline batteries) is used to measure pH. The cell generates an EMF (electromotive force or 'voltage') in proportion to hydrogen ion concentration. $PaCO_2$ is measured by a similar electrode, which is immersed in a bicarbonate buffer solution. This effectively measures the $PaCO_2$ as hydrogen ion concentration.

A polarographic cell is used for the measurement of PaO_2 and incorporates an electrode system the resistance of which varies with oxygen concentration. The cell is energized to 0.6 V and the oxygen to which the cell is exposed takes part in a chemical reaction so that the current flowing is proportional to the oxygen concentration.

Within the blood gas analyser all these electrodes (and any other ion-specific electrodes) are exposed to a common channel along which the blood sample is sucked. The small size of this channel means that less than 0.5 ml of blood is needed but the blood is prone to clot within the machine unless it is heparinized.

RECOMMENDED READING

Moyle JTB, Davey A 1998, Ward's Anaesthetic Equipment 4th edn. WB Saunders, London.

11

SCIENTIFIC PRINCIPLES IN RELATION TO ENDOSCOPIC, LASER AND RADIOLOGICAL EQUIPMENT

G. Grice

INTRODUCTION

Endoscopes, lasers and radiological equipment all utilize the harnessing and manipulation of the physical properties of the electromagnetic spectrum, especially light. Although they have become commonplace in operating theatres, the rapid development of technology in the latter part of this century has greatly increased the scope of surgical practice. Most of this technology has been developed in other fields and then adapted for medical use later. In practice, the application of such technology greatly improves surgical technique and allows much more information to be gathered and utilized by the operation of ever more sophisticated hardware. The rapid increase in its use has not only had the benefit of safer and more successful surgery but has also expanded the range of procedures available. A more recent consideration is the trend towards less invasive and non-invasive surgery where such technology, although initially very expensive, can greatly benefit patients by involving them in less trauma and thus decreasing the time spent in hospital. This also reduces the cost of treatment.

THE ELECTROMAGNETIC SPECTRUM

Having briefly placed these particular tools into context as far as their use in surgery is concerned, we can now examine the underlying scientific and technological principles involved in their use.

To fully appreciate the fundamentals of the electromagnetic spectrum we must understand a little about particle physics, quantum theory and the theory of special relativity. Although the in-depth examination of these subjects is essential to the pure physicist it can be a little daunting to those of us who merely use the technology. However, if we are to understand how these tools work it is first important to examine the behaviour and characteristics of light. Light is the medium by which visual information about the universe is transmitted via the eye to the brain. This is what we all know and experience as visual light but it occupies only a small area within the spectrum of electromagnetic energy (Fig. 11.1).

The primary source of electromagnetic energy is radiation that is emitted from the sun and the stars as a product of nuclear fusion. This process is essentially the conversion of matter into energy, due to the reaction and fusion of the nuclei of predominantly hydrogen atoms. The energy released in such reactions is enormous and fundamentally supports the biological life on our planet. Developments this century have

enabled man to duplicate the release of nuclear energy for both constructive and destructive ends.

Other sources of electromagnetic radiation mainly involve the electronic forces surrounding the nucleus of an atom. An example of the production of radiation is the chemical reaction of burning material, which produces a flame, or the passing of an electric current through a narrow metal filament (electric light bulb). The electromagnetic radiation produced by such sources is the result of the absorption and transmission of energy at the atomic and molecular level of matter, without altering or releasing the huge amounts of energy within the nucleus of the atom. Energy produced in such processes emanates in a random manner from different parts of the electromagnetic spectrum, travelling as waves and identified by its wavelength and frequency (Fig. 11.2). Most of the energy that our bodies sense is broadly heat and light but other parts of the spectrum may be detected, identified and utilized by instruments of technology.

THE ATOM

The smallest packet of electromagnetic energy is called a *photon*. Atoms have a positively charged nucleus orbited by negatively charged electrons, the number of which determines the characteristics of the element. An *element* is the smallest number of atoms that can exist in a stable form by themselves. Thus two atoms of hydrogen form the element hydrogen (H_2) and there is one atom of helium in the element helium (He). In a normal state the charge on the nucleus of an atom is balanced by the electron charge and this is called the *ground state*. When the electrons are allowed to absorb electromagnetic energy (photons) they jump to a higher orbit, said to be the *excited state*. The atom then returns to its ground state and during the process spontaneously and randomly emits photons. In this way, it can be said that photons are transmitted as messenger packets of energy (Fig. 11.3).

THE TRANSMISSION OF ELECTROMAGNETIC RADIATION

As previously stated, electromagnetic energy is transmitted in waves and its wavelength and frequency identify the type of radiation. Wavelength is measured in *nanometres* (0.000,000,001 m or one thousand millionth of a metre) and the frequency is measured in hertz (Hz) or cycles per second. The speed or velocity at which a wave is transmitted is a product of the wavelength and the frequency, so that if wavelength increases, its frequency decreases and vice versa.

ELECTROMAGNETIC SPECTRUM

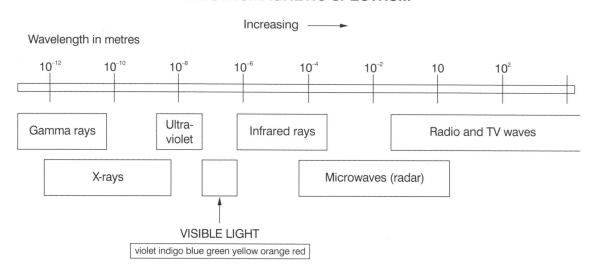

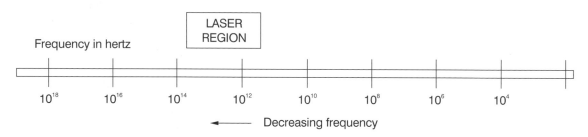

Figure 11.1   The electromagnetic spectrum.

The characteristics of a wave are dependent on the source and the medium through which it is being transmitted. Electromagnetic energy can travel through a vacuum (space) at a constant velocity of 186,282 miles per second, i.e. the speed of light. When it encounters matter (the atmosphere or water), which can absorb

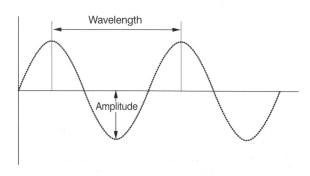

Figure 11.2   Characteristics of the electromagnetic waveform.

some or all of the energy, it is transmitted in the form of waves. The characteristics of these waves will then be dependent on the type of matter through which they are travelling, i.e. gas, liquid or solid. Electromagnetic wavelengths will only transmit through certain mediums, i.e. X-rays will transmit through flesh and bone but not lead, while visual light will transmit through glass but not a brick wall. The behaviour and interaction of light is thus a complex affair but there are some physical laws and properties that can be applied. Wave transmission can be reflected, refracted or diffracted and can exhibit interference.

REFLECTION

Light originates from primary sources such as the sun, a burning flame or a light bulb, which we visualize directly. It also reflects off surfaces, enabling us to see the object in question. Reflection of light (Fig. 11.4) depends on the type and surface of an object. Smooth, flat, polished surfaces reflect parallel rays of light which

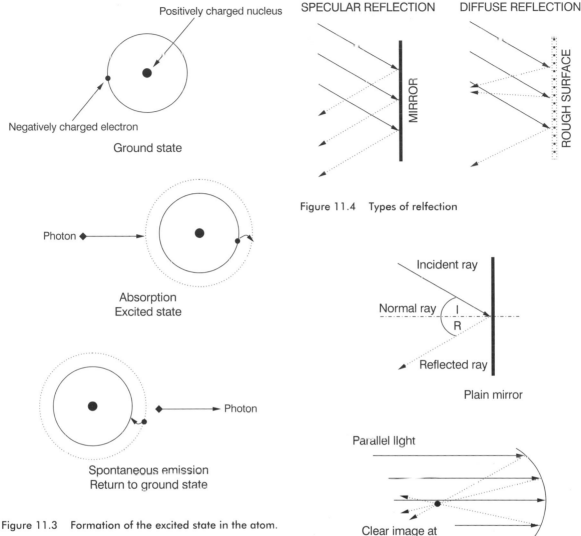

Figure 11.3   Formation of the excited state in the atom.

Figure 11.4   Types of relfection

Figure 11.5   Light reflection from a mirror

remain parallel (*specular reflection*) while rough, uneven surfaces reflect parallel rays in different directions (*diffuse reflection*). A flat, polished surface, i.e. a mirror, reflects light in a uniform way and demonstrates the laws of reflected light (Fig. 11.5), which are

1. The incident ray, the reflected ray and the normal ray are all in the same plane.
2. The angle of incidence is equal to the angle of reflection (i = r).

A ray of light will reflect in the same way from a curved mirror, except that for each ray the norms will be different. Parallel light from a distant object will produce a clear image at the focal length of a concave curved mirror (Fig. 11.5). In this way images can be manipulated by reflecting rays of light from different shaped mirrors.

REFRACTION

Light waves passing from one medium to another, e.g. from air to water or glass, change direction (bend) and this is called refraction (Fig. 11.6). Refraction is caused by a change in speed of the transmission of light while the angle of refraction is dependent on the medium. The latter is constant for a particular substance and is known as the *refractive index*. This property of light is the basis for manipulating images through lenses and is used in the production of optical devices.

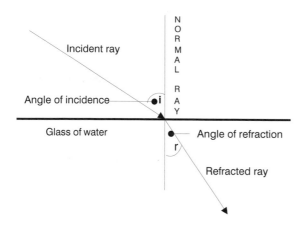

Figure 11.6   Refraction

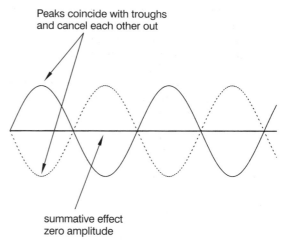

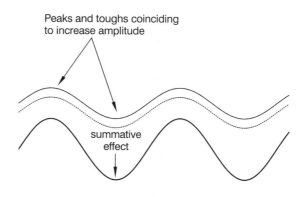

Figure 11.7   Interference (Courtesy of Dr Paul Atherton)

DIFFRACTION

Light diffracts when passing through a small aperture. It bends and becomes diffuse, producing an image that has light and dark rings surrounding it (the so-called Newton's rings). The reader should consult a standard physics textbook for a more detailed description.

INTERFERENCE

Electromagnetic waves are capable of interfering with each other. If two waves are 'in phase' their troughs and peaks coincide with each other, the wave energy summates and the amplitude of the combined wave is increased. If two waves are 'out of phase' they tend to cancel each other out and there is a decrease in overall amplitude. If two identical waves are exactly out of phase the resulting amplitude will be zero. This is illustrated in Fig. 11.7.

Having examined the fundamental properties of electromagnetic waves we should be able to understand how these properties are utilized in our technological instruments.

ENDOSCOPES

The basic principles underlying the use of endoscopes involve the science of optics, which started with the invention of the telescope. Light is used to illuminate the object to be viewed, thus allowing it to be seen and interpreted by the human brain. Optical lenses are used to manipulate the returning light in order to produce an enhanced and clearly focused image of that object. Endoscopes may be classified as rigid or flexible.

RIGID ENDOSCOPES

Rigid endoscopes vary from simple metal tubes with a light source at the distal end to operating telescopes that can enlarge, reduce or bend the image and are used to perform complex surgical procedures in enclosed areas of the body. The anatomy and position of the internal organ or bodily orifice that is to be examined will determine the design of the simple endoscope. Examples include the oesophagoscope, sigmoidoscope and laryngoscope. These instruments are used for examination under direct vision and the field of vision is limited to the area immediately in front of the end of the endoscope. They have changed very little over the years except for the way that the light, originating from an electric lamp, is delivered to the subject. Until relatively recently, a "light carrier" consisted of a metal tube with an internal wire connected to a bulb at the distal end of the carrier. The carrier would be inserted down the endoscope, illuminating the area immediately around the light source, which became hot with use. The power source was either a battery or transformed mains current. Today, almost universally, light carriers consist of optical fibres through which light is transported and which deliver a cold, more powerful, reliable and even illumination.

Fibreoptic transmission of light is dependent on the phenomenon of *total internal reflection*. Light reaching a glass–air or similar interface will either be refracted or internally reflected. If the light strikes the glass–air junction at an angle greater than 42° it will be totally reflected (Fig. 11.8). Optical fibres are long strands of glass bundled together to produce a fibreoptic cable. All the strands transmit light because as the light travels along the glass fibre the rays strike the surface at an angle greater than the critical angle of 42°. The rays are therefore reflected totally, cannot escape through refraction and remain within the glass fibre. Thus the light travelling along these cables not only illuminates the object but can be used to transmit all kinds of images as information.

More sophisticated rigid endoscopes such as arthroscopes and laparoscopes are inserted surgically into joints and cavities, producing an enhanced image using lenses and prisms. The image may be viewed directly through the endoscope or displayed via a small camera onto a television screen. This particular development has facilitated so-called "keyhole surgery", which is far less invasive and the ability to televise such procedures greatly enhances the teaching of this surgical technique.

FLEXIBLE ENDOSCOPES

Flexible endoscopes, as the name suggests, can bend and flex within the orifices, lumina and tracts of the body. The main difference is that the flexible endoscope has the ability to transmit an image as well as light along optical fibres, thus enabling the tube to bend considerably without compromising the performance of the instrument. (This also permits a much more thorough examination with less chance of missing pathology.) Flexible endoscopes may be linked to television and recording equipment, enabling review and of course opportunities for teaching. They can be much longer than rigid endoscopes and are fitted with channels for suction, blowing, irrigation and biopsy depending on the type of endoscope. The advent of flexible endoscopes has enabled the use of some types of laser, transmitted down the optical fibres, especially in the field of gastrointestinal treatment when bleeding can be accu-

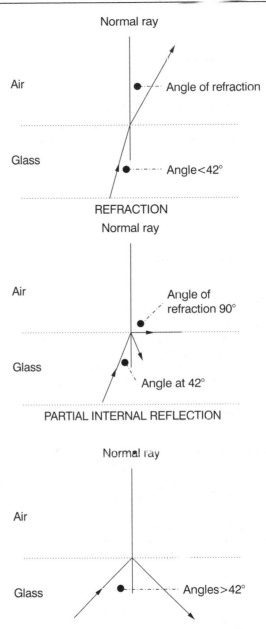

Figure 11.8   Fibreoptic transmission of light.

rately and safely coagulated within the alimentary tract.

THE LASER

Laser is an acronym for **L**ight **A**mplification by **S**timulated **E**mission of **R**adiation and to understand how it works, we must look at each component.

LIGHT

The light in a laser is that part of the electromagnetic spectrum that extends from the near infrared to the near ultraviolet and includes visible light (see Fig.11.1).

STIMULATED EMISSION

In the normal course of events atoms spontaneously emit photons when absorbing energy such as light or heat (see Fig. 11.3). With stimulated emission, specific atoms such as carbon dioxide (the *lasing medium*) are pumped by a high-energy source so that more of the atom's electrons are in a higher orbit (Fig. 11.9) and this is called *population inversion*. More atoms will then return to a ground state and will emit more photons that collide with other photons, causing a stimulated chain reaction. The outcome is an emission of photons of identical wavelength producing monochromatic light. Because all the wave fronts are in phase (coherent), the beam remains parallel (*collimated* or in the same direction) and concentrated over long distances. Control and focusing are relatively easy to achieve using mirrors or, in most cases, fibreoptics.

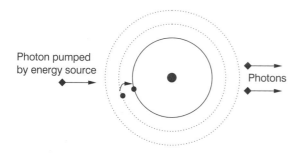

Figure 11.9   Stimulated emission

AMPLIFICATION

Amplification takes place within the tube containing the lasing medium (the *resonating tube* or *optical cavity*). Mirrors are placed at each end of the tube so that photons reflect back and forth through the lasing medium, stimulating more atoms to release more photons, thus amplifying the effect (Fig. 11.10). One of the mirrors allows a beam of laser light to escape from the tube and this is delivered via optical devices (mirrors, fibreoptics) to the objective.

RADIATION

Radiation refers to that part of the electromagnetic spectrum (near infrared to near ultraviolet) that produces a laser beam, which can be used to vaporize tissue accurately and precisely. The wavelength and type of beam produced are dependent on the medium used and this medium can vary from gases, such as carbon dioxide and helium/neon, to a liquid dye or a solid such as ruby. Each medium produces a different wavelength of light that has different properties and uses in surgery.

The *carbon dioxide laser* produces a powerful (40 watts output) invisible infrared beam, focusing on a small area (0.9–1.7 mm) and is useful for vaporizing tissue cells in surface lesions. Penetration is minimal due to the wavelength of light being readily absorbed by water, which is the main constituent of the cells. This laser is ideal for the bloodless excision of small lesions when minimal damage to surrounding and underlying tissue is required. The only drawback is that currently the beam cannot be transported through fibreoptic cables and can only be used in direct line of sight, transported by a cumbersome articulated arm. Carbon dioxide lasers are mainly used in ENT, maxillofacial surgery inside the mouth and in gynaecological surgery for surface ablation of the cervix.

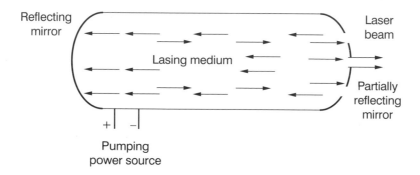

Figure 11.10   Resonating tube

The *argon laser* produces a visible blue/green light and is most suitable for coagulation, due to the wavelength being readily absorbed by the haemoglobin in red blood cells. Because the beam will travel through the lens and body of the eye without damaging them, it is ideal for targeting the blood vessels and tissue of the retina. Argon lasers are widely used in the treatment of diabetic retinopathy. An argon laser beam can be transmitted by way of flexible fibreoptics and produces a beam with a spot size of 50–100 micrometers, but with a smaller power output of 5 watts. Argon lasers are also used to photocoagulate gastrointestinal bleeding by introducing the fibreoptic cable down a flexible gastroscope. A power output of up to 20 watts is available for this purpose.

The *dye laser* produces laser light across the spectrum of visible light by simply changing to a different dye and this allows it to be tuned to the required wavelength. The only drawback is that the power output is relatively low (10 watts). Because the blood vessels within the skin are selectively destroyed without undue surface scarring, it is most useful in the photocoagulation of skin blemishes such as port-wine stains.

The *Nd-YAG laser* is the only common surgical laser using a solid medium. This consists of a crystal rod composed of yttrium, aluminium and garnet infiltrated with neodymium. The energy used to stimulate the laser light is usually provided by a krypton arc lamp. It is the most powerful surgical laser (up to 100 watts) and its wavelength is in the near infrared. The beam can be transmitted by fibreoptic cable and a low-power helium/neon laser aiming beam of visible light is also transmitted along the same fibres. Carbon dioxide lasers use the same guidance system. This wavelength is deeply absorbed in tissue without being colour specific. At a higher power level, the absorption is over a larger area at a lower temperature and it can therefore be used to treat larger areas without causing damage to underlying or surrounding tissue. This laser is less precise than the carbon dioxide laser but can be used in a wider range of surgical procedures such as cataract removal, debulking brain tumours and destroying renal and gall stones. The laser may also be used via an endoscope.

HEALTH AND SAFETY

Because lasers emit potentially harmful radiation, their use is limited to authorized and approved personnel who have undertaken a special training course. Each hospital must produce local rules for the safe use of lasers and a copy of these rules must not only be kept in the theatre office but also must be attached to the laser in question. As an illustration, the following should be included in any rules written for the use of the SLT CLMD YAG laser.

Hazards

The red aiming beam does not present a hazard except in the case of prolonged exposure. Staff should not stare into the beam; the normal blink reflex will keep the exposure of any accidental exposure to a safe minimum.

The invisible radiation beam produced by the YAG laser is much more powerful and hazards associated with it are as follows:

The eye is the critical organ for damage. Radiation at this wavelength (1064 nm) is mainly absorbed at the retina and can cause damage leading to impaired vision.

Hazards to the skin (particularly uncovered areas of skin) range from various photochemical effects to severe burns.

Fire, emission of toxic gases and explosion may result if unsuitable materials are exposed to the beam. Examples include drapes, clothing, plastic instruments and tubing, flammable anaesthetics and skin preparations.

Reflective surfaces may redirect the beam along unexpected paths and reflective curved surfaces may refocus this beam, thus causing hazardous conditions outside the normal beam path.

Administrative precautions

The employer is ultimately responsible for all protection measures and for the protection of all workers (whether or not they are employed by the trust), patients and members of the public on their premises.

In consultation with the Head of Department and the Laser Protection Adviser (by law each geographical area must have a Laser Protection Adviser), the Trust must appoint a Laser Safety Officer from amongst the staff regularly working with the particular laser. Appointments and terminations of employment must be in writing.

The Head of Department is responsible for ensuring that the safety measures recommended in the rules are implemented but the Laser Safety Officer has a direct responsibility for:

1. The safe custody of the key to operate the laser.
2. The register of authorized operators.

3. Ensuring that the safety measures laid down in the local rules are carried out at all times.

The Laser Safety Officer may obtain assistance and advice from the Laser Protection Adviser at any time but must seek this advice if there are major changes to the laser or the working conditions.

The names of the authorized operators must be kept in a register and these individuals must satisfy themselves that all those present, including visitors, are fully aware of the hazards and precautions to be followed. They must also sign the register to indicate that they have read and understood the local rules.

The laser may only be used in an area approved by the Laser Protection Adviser and the Laser Safety Officer. This laser controlled area must have warning lights at each entrance and no person should be in the room during use unless their presence is required.

If there is any suspected overexposure to the main therapeutic beam, the Head of Department must request the Laser Protection Officer to investigate the circumstances. Any recommendations will be included in the subsequent report. If the eyes were affected, an immediate ophthalmic examination must be arranged.

Equipment design

All medical lasers must incorporate a number of safety features. The local rules should have an appendix listing the safety features and their operation and all operators must be familiar with these features.

If there is any possibility of exposing tubes containing oxygen, nitrous oxide or other oxidizing anaesthetic agents to the beam, they must be protected by wrapping them with aluminium tape or by using specially designed tubes with a metallic surround. Extreme care must be taken to avoid the risk of ignition of flammable materials.

Personal protection

Unless appropriate filters are included in the viewing optics, any person viewing the procedure via an endoscope must wear safety glasses at all times while the laser is in READY mode.

If the beam is not completely enclosed within the patient or the external power meter, it is essential that all staff in the laser controlled area wear appropriate safety glasses while the laser is in READY mode. The patient must wear protective glasses if there is any possibility of eye exposure from the laser. Protective glasses must be marked with their optical density at the relevant wavelengths and provide adequate protection from brief exposure but are not designed to protect from prolonged exposure. Protective glasses designed for use with other types of laser are not suitable and MUST NOT be used.

Operating procedures

1. Check that all entrance doors are either bolted or fitted with suitable warning signs. Check that the warning lights outside the main doors are illuminated.
2. Carry out the 'switch on' procedure according to the manufacturer's instructions and calibrate the fibre.
3. Verify that the red aiming beam is present. If it is not, treatment MUST NOT PROCEED.
4. Check that all present are wearing protective glasses as necessary. Check that any suction or smoke evacuation equipment is working.
5. Set the desired power level and exposure time and ensure that the fibre is correctly positioned. Select READY, announce that the treatment is about to begin and proceed, using the footswitch.
6. During any pause in treatment, STANDBY must be pressed to disable the footswitch.
7. When the treatment is completed switch OFF with the key before removing the fibre or endoscope.
8. At the end of the session the key must be removed and returned immediately to the custody of the Laser Safety Officer.

RADIOLOGICAL EQUIPMENT

X-RAYS

X-rays are invisible, are situated at the shorter wavelength end of the electromagnetic spectrum (see Fig. 11.1) and are produced by accelerating electrons in an X-ray tube (Fig. 11.11). The electrons are induced to accelerate through the high vacuum tube by heating a metal filament (the cathode) with a very high voltage (30–100 Kv). Electrons, forced from the metal atoms by the high voltage, are focused into a beam that is aimed towards a target, the anode, which is a high melting point metal such as tungsten. Ninety-nine per cent of the electron beam's energy produces heat, which is dissipated by pumping oil through a copper rod containing the target metal. The remaining energy is emitted as X-rays through a window in the lead-lined tube. X-rays thus produced are penetrating

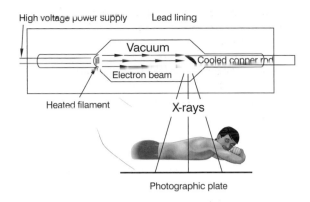

Figure 11.11   X-ray tube.

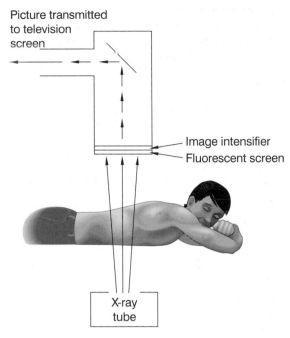

Figure 11.12   The image intensifier.

electromagnetic radiation that is absorbed by matter at differing rates depending on the density of that matter. The X-ray tube is lead lined because the X-ray radiation is unable to penetrate this medium.

Use of X-rays

X-rays are mainly used within the operating theatre as a diagnostic tool but also have a therapeutic use in the treatment of cancer. The penetrating power of X-rays is dependent upon the input voltage, so the shorter wavelengths can be used to destroy cancer cells while longer wavelengths are used for diagnostic purposes.

X-rays react with a photographic film in much the same way that light does and, after passing through the body tissue, produce a contrasting picture on a photographic plate. The production of this shadowy picture of the structures inside the body is possible because body tissues absorb electromagnetic energy at different rates.

The most common piece of equipment that utilizes X-rays in the operating theatre is the image intensifier (Fig. 11.12). Instead of using a photographic plate, the X-rays are passed through a screen coated with zinc sulphide, causing it to produce fluorescence. This screen converts the shorter wavelength X-rays into longer wavelength visible radiation, thus allowing us to actually see a picture, which is then transmitted onto a television screen.

The advantages of this system are the convenience of 'real-time' viewing together with the lower level of radiation that is needed. Image intensifiers are used in surgery when information is required before proceeding further but they are also able to take conventional X-ray pictures.

HEALTH AND SAFETY

All X-rays are dangerous and must therefore be strictly controlled and monitored when radiological equipment is in use.

Administrative precautions

The administrative arrangements are exactly the same as described for the laser and include a Radiation Protection Adviser and a Radiation Protection Supervisor. Ultimate responsibility lies with the Chief Executive of the Trust, through the Clinical Director of Radiology.

All clinicians who direct medical exposure to ionizing radiation must receive adequate training under the Protection of Persons Undergoing Medical Examination or Treatment 1998 regulations. Everyone who is potentially exposed to ionizing radiation must also wear a radiation-monitoring device under their protective clothing.

Radiation protection within the operating theatre

The local rules are very extensive and cover working within and outside the X-ray department. This chapter will therefore only give a summary of the rules involving the use of X-rays within the operating theatre.

1. X-ray equipment must only be operated by a radiographer and directed by an appropriately trained clinician.
2. All doors leading to the X-ray area must have a warning notice stating that X-rays are in use.
3. A controlled area will exist for 2 metres around the irradiated area of the patient and the X-ray tube, together with everywhere that is in direct line of the primary beam or is designated by the radiographer.
4. Only essential staff will remain in this controlled area when X-ray equipment is in use.
5. Any member of staff who is, or suspects that she is, pregnant must wear a lead rubber apron at all times when X-rays are in use and MUST NOT be within the controlled area during X-ray exposure.
6. The patient's reproductive organs should be shielded from radiation.
7. All staff within the controlled area must wear a full-size lead rubber gown and other protection as deemed appropriate, e.g. thyroid protector and lead glasses, and a radiation-monitoring badge, which should be worn on the front of the trunk at waist level beneath the lead gown.
8. If a person needs to hold any part of the patient they must also wear lead lined rubber gloves.
9. All other staff should leave the controlled area and stand behind a lead-lined protective screen during exposure. This screen must be at least 2 metres from the irradiated area and out of direct line of the primary beam.
10. Because the radiation protection badges are used by more than one surgeon, anaesthetist, scrub person, etc., a register must be kept of the users on each occasion.
11. The radiation protection badges are checked monthly by the Radiation Protection Officer.

In summary, electromagnetic radiation is a most useful medical tool but, because the radiation is potentially dangerous, it must be used within strictly controlled safety guidelines.

RECOMMENDED READING

Local rules for the safe use of lasers.

Local rules for radiation safety in diagnostic radiology.

12

PHARMACOLOGICAL PRINCIPLES OF DRUG ADMINISTRATION

E. Whelan

WHAT ARE DRUGS?

A drug is a chemical agent introduced into the body with the aim of producing some form of biological response. Such agents may vary in size and complexity, from small molecules consisting of a few atoms to very large complicated molecular structures. Some drugs, such as antibiotics, are given with the intention of curing a particular disease process while others may act to prevent the complications of a disease, as in the case of antihypertensive agents used in the treatment of high blood pressure. It is also possible for drugs to relieve the symptoms of a disease without affecting the disease process itself, as is seen in the treatment of pain with analgesics. Finally, in some cases, the drug is given as a replacement for a deficiency of an agent that is produced naturally in the body as occurs, for example, in the use of insulin to treat diabetes mellitus.

Although there are numerous classes of drugs with many modes of action it is possible to consider two broad ways in which drugs may affect the body's biological responses. First some drugs act by enhancing, facilitating or increasing a normal biological function. An example is digoxin, a drug used to increase the force with which cardiac muscle contracts in patients with heart failure. In contrast, many drugs work by blocking or inhibiting normal biological functions. Thus, local anaesthetic agents act by blocking the transmission of impulses along nerve cells.

HOW DO DRUGS WORK?

There are three main ways by which drugs act in the body to produce biological changes. First, they can act by binding to receptors. Second, they may inhibit the action of enzymes and, finally, they may block the passage of ions across cell membranes. Most drugs act by one of these three mechanisms.

WHAT ARE RECEPTORS?

Receptors are complex protein molecules located in cell membranes. When a drug molecule binds to a receptor, a *drug–receptor complex* is formed. This process of binding and complex formation stimulates a series of biochemical reactions within the cell and these reactions culminate with the production of the desired effect (Figure 12.1). For example, adrenaline binds to receptors on the membranes of smooth muscle cells, which are found in the walls of small blood vessels. The biochemical changes produced in the cell as a result of this binding produce contraction of the muscle cell. Drugs binding to receptors in this manner,

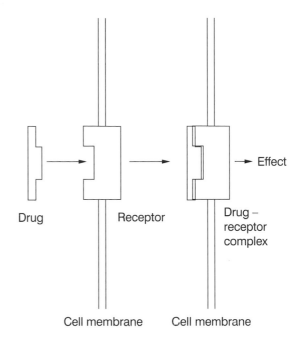

Figure 12.1   The drug–receptor complex.

producing a positive effect, are called *agonists*. There is an alternative means of drug binding to receptors to produce a biological effect and these drugs, called *antagonists*, bind to cell receptors but do not produce any changes within the cell as a result. Other agonist drugs, however, cannot bind to the receptor while the antagonist drug is bound to it and the antagonist thus acts to block the action of an agonist which is already present (Figure 12.2). The most commonly seen example of this is the action of neuromuscular blocking agents such as atracurium. Atracurium binds to receptors on the membrane of skeletal muscle cells but does not produce contraction. Acetylcholine molecules, which are released from nerve endings, cannot bind to the receptors and thus cannot cause the muscle cell to contract. Atracurium in this way blocks the agonist action of acetylcholine.

HOW DO SOME DRUGS ACT ON ENZYMES?

Enzymes are protein molecules that act as catalysts for specific biochemical reactions: that is, substance A may be changed into substances B and C by the action of an enzyme without the enzyme undergoing any change itself. The speed of the reaction, in this case $A \rightarrow B + C$, is changed by the activity of the enzyme but the reaction would take place even if the enzyme were absent. Many of the body's important biochemical

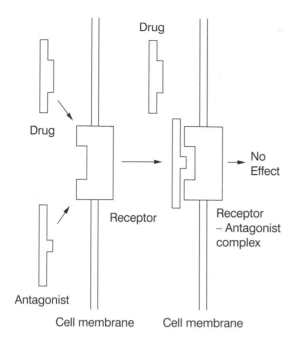

Figure 12.2   How the antagonist blocks the action of the agonist.

pathways are controlled by the action of a series of enzymes. Some drugs exert their effect by inhibiting the action of one or more enzymes in a particular biochemical pathway and thus prevent the formation of the end products of the pathway. For example, aspirin produces its analgesic effect by inhibiting the action of the enzyme prostaglandin synthetase. This action reduces the production and release of the prostaglandin molecules that produce painful sensations. Similarly, neostigmine inhibits the action of the enzyme acetylcholinesterase, which is responsible for the breakdown of acetylcholine. Inhibiting the enzyme causes an accumulation of acetylcholine molecules that can then overcome the effects of a neuromuscular blocking agent.

HOW DO DRUGS ACT ON MEMBRANE IONIC CHANNELS?

Some specialized cells, e.g. peripheral nerves, function by transmitting a mild electrical impulse down the body of the cell, which then causes the release of transmitter molecules from the end of the cell. This electrical impulse is generated by the passage of ions (charged particles) in both directions across the cell membrane and specific channels exist in the membrane to allow the passage of such ions. Some drugs act by blocking these *ion channels*, thus preventing

the generation of an electrical impulse. Local anaesthetic agents work in this way, as will be explained in Chapter 14.

HOW DO DRUGS ENTER THE BODY?

The process by which drugs enter the body is referred to as *absorption*. There are several routes of absorption commonly used in operating theatre practice. The basis of most routes, however, is the introduction of a drug into a particular region of the body. This drug is then absorbed into blood as it flows through this area. In this way the drug enters the general circulation and is distributed throughout the body.

The *oral* route is used for the administration of many drugs with absorption occurring across the mucosal surfaces of the stomach and small intestine and hence into the circulation supplying these structures. Some drugs do not readily cross these mucosal surfaces and are therefore poorly absorbed via this route. Changes in gastric emptying rates, other substances already present in the stomach and diseases of the stomach and intestines may also limit absorption. In such situations an alternative route should be used.

Some drugs can be given via the *rectal* route, which may be adopted if the oral route cannot be used or if it is necessary to avoid the passage of the drug through the liver before entering the general circulation.

The *intravenous* route is most commonly used in anaesthetic practice, the drug being injected directly into a vein and thus immediately entering the circulation. The onset of drug action occurs rapidly, as can be seen from the swift effect of an intravenous bolus injection of an anaesthetic agent such as thiopentone. Other drugs may be given slowly, often over a period of many hours, as an infusion via the intravenous route. Narcotic analgesics may be given in this way to provide lasting analgesia during the postoperative period.

Drugs given by the *intramuscular* and *subcutaneous* routes are removed from the site of injection by the local blood flow through the site. This results in a slower onset of action than that of the intravenous route, particularly if there is reduced peripheral blood flow as might occur in a cold or shocked patient. These routes are often used as an alternative to the oral route if, as in the case of insulin, the drug will be destroyed in the stomach and intestines before it can be absorbed.

The anaesthetic gases and vapours are given by *inhalation*, with absorption occurring from the pulmonary alveolus into the pulmonary circulation and thence to the general circulation. As a large area of the pulmonary blood flow is exposed to the drug, absorption by this route is relatively rapid and this is utilized in the treatment of asthma using inhalers and nebulizers.

Less commonly used routes include the *epidural* and the *transdermal* routes of absorption. Drugs such as local anaesthetic agents and analgesics are given into the epidural space and act directly on nerves within the space. With the latter route, drugs such as glyceryl trinitrate and hormone replacements are absorbed from the skin into blood vessels directly beneath it.

Absorption may also occur from the mucous membranes as with drugs instilled into the eye and in the sublingual and vaginal routes. The various routes of drug absorption are shown in Figure 12.3.

HOW DO DRUGS REACH THEIR SITES OF ACTION?

Following absorption, drugs are carried around the body in the general circulation from which they enter into the tissues, some of which include their sites of action. This process is generally called *drug distribution*. In most circumstances drugs move between sites by a process of *diffusion*, in which movement is from an area of high drug concentration to an area of lower drug concentration, i.e. down a concentration gradient. Movement continues down this gradient until the concentrations are equal at both sites and equilibrium is reached.

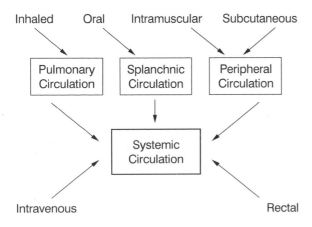

Figure 12.3   Routes of absorption

The initial part of this process involves the distribution of drug throughout the systemic circulation. Blood flow, however, does not occur evenly throughout the body; there are certain organs such as the brain, liver and heart which receive proportionally more blood flow than peripheral tissues such as fat and muscle. The vessel-rich organs are therefore exposed to drug more rapidly than the vessel-poor tissues.

Some drug travels in the circulation dissolved in plasma but in many cases most of the drug travels bound to plasma proteins such as albumin and α-1-glycoprotein. To leave the circulation, such drugs must first be freed from protein binding and then dissolve in plasma. The next step is the diffusion of the drug out of the circulation and into the tissues. To achieve this step, drugs must cross cell membranes, which constitute a barrier to drug diffusion. Such membranes are typically made of complex arrangements of phospholipid molecules and drugs vary in their ability to cross such an obstacle. Drugs that are naturally lipid soluble will cross membranes more readily than those that are water soluble and drugs that are ionized (electrically charged) do not penetrate membranes as easily as those do that are non-ionized. For many drugs the pH (degree of acidity) of the site at which drug is diffusing will alter the degree to which a drug is ionized, since many drugs can exist both as ionized and non-ionized forms. Finally, drugs that are large molecules do not cross membranes as easily as those that are of a smaller size.

IS THERE A SIMPLE WAY OF DESCRIBING THE PROCESS OF DISTRIBUTION?

Yes. In many cases drugs behave as if the body is made up of two or more *compartments*, a two-compartment model being shown in Figure 12.4. Each compartment represents a group of tissues and organs rather than an individual anatomical structure. Drug is introduced into the central compartment, which includes the systemic circulation and vessel-rich organs, and distribution in this compartment thus occurs rapidly. Drug then diffuses down a concentration gradient from the central compartment into the peripheral compartment, which includes the vessel poor group of tissues. Distribution into this compartment therefore occurs more slowly than in the central compartment. Diffusion continues in this direction until the concentrations in both compartments are equal and equilibrium is reached.

Drugs may exert their effects in either or both compartments. For some drugs it is the movement of drug into the peripheral compartment that limits its

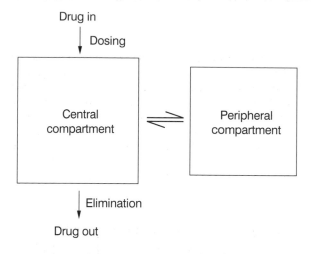

Figure 12.4   The two-compartment model.

effect in the central compartment. For example, thiopentone is rapidly distributed in the central compartment (including the brain), producing high concentrations soon after injection. The distribution of the drug into the peripheral compartment reduces thiopentone concentrations in the central compartment and thus reduces its effect until the patient regains consciousness.

Once equilibrium between the compartments has occurred, drug is removed from the central compartment by processes of *elimination*, which will be described later. This causes the drug concentrations in the central compartment to fall below those in the peripheral compartment and the diffusion process is reversed, with drug now moving from the peripheral compartment into the central compartment, where it is then subjected to elimination processes. This continues until the entire drug is removed from both compartments.

WHAT IS MEANT BY THE PHARMACOKINETICS OF A DRUG?

Pharmacokinetics is the study of the action of the body on the drug. It involves the numerical description of the processes of absorption, distribution, metabolism and elimination of drugs so that the behaviour of different drugs can be compared or the behaviour of a single drug in differing clinical situations can be described.

It is possible to measure the plasma concentration of many drugs. A series of such measurements can thus be made after drug administration showing an initial rise in plasma concentrations followed by declining levels as the drug is distributed and eliminated. A typical plasma concentration–time curve is shown in Figure 12.5. The initial steep decline in concentration is caused by the distribution of drug into the peripheral compartment and the second, more gradual decline in concentration is a result of the processes of elimination. Such data can be analysed mathematically into a set of numerical pharmacokinetic values. The volumes of the central and peripheral compartments can be calculated and are usually referred to as *volumes of distribution*. Such values can indicate the lipid solubility, tissue solubility and protein binding of the drug.

Values for drug *half-life*, which is the time taken for the plasma concentration of the drug to decrease by 50%, can also be derived. As can be seen from the graph the half-life due to processes of distribution is shorter than the half-life due to elimination processes. It is usual, therefore, to describe both distribution and elimination half-lives.

Finally, drug *clearance* can be calculated. This is the volume of fluid, usually plasma, that is completely cleared of drug in a given time period. In general, clearance values reflect the sum of all elimination processes and therefore indicate the rate at which the drug is eliminated from the body. Drugs with high clearance values will be eliminated quickly and those with low values will be eliminated slowly.

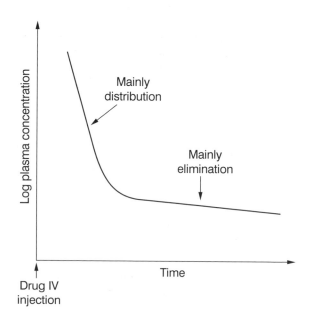

Figure 12.5   Typical plasma concentrattion–time curve.

HOW ARE DRUGS REMOVED FROM THE BODY?

The process by which drugs are removed from the body is collectively referred to as *elimination*. In a small number of cases drugs may remain unaltered by the body and are eliminated via their route of administration. The volatile anaesthetic agents, for example, are almost exclusively eliminated via the respiratory tract without previous modification within the body.

Most drugs, however, are subjected to some form of chemical alteration before elimination. Such changes are generally called processes of *metabolism* and aim to change the structure of drugs to produce a molecule that is easier to eliminate than the parent drug molecule. In particular, drug metabolism aims to convert drugs that are highly lipid soluble into compounds (*metabolites*) that are watersoluble. In most cases drug metabolism also has the effect of reducing or abolishing the biological activity of the parent drug. Sometimes, however, metabolites may have some biological activity and are thus called *active metabolites*.

Most drug metabolism takes place in the liver although some drugs are metabolized in the kidney, gut, lung or plasma. Two types of chemical reactions take place in the liver to metabolize drugs: *Phase 1* and *Phase 2* reactions. Phase 1 reactions are carried out by a specific enzyme system in the liver cell called the cytochrome P-450 system. This enzyme system produces oxidation, reduction or hydrolytic alterations in the drug molecule but does not combine that molecule with others. Phase 2 reactions, in contrast, are achieved by combining the molecule produced by the Phase 1 reaction with another molecule. The resulting larger molecule is more water soluble than the drug molecule and is thus more easily eliminated. This process is called conjugation and is controlled by a second series of liver enzymes. Some drugs bypass Phase 1 reactions completely and are entirely metabolized by Phase 2 reactions.

HOW DO METABOLITES LEAVE THE BODY?

Most metabolites and the few drugs that are not metabolized are eliminated either in urine or bile or in both. In general, larger metabolite molecules tend to be eliminated in bile and smaller molecules in urine. In the kidneys drugs may be eliminated by passive filtration in the renal glomerulus or by active secretion in the proximal renal tubule or by diffusion out of the distal renal tubule. The elimination of drugs in bile is generally less important than that occurring in the kidney and results from the active secretion of metabolite molecules into bile by liver cells. The major pathways of metabolism and elimination are summarized in Figure 12.6.

WILL ALL PATIENTS REACT IN THE SAME WAY TO THE SAME DRUG?

No. There is wide variation in patients' responses to drugs and their absorption, distribution and elimination. Factors such as youth, old age, sex, genetic make-up and pregnancy are all naturally occurring states that may result in an altered drug response. Environmental factors such as tobacco and alcohol usage may also affect such responses, as may the administration of more than one drug simultaneously (drug interaction). Finally cardiac, liver and renal disease may produce complex physiological changes that affect drug action and disposition in such individuals.

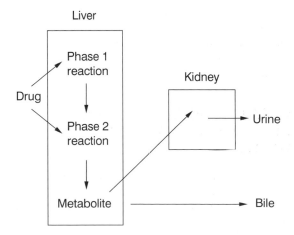

Figure 12.6   Major pathways of metabolism and elimination

13

THE PHARMACOLOGY OF DRUGS USED IN GENERAL ANAESTHESIA

E. Whelan & H. Davies

INTRODUCTION

WHY ARE SO MANY DRUGS INVOLVED IN ANAESTHESIA?

In the early days of the development of anaesthesia, a single anaesthetic agent such as ether or chloroform was used throughout the operation. The agent would be used to both induce and maintain anaesthesia and would be administered in most types of surgery. This situation was complicated by the side effects of the anaesthetic agents, which would be dangerous if large doses were used. As the development of new anaesthetic agents progressed, it became apparent that it was possible to use several agents to provide anaesthesia, thus limiting the dose of any single agent. This *balanced anaesthesia* is based on the use of several agents, each of which is given to achieve a particular component of the desired anaesthetic effect.

WHAT IS THE TRIAD OF ANAESTHESIA?

The concept of a 'triad' of anaesthesia was developed to describe the three basic requirements of an anaesthetic that must be achieved during anaesthesia to ensure a successful outcome. These three conditions are:

1. Hypnosis.
2. Analgesia.
3. Relaxation

and are provided by the use of a 'balanced' combination of anaesthetic and other agents.

Hypnosis is the general term used in this context to describe alterations in the patient's consciousness. In the case of general anaesthesia, this obviously means the patient is rendered unconscious. During operations performed under local anaesthesia, however, a sedative may be given to produce a state of drowsiness and this effect is also included under the general 'hypnosis' part of the triad.

The *analgesia* component of the triad has two related meanings. It refers to the use of drugs and other techniques that ensure the patient recovers with as little pain as possible and also to the suppression of physiological reflexes that occur following surgical stimulation. A penetrating wound, such as a surgical incision, would cause a complex series of physiological responses if made in a conscious subject, including a dramatic increase in heart rate and blood pressure, hyperventilation, sweating and vomiting. The 'analgesia' component of the triad comprises those drugs and manoeuvres designed to limit these physiological responses to surgical stimulation. In many situations, this reflex suppression is achieved by the use of powerful narcotic analgesics.

The '*relaxation*' component of the triad refers to the need for the reduction or elimination of muscle tone, which can be retained even when the patient is deeply unconscious. While this may be of limited importance during some types of surgery, it is especially necessary during intraabdominal and similar surgery and also to assist some anaesthetic procedures, such as endotracheal intubation.

The idea of a 'triad' of anaesthetic components that are integrated into a balanced anaesthetic can be illustrated by the use of some examples. Consider a patient having simple dental extractions under general anaesthesia. Anaesthesia is induced with intravenous thiopentone and the patient then breathes a mixture of nitrous oxide, oxygen and sevoflurane. A paracetamol suppository may also be inserted while the patient is asleep. Thiopentone, sevoflurane and nitrous oxide provide the 'hypnosis' part of this general anaesthetic while nitrous oxide and paracetamol provide the 'analgesia' component. As the need for muscular relaxation is limited in this context, no specific relaxant drugs are given and the 'relaxation' component is supplied by the combination of all the agents used.

In contrast, consider a patient having an appendicectomy. Anaesthesia is induced with intravenous thiopentone and the muscle relaxants, suxamethonium and later atracurium, and the narcotic analgesic alfentanil are also given at this time. The patient's lungs are then ventilated with nitrous oxide, oxygen and a volatile agent, e.g. sevoflurane. At a later stage morphine is given intravenously and the muscle relaxation is reversed at the end of the operation. Further morphine is given during recovery. In this anaesthetic, thiopentone, nitrous oxide and sevoflurane provide the 'hypnosis' component, with a small contribution from the narcotic analgesics. The 'analgesia' component is provided by the alfentanil (a powerful suppressant of reflex responses to traumatic stimuli), the morphine and the nitrous oxide. 'Relaxation' is achieved by the use of the muscle relaxants suxamethonium and atracurium. This example shows how each component of the triad is provided by one or more specific agents and also how some agents may have more than one 'triad' effect.

The final example involves a patient having a leg operation under spinal anaesthesia, in which the activity of the sensory and motor nerves of the lower body is blocked, with intravenous midazolam used to provide some sedation and amnesia during the operation. In this example, the 'analgesia' and 'relaxation' components of the triad are both provided by the spinal anaesthesia, while the 'hypnosis' is supplied by the midazolam. It also shows that the concept of the triad of anaesthesia is not limited to general anaesthetic techniques.

The triad properties of agents commonly used in anaesthesia are shown in Table 13.1.

The major groups of drugs encountered in anaesthetic practice will now be reviewed.

VOLATILE ANAESTHETIC AGENTS AND ANAESTHETIC GASES

ABSORPTION AND ELIMINATION

The volatile anaesthetic agents (halothane, enflurane, isoflurane, sevoflurane and desflurane) and the anaesthetic gas nitrous oxide enter the body via the lungs. Although the mechanism whereby anaesthesia produced is not known precisely, it is clear that the main site of action is in the brain. These agents must therefore be distributed from their source in the anaesthetic apparatus into alveoli within the lungs. They dissolve in the fluid lining the alveoli, pass into the pulmonary venous blood, which then leaves the pulmonary circulation and returns to the left atrium and from there blood flows into the left ventricle. This ventricle pumps arterial blood via the aorta into the cerebral circulation and thus the anaesthetic agent passes into its site of action in the brain. The pathway of the absorption of anaesthetic agents and gas is shown in Figure 13.1.

During the induction of anaesthesia, anaesthetic agents move from areas of high concentration to areas of lower concentration. This phenomenon is called *movement down a concentration gradient* and is similar to the process whereby water flows down pipes from areas of high water pressure to areas of lower pressure. In biological systems, the concentration of a substance in these circumstances is referred to as its *partial pressure*. During induction the partial pressure of anaesthetic agent in the alveolus is higher than the partial pressure in blood and the agent therefore passes into the blood. Similarly, the partial pressure of the agent in

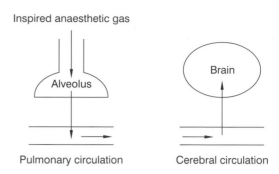

Figure 13.1   The absorption of volatile anaesthetic agents and gases.

blood is higher than that in the brain and the agent passes into the brain where it exerts its effect.

It is obvious that the partial pressures in blood and brain will be very low at the beginning of induction and absorption of anaesthetic agent is rapid because of the high partial pressure gradients. As the process proceeds, however, the partial pressures of the agent in blood and brain increase until they are equal to that in the alveolus. This is called the *state of equilibrium* and no further absorption of agent occurs because there are no remaining pressure gradients. In practice, a state of equilibrium is rarely produced. Agents that rapidly produce a high partial pressure in the alveolus tend to induce anaesthesia most quickly, since the alveolar partial pressure is effectively the 'driving force' leading to the absorption of the agent.

When the supply of anaesthetic agent from the anaesthetic machine is stopped, the process reverses. Respiration reduces the partial pressure of the agent in the alveolus so that its passage is from blood into the alveolus. The partial pressure of the agent in blood is thus reduced below that in the brain, so that

Table 13.1 The contribution of anaesthetic drugs to the triad of anaesthesia

	Hypnosis	Analgesia	Relaxation
Nitrous oxide	++	++	0
Volatile anaesthetic agents	+++	0	+
Barbiturate IV agents	+++	0	0
Propofol, etomidate	+++	0	0
Ketamine	+++	++	0
Muscle relaxants	0	0	+++
Narcotic analgesics	+	+++	0

anaesthetic agent passes from the brain into blood and the system of pressure gradients is thus reversed, the anaesthetic agent being gradually eliminated via the lungs, as illustrated in figure 13.2. Although respiratory elimination is the main mechanism for ridding the body of volatile anaesthetic agents and gases, some agents also undergo limited metabolism in the liver. The importance of this liver transformation in the case of halothane is described below.

MINIMUM ALVEOLAR CONCENTRATION (MAC) OF A VOLATILE AGENT OR GAS

The MAC of a volatile anaesthetic agent or gas is the minimum concentration of the agent in the alveolus that produces immobility in 50% of subjects exposed to a standard surgical stimulus. It is therefore a measure of an agent's 'strength' or, as it is more commonly put, its *potency*. MAC values can thus be used to compare the potencies of different agents. An agent with a high MAC value will require a greater concentration to achieve a given depth of anaesthesia than one with a low MAC value. The MAC values for the agents described below are:

- Halothane 0.7%
- Enflurane 1.7%
- Isoflurane 1.2%
- Sevoflurane 1.9%
- Desflurane 6%
- Nitrous oxide 105%.

Halothane is thus the most potent and nitrous oxide the least. MAC values such as these are averages produced by examining a large number of 'normal' subjects. In certain situations, the MAC value may be altered; for example, increasing age, pregnancy, hypothermia and other drugs may all reduce the MAC of a particular agent.

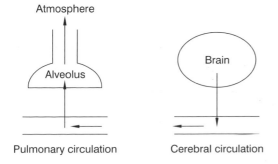

Figure 13.2   The elimination of volatile anaesthetic agents and gases

SPEED OF INDUCTION AND RECOVERY FROM ANAESTHESIA

The speed of induction of anaesthesia is determined by a complex set of pharmacological and physiological factors but the solubility of the agent in blood plays an important part. Very soluble agents are rapidly absorbed into the blood from the alveolus, thus preventing the build-up of the alveolar 'driving pressure' described above. Such soluble agents also tend to stay dissolved in blood rather than diffusing rapidly into the brain. Soluble agents are therefore slower at producing anaesthesia than those that are more insoluble. In order of increasing solubility (and thus decreasing speed of induction), the anaesthetic agents may be ranked as nitrous oxide, desflurane, sevoflurane, isoflurane, enflurane and halothane. The speed of induction may also be affected by individual patient characteristics such as changes in pulmonary ventilation or cardiac output.

PROPERTIES OF AN IDEAL VOLATILE ANAESTHETIC AGENT OR GAS

The properties of the ideal anaesthetic agent would be as follows:

- Stable under normal storage conditions, with a long shelf-life.
- Non-flammable and non-explosive under standard hospital conditions.
- Possessing a low MAC (small amounts would be needed to produce anaesthesia).
- Possessing a low solubility in blood (rapid induction and recovery from anaesthesia).
- Non-irritant to the airways.
- No respiratory or cardiovascular effects.
- Good analgesic properties.

The commonly used volatile anaesthetic agents and the anaesthetic gas, nitrous oxide, are described in detail below. It will be seen that, although the more recently developed agents have advantages over the longer-standing agents, none of them can be considered to be 'ideal.'

NITROUS OXIDE

Nitrous oxide is a gas with a boiling point of $-88°C$ and is stored as a liquid under pressure in steel cylinders at a pressure of 5000kPa (50 atmospheres). The space in the cylinder above the liquid is occupied by gaseous nitrous oxide, which escapes when the cylinder valve is opened, and is then replaced with further gas from the liquid. This continuing process of vaporization uses energy and causes the cylinder to cool. Nitrous oxide is heavier than air and less soluble than other inhalational agents.

The MAC of nitrous oxide is 105% v/v at atmospheric pressure, which indicates that the gas alone cannot produce surgical anaesthesia, since it is necessary to use oxygen in combination with the gas. The low potency is a result of the gas having low lipid solubility. In clinical practice, nitrous oxide is therefore used in a mixture with oxygen to augment the actions of other inhalational agents, intravenous anaesthetics and narcotic analgesics. Unlike other inhalational agents, nitrous oxide is a powerful analgesic and may be used as a sole analgesic agent. Entonox, for example, is a mixture of equal volumes of nitrous oxide and oxygen and is used to provide analgesia during childbirth.

Induction and recovery from nitrous oxide anaesthesia are both rapid. Due to its low blood solubility, the concentration of the gas in the alveolus rises rapidly. Despite this relatively low solubility, nitrous oxide is more soluble than nitrogen and oxygen and crosses cell membranes faster than these gases. This has important effects during induction and recovery from nitrous oxide anaesthesia. During induction, nitrous oxide leaves the alveolus more rapidly than oxygen, in effect leaving an increased concentration of oxygen in the alveolar gas. During recovery, when nitrous oxide concentrations in the alveolus are lower, nitrous oxide diffuses into the alveolus faster than oxygen, effectively reducing the alveolar oxygen concentration. Additional inspired oxygen is thus required during recovery to prevent this *diffusion hypoxia* developing. Nitrous oxide also enters spaces containing oxygen and nitrogen more rapidly than these two gases can leave the spaces. Nitrous oxide, therefore, diffuses rapidly into pneumothorax spaces and air emboli and causes a dangerous increase in their volume. Its use is thus contraindicated in patients with these conditions. The gas also diffuses rapidly into the cuff of an endotracheal tube, causing the pressure within the cuff to rise. Nitrous oxide diffusion into the bowel and the middle ear results in its use being avoided in some operations involving these sites.

Nitrous oxide is a non-irritant gas and its use is not usually associated with coughing, breath holding or laryngeal spasm. Nitrous oxide anaesthesia causes an increase in respiratory rate and a decrease in tidal volume, such that the minute volume is relatively unchanged and $paco_2$ levels remain stable. Using it in combination with other inhalational agents tends to limit the respiratory depressant effects of the latter. Nitrous oxide / oxygen mixtures used during anaesthesia cause the 'wash-out' of nitrogen from the lung. This effect may cause areas of pulmonary collapse to occur during the postoperative period.

When used without other drugs, nitrous oxide tends to be a cardiovascular depressant, causing a decrease in cardiac output and heart rate. A simultaneous increase in peripheral resistance, however, means that the arterial blood pressure tends to remain stable. The addition of other inhalational agents or narcotic analgesics produces a more complex series of cardiovascular responses. The gas also increases cerebral blood flow and intracranial pressure, while maintaining the responsiveness of the cerebral circulation to carbon dioxide.

Nitrous oxide can have serious effects on bone marrow function, with prolonged exposure to the gas reducing the production of red blood cells, white blood cells, and platelets. This megaloblastic anaemia is a result of nitrous oxide inactivating vitamin B_{12}, which is one of a series of substances responsible for DNA synthesis. Serious bone marrow suppression occurs following exposure to anaesthetic concentrations of nitrous oxide for over 24 h, with the severity being proportional to the length of exposure and recovery taking several days following discontinuation of the gas. Environmental exposure to nitrous oxide does not cause these effects if the concentration is less than 450 parts per million (ppm) and an operating theatre with efficient scavenging should have concentrations less than 50 ppm. The gas has also been shown to produce foetal abnormalities in animals, probably as a result of its effect on DNA synthesis. There is little evidence that this occurs in humans exposed to nitrous oxide during early pregnancy, either during anaesthesia or environmentally.

HALOTHANE

Halothane, a fluorinated hydrocarbon, is a colourless liquid with a boiling point of 50.3°c. It is non-flammable, non-explosive and dissolves in rubber, but it decomposes when exposed to light and is thus stored in amber bottles containing 0.01% thymol. Halothane is relatively insoluble in blood, rapidly inducing anaesthesia, and has a relatively high lipid solubility, making it a potent anaesthetic agent. Anaesthesia can be induced with a concentration of 2–4% and 0.5–1% is usually required for maintenance.

Halothane is a respiratory depressant and, although respiratory rate increases, a simultaneous decrease in tidal volume causes a reduced minute volume together with an increase in $PaCO_2$. The extent of this respiratory depression is dependent on the concentration of the agent used and may be severe at high concentrations. The agent, however, is a good bronchodilator and is useful in patients with asthma.

Halothane has significant cardiovascular effects. The combination of increased vagal activity, inhibition of sinoatrial node discharge and delayed atrio-ventricular conduction leads to the production of sinus bradycardia or an atrioventricular junctional rhythm. Myocardial contractility is reduced, causing a fall in cardiac output, and there is also a decrease in total peripheral resistance, the combination of which usually results in a reduction of systemic arterial blood pressure. Cardiac arrhythmias are also seen during halothane anaesthesia, particularly if adrenaline or other catecholamines are administered, e.g. to produce vasoconstriction at the operation site. Sudden increases in naturally occurring adrenaline and noradrenaline, as may occur during surgical and anaesthetic stimuli, will have a similar effect. Other systemic changes, such as acidosis, hypokalaemia, alkalosis, hypocalcaemia and hypertension may also be precipitating factors. The arrhythmias produced, if allowed to progress, may include life-threatening forms such as ventricular tachycardia and ventricular fibrillation.

Halothane induces cerebral vasodilatation, causing an increase in cerebral blood flow and a decrease in cerebral resistance. These changes often result in an increase in intracranial pressure, which is undesirable in neurosurgical anaesthesia. Cerebral oxygen requirements are usually reduced.

Other effects of halothane include a mild decrease in renal function, uterine relaxation and a reduction in liver blood flow. The effects of non-depolarizing muscle relaxants are potentiated by halothane anaes-thesia, although halothane itself has no neuro-muscular blocking properties.

One of the most important complications of halothane anaesthesia is halothane-induced liver damage, which may also be called *halothane hepatotoxicity* or *halothane hepatitis*. In most cases this liver damage is a mild, tran-sient condition that may be caused by mild hypoxia of the liver cells during the perioperative period and is only detected by biochemical testing. In a small number of cases (approximately 1 in 10,000 administra-tions) halothane produces a severe form of liver failure, which is fatal in more than 50% of cases. It seems that this liver failure is more likely to occur in patients who have had repeated exposures to halothane, particularly if the period separating expo-sures is less than 28 days. It is also more common in females and obese patients but is less common (but not unknown) in children. The exact mechanism of such liver damage has not been determined but it is probably related to the fact that 25% of halothane in the body is eliminated by metabolism in the liver. Other volatile anaesthetic agents have much less hepatic metabolism. There is evidence that a metabolite of halothane binds to certain proteins in liver cells. This newly formed

complex is then detected by the immunological system, which interprets it as being 'foreign' and mounts a destructive immunological response to the liver cells. A similar response has been described in the case of enflurane but is thought to be much less frequent.

Isoflurane, sevoflurane and desflurane do not appear to cause liver damage.

ISOFLURANE

Isoflurane is a colourless liquid with a boiling point of 48.5°C. It is less soluble in blood than halothane and enflurane, allowing rapid induction and recovery from anaesthesia. It is less lipid soluble than halothane and concentrations of up to 5% may be needed for induction, with maintenance concentrations of 1–2 % usually required.

The respiratory effects of isoflurane are similar to those of halothane and enflurane, with an increased respi-ratory rate, decreased tidal volume and decreased minute volume. It also has a pungent smell, which occasionally causes upper airways irritation. It is, however, a mild bronchodilator.

The effects of isoflurane on the cardiovascular system are less pronounced than those of halothane and enflurane. In general, an increase in heart rate occurs and the cardiac output is often maintained at preanaesthetic levels. Marked peripheral vasodilatation is common, however, and can cause a reduction in systemic blood pressure. Cardiac arrhythmias are infrequently induced during isoflurane anaesthesia. In patients with coronary artery stenosis, it is possible that isoflurane anaesthesia causes coronary blood flow to be directed away from the area supplied by the diseased artery. This further reduces oxygen delivery to this area of heart muscle and, as a result, isoflurane should be used cautiously in patients with severe ischaemic heart disease.

Isoflurane dilates the cerebral circulation, causing an increase in cerebral blood flow. It does not, however, stimulate seizure activity on the EEG and may therefore be used in epileptic patients. Like halothane and enflurane, it potentiates the effects of non-depo-larizing muscle relaxants and also causes relaxation of uterine muscle. Liver and renal damage due to isoflurane anaesthesia, are extremely rare.

ENFLURANE

Enflurane is a colourless liquid with a boiling point of 56.5°C. It is relatively insoluble in blood, so induction and recovery from anaesthesia are rapid. It is, however, less lipid-soluble than halothane and so a higher concentration of the agent is required to achieve a given depth of anaesthesia. Concentrations of over 5% are needed for induction, followed by 1–3 % for maintenance.

Enflurane has similar respiratory effects to those of halothane, with an increase in respiratory rate coupled to a decrease in tidal volume. The overall decrease in minute volume causes an increase in $PaCO_2$. Enflurane is also a mild bronchodilator.

The effects of enflurane on the cardiovascular system are, like halothane, largely depressant with myocardial contractility and cardiac output falling during anaesthesia. Unlike halothane, however, there is typically an increase in heart rate. Enflurane is also a more potent dilator of peripheral blood vessels. A fall in both peripheral resistance and cardiac output produces a significant fall in the systemic blood pressure, particularly during deep enflurane anaesthesia, and it is more common in the elderly patient. Cardiac arrhythmias are occasionally seen during enflurane anaesthesia but are less frequent than those associated with halothane.

Enflurane produces cerebral vasodilatation, with an increase in cerebral blood flow resulting if the systemic blood pressure is maintained. Enflurane anaesthesia also causes abnormal electrical activity in the brain. In some cases, the resulting electroencephalograph (EEG) changes are similar to those seen in epilepsy. Although these changes do not appear to have any persisting effects, enflurane is usually avoided in individuals with epilepsy and similar conditions.

Unlike halothane, enflurane has a low level of metabolism in the liver (approximately 2%) and, as discussed above, liver damage as a result of enflurane metabolism is extremely rare. One of the metabolic products of enflurane is the fluoride ion, which can cause reversible renal damage if present in sufficient concentration. Although concentrations of fluoride ions are generally too low following enflurane anaesthesia to produce any renal effects, the agent is generally avoided in patients with renal disease.

Enflurane, like halothane, potentiates the action of non-depolarizing muscle relaxants. It also relaxes uterine smooth muscle and reduces intraocular pressure.

SEVOFLURANE

Sevoflurane is a colourless liquid with a boiling point of 58.5°C. Although it is generally stable, it may decompose when exposed to strong bases such as soda lime, producing toxic breakdown products. This effect is most likely to occur during prolonged low-flow anaesthesia.

Sevoflurane is relatively insoluble, so induction and recovery from anaesthesia are accordingly rapid. Concentrations of 4–6 % are typically needed for induction of anaesthesia, with 1–3 % providing maintenance of anaesthesia.

Sevoflurane depresses respiratory function in a manner similar to other volatile agents. Respiratory rate increases, tidal volume decreases and overall there is a decrease in minute volume. The ventilatory response to increased carbon dioxide tensions is obtunded. A major advantage of sevoflurane is its lack of an irritating odour. This feature makes the agent suitable for induction of anaesthesia, particularly in children.

Sevoflurane anaesthesia produces a reduction in blood pressure as a result of peripheral vasodilatation. Increased heart rates are not often seen and changes in arrhythmias are uncommon, even if catecholamines such as adrenaline are administered simultaneously. Increases in cerebral and coronary blood flow may occur during sevoflurane anaesthesia, probably as a result of vasodilatation within these regional circulations.

Approximately 3% of inhaled sevoflurane is converted by the liver to organic and inorganic fluoride compounds. This conversion may be increased if the action of the liver enzyme responsible is increased by agents such as alcohol.

DESFLURANE

Desflurane has recently been introduced into UK anaesthetic practice. Its chemical structure is similar to that of isoflurane but it has markedly different properties. In particular, its low boiling point (23.5°C) and its vapour pressure (669 mmHg at 20°C) mean a specially heated and pressurized vaporizer is necessary for its clinical usage. It is, however, an extremely stable agent. Desflurane is relatively insoluble compared to other volatile agents, so induction and recovery from anaesthesia are extremely rapid. Typically, concentrations of 6–9% are needed for induction and 3–5% for maintenance of anaesthesia.

Desflurane has effects on respiratory function that are similar to those of other volatile anaesthetic agents. An increase in respiratory rate and decrease in tidal volume result in an overall decrease in minute volume and the respiratory response to increasing carbon dioxide tensions is inhibited. The agent has a particularlypungent smell and may cause significant airway irritability. This feature limits its use in the induction of anaesthesia.

Desflurane is a potent vasodilator, an effect that induces a reflex increase in heart rate. This combination of effects tends to maintain cardiac output because the agent does not significantly inhibit cardiac contractility. Changes in cardiac rhythm, even during catecholamine usage, are rarely a result of desflurane. Cerebral vasodilatation may result in an increase in cerebral blood flow and there may also be a similar increase in the coronary circulation.

There is effectively no metabolism of desflurane under normal conditions and the agent is eliminated unchanged. This means that liver and renal damage are extremely unlikely following its use.

INTRAVENOUS ANAESTHETIC AGENTS

WHAT ARE INTRAVENOUS ANAESTHETIC AGENTS AND HOW DO THEY WORK?

Intravenous anaesthetic agents generally produce unconsciousness in one arm–brain circulation time. They may be used to induce anaesthesia prior to maintenance with anaesthetic gases, vapours and opioid agents or they may be used as the sole anaesthetic agent during short surgical procedures. Some may also be given by infusion to produce *total intravenous anaesthesia*.

An intravenous injection of such an agent is initially distributed, via the systemic circulation, to the brain (the drug's action in the brain produces unconsciousness) and other organs in the 'central compartment.' The drug is then redistributed to one or more peripheral compartments and its concentration in the brain falls to the point at which consciousness returns. This occurs while there is still a substantial amount of drug remaining in the body, the processes of elimination being much slower than those of redistribution are. Recovery from intravenous anaesthesia is thus due to redistribution of the drug rather than its elimination.

The ease with which an intravenous agent reaches the brain and has its effect will be governed by several factors. First, cerebral blood flow will determine the rate at which the agent is delivered to the brain. Second, the degree of ionization of the drug will influence penetration of the brain, since only unionized drug will cross cell membranes. Similarly, the lipid solubility of the drug will affect its rate of transfer into the brain because highly lipid-soluble agents cross cell membranes rapidly. Finally, the degree to which the drug is bound to plasma proteins will be influential, because only unbound drug is free to cross cell membranes.

PROPERTIES OF AN IDEAL INTRAVENOUS ANAESTHETIC AGENT

Properties of the ideal intravenous agent should include:

- Rapid and smooth production of anaesthesia within one arm–brain circulation time.
- Predictable duration of anaesthesia.
- Recovery from anaesthesia, which would ideally be free from sedation, nausea and vomiting.
- Pain-free injection.
- No associated involuntary muscle movements.
- Minimal effects on the major organ systems, including the cardiovascular, respiratory and central nervous systems.
- No accumulation in the body, so that it could be used by infusion if needed.
- No histamine release or anaphylaxis.

There are five intravenous anaesthetic agents currently in use in the UK: thiopentone, methohexitone, etomidate, propofol and ketamine. The main features of these agents will now be reviewed to illustrate how each differs from the hypothetical ideal agent.

THIOPENTONE AND METHOHEXITONE

Thiopentone and methohexitone are members of a group of drugs based on the barbituric acid molecule and are thus *barbiturate anaesthetic agents*. Alterations to the structure of the basic barbiturate molecule produces anaesthetic agents that vary in their onset of action, speed of recovery and incidence of excitatory phenomena but thiopentone and methohexitone are the only two such anaesthetic agents now used in clinical practice.

Sodium thiopentone is supplied as a pale yellow powder, which is dissolved in water to produce a 2.5% w/v solution; 6% sodium carbonate is added to increase the solubility and this makes the solution highly alkaline (pH 10.5). A standard intravenous dose of the drug produces unconsciousness rapidly and without muscle excitation. Increased sensitivity of the laryngeal and pharyngeal reflexes may be noticed soon after induction and at low plasma concentrations, increased sensitivity to painful stimuli may occur.

Thiopentone has anticonvulsant properties and is thus suitable for use in patients with epilepsy and similar conditions. The drug reduces both the rate of metabolism and the oxygen consumption of the brain. It also produces constriction of the cerebral circulation, causing a reduction in cerebral blood flow. These features have made it a useful agent in neuroanaesthesia and in the intensive care management of patients with head injuries and intracranial pathology.

Thiopentone usually produces a decrease in arterial blood pressure after induction of anaesthesia and this is probably due to increased peripheral pooling of blood, which reduces the venous return to the heart and thus causes a fall in cardiac output and blood pressure. A reflex tachycardia follows, with the net effect being a fall in blood pressure and increase in heart rate following induction of anaesthesia. These cardiovascular effects make thiopentone an agent that should be used cautiously in patients with cardiac disease or systemic hypotension.

Thiopentone is also a respiratory depressant and a few deep breaths, followed by a period of apnoea, usually follow injection. Respiration then returns with a reduction in tidal volume and rate, both of which may also be influenced by other drugs, such as relaxants or opioids, given at the same time. The respiratory depressant effect of thiopentone occurs by inhibition of the respiratory control sites in the brainstem, including a decreased sensitivity to carbon dioxide occurring at these sites.

Intravenous injection of thiopentone is painless but accidental injection of the agent into an artery causes intense spasm of the artery, with cessation of the circulation in the area supplied by the artery. The spasm may be followed by the deposition of thiopentone crystals in smaller vessels in the arterial tree. Severe ischaemic damage may result if treatment with vasodilators, heparin and sympathetic nervous blockade is not rapidly instituted. This complication was more frequent when 5% thiopentone was used.

Thiopentone occasionally causes histamine release but very rarely produces a severe anaphylactic reaction (approximately once per 20,000 administrations). It is contraindicated in patients with porphyria, an inborn error of metabolism, in whom it may produce an acute exacerbation of the disease.

Methohexitone is supplied as a white powder, which is dissolved in water to produce a 1% w/v solution. Like thiopentone, the solution is highly alkaline, with a pH of 11. A standard intravenous dose produces anaesthesia rapidly but, unlike thiopentone, it is often associated with excitatory side effects. These include muscle movements, tremor, rigidity, coughing and hiccuping. Pain at the site of intravenous injection occurs frequently. Clinical recovery from anaesthesia is typically faster than that from thiopentone.

The central nervous system effects of methohexitone are similar to those of thiopentone, except for its ability to produce convulsant activity in patients with a history of epilepsy. It is, therefore, not used in patients who have this condition. Arterial hypotension, a reduced cardiac output and an increased heart rate also occur following methohexitone administration, although these cardiovascular effects may be less marked than those produced by thiopentone. Methohexitone also has a similar central depressant effect on respiration. Severe anaphylactic reactions to the drug are rare and it is probable that accidental intra-arterial injection has less dangerous effects than those seen following thiopentone.

PROPOFOL

Propofol is derived from the phenol molecule and is almost insoluble in water. It is therefore supplied as a 1% w/v emulsion containing soya bean oil and purified egg lecithin. A standard intravenous dose produces rapid loss of consciousness, with recovery within 4–6 min. The speed and quality of the recovery, which are both more favourable than those of the barbiturate agents, have led to propofol becoming popular in anaesthesia for day case surgery and short procedures. Using other anaesthetic agents at the same time, however, reduces these benefits. The agent's pharmacokinetic profile also suggests that it does not readily accumulate in the body after repeated dosing and is thus suitable for use by infusion. It has thus become popular in total intravenous anaesthetic regimens and is also used in subanaesthetic doses to provide sedation in intensive care units and during regional anaesthesia.

Pain on injection is more common than with thiopentone and involuntary muscle movements sometimes occur. Severe muscular spasms, and possibly convulsions, have been associated with the use of propofol and it is thus not used in patients with epilepsy, although this is currently under debate. There appears to be a lower incidence of postoperative nausea and vomiting following induction with propofol than following other intravenous agents. Severe anaphylactic reactions to propofol have been reported and it should be avoided in patients who have an allergy to egg protein.

Propofol's cardiorespiratory effects are similar to those produced by the barbiturates. A decrease in arterial blood pressure and cardiac output typically occurs following administration, with a variable change in heart rate. These effects are mainly caused by peripheral vasodilatation. Respiratory depression is common following induction of anaesthesia and may be more pronounced than that seen with thiopentone. A decrease in tidal volume and increase in respiratory rate usually proceed a period of apnoea.

ETOMIDATE

Etomidate is an imidazole derivative and is supplied as a 0.2% w/v solution which contains 35% propylene glycol. Intravenous injection of a standard induction dose rapidly produces unconsciousness, with recovery occurring 7–14 min later. It induces spontaneous muscle movements, often myoclonic, in a large proportion of patients. In addition, it frequently causes pain on injection and postoperative nausea and vomiting appear to be more common than with other intravenous anaesthetic agents.

Unlike the barbiturate anaesthetics and propofol, etomidate has a limited effect on the cardiovascular system, with small decreases in peripheral resistance and blood pressure occurring in some cases. This property has led to its use in patients with cardiac disease and systemic hypovolaemia. Etomidate reduces intracranial pressure, cerebral metabolism, cerebral oxygen consumption and cerebral blood flow. It also produces respiratory depression, including reductions in respiratory rate and tidal volume, but these effects are less than those produced by barbiturate agents.

Etomidate has the unusual effect of inhibiting the production of the steroids cortisol and aldosterone in the adrenal gland. This effect is most marked when it is given by infusion and is due to the inhibition of key enzymes responsible for the adrenal synthesis of these hormones. Although the effect also occurs following a single dose of the agent, it is not thought to be of clinical importance in most situations. Etomidate is, therefore, not used by infusion and is available only for the induction of anaesthesia.

KETAMINE

Although it is classified as an intravenous anaesthetic agent, ketamine differs markedly from the agents already described. Chemically, it resembles phency-clidine and cyclohexamine and is readily water soluble. It can be administered by both the intravenous and intramuscular routes and is therefore supplied in three concentrations: 10, 50 and 100 mg/ml. These solutions are highly acidic, with pH ranging from 3.5 to 5.5.

Unlike other induction agents, unconsciousness is not achieved in one arm–brain circulation time. The quality of anaesthesia also differs from the other agents in that ketamine produces a state called 'dissociative anaesthesia,' characterized by profound anterograde amnesia and a cataleptic state. The patient's eyes may remain open and coordinated muscle movements often occur spontaneously. Depending on the initial dose used, recovery from this state may be slow.

Ketamine, unlike other intravenous agents, stimulates the cardiovascular system. Increases in systemic and pulmonary blood pressure, cardiac output and heart rate all follow administration. Central nervous system stimulation and peripheral action on cardiac adrenoreceptors probably cause these effects. Respiratory changes following ketamine are mild with an occasional increase in the respiratory rate, and some bronchodilatation may also be induced. Upper airway tone is unaffected and protective reflexes remain intact.

Central nervous system stimulation also follows ketamine administration. Cerebral blood flow, cerebrospinal fluid pressure, intracranial pressure and intraocular pressure all increase, thus making ketamine an unsuitable agent for use in patients with intracranial and intraocular disease. Unlike other agents, ketamine has powerful analgesic properties, which persist beyond recovery of consciousness, and subanaesthetic doses may be used in analgesic regimes.

Psychological disturbances during emergence from ketamine anaesthesia are a major problem with the agent. These emergence phenomena may last for up to 24 h and include vivid dreams, visual and auditory hallucinations and delirium. Adults are more often affected than children and women more often than men. Preoperative treatment with benzodiazepines such as diazepam reduces the frequency of this side effect.

Ketamine has limited use in clinical practice. Its analgesic and cardiorespiratory effects make it useful as a sole anaesthetic agent in isolated sites. It has also been advocated for induction of anaesthesia in hypovolaemic patients. Subanaesthetic infusions are used in some centres to provide sedation and analgesia during surgery under regional blockade and during the postoperative period. Its use as an anaesthetic agent, however, should be avoided in patients with cardiac disease, hypertension, intracranial disease and psychological disturbances.

MUSCLE RELAXANTS

VOLUNTARY MUSCLE CONTRACTION

Voluntary muscle is composed of many long, thin cells called muscle fibres. The fibres contain a complex system of protein filaments which, under the stimulus of a motor nerve (described below), slide across each other, causing the fibre to contract. The combined effect of all the muscle fibres contracting is the contraction of the whole muscle. All voluntary muscles have a motor nerve supply, which begins in the spinal cord and consists of many motor neurones. The motor neurone splits as it enters the muscle, ending in a large number of nerve terminals. Each nerve terminal lies in a fold of the external surface of a single muscle fibre, an area called the *motor endplate*.

Each nerve terminal contains a number of small, mobile pockets of cell membrane called *synaptic vesicles*. These contain stores of the neurotransmitter *acetylcholine*. In response to a nerve impulse, the synaptic vesicles fuse with the nerve cell membrane and acetylcholine molecules are released into the gap between the nerve ending and the muscle fibre (the *synaptic cleft*). The acetylcholine molecules then diffuse across the cleft and bind to specific acetylcholine receptors in the muscle fibre membrane. A number of small channels in the muscle fibre open as a result of this transmitter/receptor binding, allowing ions to pass into the fibre and change the resting potential of the fibre membrane. (under resting conditions there is a potential difference of −90 mV across the cell membrane.) A wave of depolarization, thus generated, spreads down the muscle fibre, triggering the chemical interactions that result in muscle contraction.

After binding to an acetylcholine receptor, the acetylcholine molecule is then broken down by the action of the enzyme *acetylcholinesterase*, which lies on the muscle fibre membrane close to the acetylcholine receptors. Choline and acetate molecules formed by this breakdown then diffuse away and some re-enter the nerve terminal to be included in the production of further acetylcholine. The mechanism of neuromuscular transmission is illustrated in Figure 13.3.

PHARMACOLOGICAL NEUROMUSCULAR BLOCKADE

There are two types of neuromuscular block that can be induced pharmacologically. The first type is called *depolarization blockade* and is induced in clinical practice with the drug suxamethonium. This drug (see below) has a structure that is similar to acetylcholine and thus binds to acetylcholine receptors, initiating a depolarization of the muscle membrane with associated muscle contraction. Suxamethonium, however, is not rapidly metabolized at the motor endplate and remains bound to the acetylcholine receptor, producing a prolonged period of membrane depolarization. Further muscle contraction cannot occur during this period of depolarization.

The second type of neuromuscular blockade is called *competitive or non-depolarizing blockade*. Drugs producing this blockade bind to acetylcholine receptors at the motor endplate but do not produce depolarization and muscle contraction. They do, however, block the action of acetylcholine at the receptor and 'compete' with acetylcholine for the receptor sites. At least 80% of the acetylcholine receptors at the motor endplate must be occupied by relaxant drug before any clinical neuromuscular block can be demonstrated.

DEPOLARIZING BLOCKADE

Suxamethonium is the only drug used in routine clinical practice to produce a depolarizing neuro-

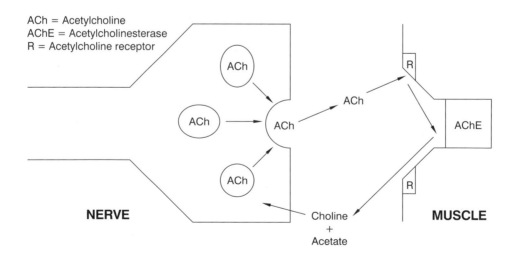

Figure 13.3   The neuromuscular junction.

muscular blockade. Its structure is that of two acetylcholine molecules joined together, which explains its ability to bind to acetylcholine receptors and produce depolarization. An intravenous dose of 1 mg/kg of the drug will typically produce neuromuscular blockade within 60 s and the block will persist for 3–6 min. Suxamethonium is not metabolized at the motor endplate by acetylcholinesterase. Its effect is ended by the drug diffusing into plasma, where it is metabolized by the enzyme plasma cholinesterase.

Side effects of Suxamethonium

Suxamethonium has several undesirable side effects. Soon after intravenous injection, muscle fasciculations of varying severity can occur. These disorganized muscle contractions may cause increases in heart rate, blood pressure, intracranial pressure and intra-abdominal pressure. Fasciculations may also be responsible for the postoperative muscle pains that many patients suffer after suxamethonium administration. Such pains occur in the neck, back and abdominal muscles, particularly in patients who have mobilized soon after surgery. A small dose of a non-depolarizing muscle relaxant given before the suxamethonium reduces or abolishes these fasciculations in many cases.

The process of muscle fibre depolarization, as described earlier, involves the diffusion of ions across the muscle cell membrane and includes the movement of potassium ions from within the cell to the extracellular fluid. In normal conditions this causes a small rise in the plasma potassium concentration. However, in patients with muscle diseases, including burns, muscle atrophy and upper and lower motor neurone lesions, severe hyperkalaemia may develop. This can cause cardiac dysrhythmias, sometimes severe enough to produce cardiac arrest. Suxamethonium is thus avoided in such patients and also in those who present with high plasma potassium levels preoperatively (for example, patients with renal failure).

Suxamethonium can also produce cardiac dysrhythmias by mimicking the action of acetylcholine on the heart, with sinus bradycardia, junctional rhythm and sinus arrest being most commonly observed. These effects are most likely to occur following the administration of a second dose of the drug when the initial neuromuscular block has worn off and is counteracted by giving atropine or glycopyrrolate. An alternative cardiovascular effect may be produced if suxamethonium mimics the effect of acetylcholine on the sympathetic nervous system, in which case increases in blood pressure and heart rate may be noted.

Increases in intragastric, intraocular and intracranial pressure are common following suxamethonium administration. In the case of the intraocular and intragastric pressures, this may be a result of the initial muscle contractions preceding neuromuscular block, while an increase in cerebral blood flow may be the explanation of the increased intracranial pressure. The drug should thus be used cautiously in patients with intracranial disease (especially those with raised intracranial pressure) and penetrating eye injuries. It is, of course, used frequently as part of a 'rapid-sequence' induction of anaesthesia, in which cricoid pressure protects against the possibility of the reflux and aspiration of gastric contents.

It has been noted that suxamethonium is metabolized in plasma by the action of the enzyme plasma cholinesterase. This is produced in the liver and patients with liver disease may have low levels of this enzyme. In this situation, the suxamethonium levels remain abnormally high due to a failure of suxamethonium metabolism and the clinical picture of prolonged neuromuscular blockade will be seen. Some individuals have a genetically determined inability to produce normal plasma cholinesterase. Some patients produce an abnormal enzyme, which is partially effective, and a moderate increase in the duration of the neuromuscular block results. In a smaller number of cases, no plasma cholinesterase is produced at all and a prolonged period of paralysis results.

Finally, it should be remembered that suxamethonium may cause severe anaphylactic shock in a small number of patients. It is also one of the agents that can trigger malignant hyperpyrexia. Both of these medical emergencies are discussed fully elsewhere.

NON-DEPOLARIZING BLOCKADE

The majority of muscle relaxants in clinical usage are non-depolarizing muscle relaxants (ndmrs). All have the same basic mechanism of action at the neuromuscular junction, as described above. There are marked differences between these drugs, however, in terms of their chemical structure, pharmacokinetic profile (including speed of onset of action, duration of action and mode of elimination) and their major side effects. Curare, alcuronium, pancuronium, vecuronium, atracurium, mivacurium and rocuronium are the NDMRs available for use clinically and each will be described briefly.

D-tubocurarine (*curare*) is the oldest and, nowadays, the least used of the NDMRs, having been introduced into clinical practice in the early 1940s. It has a slow onset of action and a long duration of neuromuscular blockade (up to 74 min following a standard dose). It is not metabolized, being eliminated unchanged in the urine (70%) and the bile (30%). Patients with renal disease may thus have a reduced ability to eliminate tubocurarine and this may result in a prolonged neuromuscular block. The drug also typically causes the systemic release of histamine, an agent that causes peripheral vasodilatation. In addition to a reduced venous return due to a loss of muscle tone, this explains the characteristic fall in arterial blood pressure that follows the injection of tubocurarine. A slight decrease in heart rate also occurs.

Alcuronium has a more rapid onset than tubocurarine but has a similar duration of action. It also is eliminated unchanged in urine (70%) and bile (30%). A fall in arterial blood pressure also occurs following injection. This is not usually a result of systemic histamine release, which occurs rarely, but is more likely to be the result of blockade of sympathetic ganglia by the relaxant. Tachycardias do not typically follow administration.

Pancuronium is a steroid-based molecule. It has a moderate onset of action but a shorter duration of neuromuscular block than tubocurarine and alcuronium. Thirty per cent of a dose is metabolized, with the remaining 70% being excreted unchanged in urine. It rarely causes systemic histamine release but, unlike tubocurarine and alcuronium, it causes a tachycardia and increase in arterial blood pressure following administration. This effect is probably due to a direct stimulation of the sympathetic nervous system and the heart.

Vecuronium has a similar molecular structure to pancuronium and a similar rate of onset of action. It has a shorter duration of action than the three NDMRs already discussed. Twenty per cent of a dose is metabolized, the remainder being excreted unchanged in bile. Adverse effects on the cardiovascular system are minimal and systemic histamine release is rare.

Atracurium has a rate of onset of action and duration of block similar to that of vecuronium. It is 95% metabolized prior to elimination and is particularly suitable for use in patients with renal and liver failure. Systemic histamine release is rare and minimal cardiovascular changes follow injection.

Mivacurium has a similar molecular structure and rate of onset as atracurium but a shorter duration of action. Similarly, systemic histamine release is rare and cardiovascular effects are minimal after administration. Unlike the other NDMRs, mivacurium is 95% metabolized by plasma cholinesterase (the enzyme also responsible for the metabolism of suxamethonium). In patients with liver disease and those with genetically determined deficiencies of plasma cholinesterase, a prolonged neuromuscular block may occur if mivacurium is given.

Rocuronium has a similar chemical structure to vecuronium but has the fastest onset of action of the NDMRs. Its duration of action is longer than that of atracurium, vecuronium and mivacurium. The drug is mainly eliminated unchanged in bile and urine and thus may have a prolonged effect in patients with renal disease. Like vecuronium, it causes minimal cardiovascular effects and rarely is associated with systemic histamine release.

REVERSAL OF NEUROMUSCULAR BLOCKADE

In the case of a depolarizing block produced by suxamethonium, there are no specific methods of reversing the block. Plasma cholinesterase metabolizes the drug and neuromuscular function returns as the concentration of suxamethonium decreases in the synaptic cleft and acetylcholine molecules can bind to their receptors to produce a muscle action potential. Mivacurium, although a non-depolarizing drug, is also metabolized by plasma cholinesterase and usually requires no specific intervention for the termination of its neuromuscular block. The other NDMRs all require specific reversal agents for reversal of the block they have produced, although some anaesthetists, in certain circumstances, will allow the effects of atracurium and vecuronium to wear off without the use of reversal agents. The two agents used to reverse a non-depolarizing block are an anticholinesterase drug in combination with an anti-muscarinic drug.

HOW DO ANTICHOLINESTERASE DRUGS WORK?

The process by which the enzyme acetylcholinesterase metabolizes acetylcholine at the neuromuscular junction has been described above. An anticholinesterase drug binds to the acetylcholinesterase enzyme on the muscle fibre membrane and prevents the enzyme from metabolizing acetylcholine. This produces an increased concentration of acetylcholine around the neuromuscular junction. Acetylcholine molecules then compete with NDMRs molecules for occupation of the acetylcholine receptors and effectively displace the NDMRs molecules from the receptors. The NDMRs molecules then re-enter the systemic circulation, are redistributed and metabolized.

Neostigmine is the most commonly used anticholinesterase drug in clinical practice. Its time to peak action following intravenous injection is approximately

6 min and its duration of action is approximately 60 min. It is both metabolized in the liver and eliminated unchanged in urine. Pyridostigmine is a similar anticholinesterase agent and may also be used for reversal of non-depolarizing neuromuscular blockade.

WHAT ARE ANTIMUSCARINIC DRUGS AND WHY ARE THEY GIVEN WITH ANTICHOLINESTERASE DRUGS?

It has previously been explained that acetylcholine is the neurotransmitter at the neuromuscular junction, an effect often called its *nicotinic* effect. It is, however, also a major neurotransmitter in the autonomic nervous system and produces bradycardia, increased salivation, increased bladder and bowel contractions and blurred vision. These effects are called its *muscarinic* effects. Antimuscarinic drugs (often called anticholinergic drugs) block these effects of acetylcholine but not the nicotinic effect at the neuromuscular junction. If an anticholinesterase such as neostigmine is given alone, acetylcholine concentrations will rise both at the neuromuscular junction and at the muscarinic sites. The neuromuscular block will be reversed but dangerous bradycardia, excess salivation, excess bowel and bladder contraction and blurred vision will also result. For this reason, an antimuscarinic agent is given with the anticholinesterase agent, so that the unwanted muscarinic effects are blocked but the reversal of neuromuscular block is unaffected.

ANTIMUSCARINIC AGENTS COMMONLY USED

The two antimuscarinic agents most commonly used in anaesthetic practice are atropine and glycopyrrolate. These drugs are used both in the reversal of neuromuscular blockade and individually in the treatment of bradycardias, and excessive salivation and as premedication agents. Both drugs block salivary secretion, increase the heart rate, relax bowel and bladder smooth muscle and dilate the pupil. It is also possible that they reduce gastric acidity. Atropine crosses the blood–brain barrier and causes sedation but glycopyrrolate has no such effect. Glycopyrrolate has a much more powerful inhibition of salivary secretions than atropine but has a less pronounced effect on heart rate and a minimal effect on pupil size.

OTHER DRUGS USED IN ANAESTHETIC PRACTICE

OPIOID ANALGESICS

The pharmacological properties of the opioid analgesics have been reviewed in detail elsewhere. When used during anaesthesia, they provide analgesia that persists into the postoperative period and may also reduce undesirable reflex responses to surgery. If used in analgesic doses, intermediate and long-acting opioids such as morphine, diamorphine and pethidine have a small effect on reflex responses and their use during anaesthesia is mainly directed at providing postoperative analgesia. Fentanyl and alfentanil are particularly potent opioid analgesics and their intraoperative use is primarily aimed at achieving stable physiological conditions by reflex suppression. Both have a shorter duration of action than morphine, with alfentanil having a shorter duration of action than fentanyl. Remifentanil, which has recently been introduced in the UK, is an ultra-short acting opioid, which is most effective when given as a continuous infusion during anaesthesia.

The side effects of most opioid analgesics are similar and include respiratory depression, cardiovascular depression and sedation, together with nausea and vomiting. Opioid analgesics exert their actions by binding to a series of opioid receptors located in brain, spinal and other tissues. Naloxone is a competitive antagonist to opioid analgesics acting at these receptors and is used to reverse the unwanted effects of the analgesics if they have been used in excess.

ANTI-EMETIC DRUGS

Postoperative nausea and vomiting (PONV) is a common and distressing complication of anaesthesia and surgery. It occurs in between 25% and 70% of patients in the postoperative period.

Who gets PONV?

PONV is more common in children, women and those with a history of motion sickness. It is also more common following abdominal operations, gynaecological surgery and the administration of various drugs, e.g. opioids, neostigmine and antibiotics.

Why do people get PONV?

Vomiting has evolved as a protective mechanism to rid the body of ingested toxins, e.g. in food poisoning. Nausea is a subjective sensation associated with the urge to vomit and to many is more unpleasant than actual vomiting. The vomiting centre, an area in the brainstem, controls vomiting. This area has much neurological input influencing its activity and, when stimulated, causes reflex muscular contractions in the gut, diaphragm and abdominal muscles to expel gut contents via the mouth. The inputs to the vomiting centre are from the gut itself (via the vagus nerve), the balance organs within the ear (vestibular apparatus) and from higher centres in the brain. Thus, if a person hears or sees someone vomiting they may feel nauseated themselves; for someone who has had PONV, even the sight of an operating theatre may make them nauseated. These effects are produced by stimulation of various receptors, the most important being acetylcholine (ACh), histamine-1 (H1) and 5-hydroxytryptamine (5-HT$_3$).

Some drugs, e.g. opioids and digoxin, have their effects via dopaminergic (D2) receptors in a second area of the brain called the *chemoreceptor trigger zone* (CTZ), which in turn feeds into the vomiting centre (see Fig. 13.4). The CTZ is a special area of the brain because, despite being part of the brainstem, it is outside the blood–brain barrier and so drugs which do not cross the blood–brain barrier may be used to stimulate or depress this area.

Nausea and vomiting may be stimulated in many ways during surgery and anaesthesia. The first report of PONV was made in 1848 (just two years after the first anaesthetic) following chloroform but it was not until the mid 1950s that antiemetic drugs were used in its treatment.

Intravenous induction agents have a variable effect on PONV. Etomidate and ketamine produce it frequently but barbiturates have less effect and propofol may even possess antiemetic properties.

Inhalational agents can all predispose to PONV but nitrous oxide is probably the commonest cause. It has both central and peripheral effects, the latter being caused by its diffusion into the gut, thus stimulating vagal pathways, and diffusion into the ear, stimulating the vestibular pathway.

Other drugs used in anaesthesia can cause PONV, especially opioids, neostigmine and certain antibiotics. Non-drug factors can also lead to PONV such as hypotension, hypoxia and pain, blowing gases into the stomach by inefficient bag and mask ventilation and surgical factors, e.g. traction on the eye during squint surgery.

Drug treatment of PONV?

There are four main groups of drugs used in the treatment of PONV:

1. Antidopaminergic drugs, e.g. droperidol, prochlor-perazine and metoclopramide.
2. Antihistamines, e.g. cyclizine.
3. Anticholinergics, e.g. hyoscine.
4. 5HT$_3$ antagonists, e.g. ondansetron.

Antidopaminergic drugs act via the CTZ and are useful in drug-induced nausea and vomiting. Droperidol is used in small doses intravenously during anaesthesia and is also mixed with morphine for use in patient-controlled analgesia. Prochlorperazine cannot be used intravenously and is most commonly prescribed as intermittent intramuscular doses but it may also be used as a suppository or a buccal preparation (placed between the upper gum and lip). Metoclopramide is useful in that it also has effects on the gut to speed up gastric emptying and is often used for this purpose as a premedication. All antidopaminergic drugs may cause uncoordinated muscular movements (called *dyskinesia*) but this is unusual in short-term use.

Antihistamines are used as antiemetics, most commonly in the form of cyclizine. This works by blocking the input from the vestibular apparatus in the vomiting centre and hence is useful in ear surgery and in those with previous motion sickness. It is used either intramuscularly or as a suppository. Side effects include sedation and dizziness.

Anticholinergics also act to block input to the vomiting centre. Despite their common use in anaesthesia, atropine and glycopyrrolate are not often used in PONV. The most commonly used drug in this group is hyoscine, which can be given intravenously, intramuscularly and as a topical patch. The side effects of anticholinergics are dry mouth, blurred vision, tachycardia and confusion (not with glycopyrrolate).

5HT$_3$ antagonists block the effects of 5HT$_3$, in both the gut and the CTZ. Ondansetron is the most frequently used and it is mostly given intravenously but may also

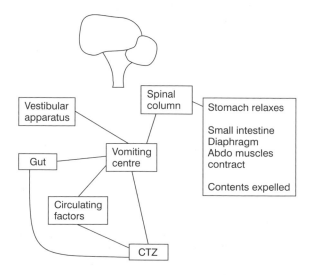

Figure 13.4 **Physiology of nausea and vomiting.**

be given intramuscularly and orally. The side effects are few but include flushing and chest pain.

BENZODIAZEPINES

The benzodiazepines form a group of drugs with similar central nervous system effects, which include sedation, anxiety reduction, muscle relaxation and convulsion suppression. Commonly used benzodiazepines include diazepam, lorazepam, oxazepam, nitrazepam, temazepam and flunitrazepam. In general medical practice the benzodiazepines are given orally to either reduce anxiety or speed the onset of sleep. In anaesthetic practice, however, a benzodiazepine is often used for premedication. The drug is given orally 1–2 h before induction of anaesthesia and acts to reduce the patient's anxiety and provide some sedation but premedication also contributes to a 'smooth' induction of anaesthesia and reduces the dose of anaesthetic agent required.

Midazolam is a benzodiazepine that is frequently used in the operating theatre. It is water soluble, unlike other drugs in this group, and can be given intravenously without causing pain on injection or venous thrombosis. It has anxiolytic, sedative, anticonvulsant and muscle relaxant properties and also affects memory, with patients being unable to remember events occurring during its duration of action. Midazolam is often used to supplement local or regional anaesthetic techniques and it is occasionally used with other intravenous anaesthetic agents and analgesics to induce anaesthesia. Excess administration may produce prolonged unconsciousness and cardiorespiratory depression. *Flumazenil* is a specific benzodiazepine antagonist, which can rapidly reverse the effects of benzodiazepines.

CARDIOVASCULAR DRUGS

During certain operations, e.g. ear surgery, it is important to keep the blood pressure reasonably low. The drugs most commonly used to do this are the β-blockers, e.g. atenolol and labetalol. These drugs block the effect of epinephrine (adrenaline) on the heart and blood vessels and reduce the heart rate and blood pressure. They also block the receptors in the lungs that keep the airways dilated and may precipitate bronchospasm in asthmatic patients. A shorter acting β-blocker, esmolol, is sometimes used as it has a very short duration of action and is particularly useful in preventing the hypertension and tachycardia seen following intubation.

During regional anaesthesia (spinal and epidural), there is a relatively high incidence of hypotension caused by dilatation of blood vessels and reduced pumping of blood back to the heart by the leg muscles. The first-line treatment of this is fluid loading but drugs are also commonly used to increase the blood pressure, particularly the *sympathomimetic agents*, ephedrine and methoxamine.

Ephedrine raises the blood pressure by increasing the output of the heart and by causing constriction of peripheral blood vessels. The first effect is predominant and a rise in heart rate is commonly seen that may be a problem in patients with pre-existing tachycardia, particularly atrial fibrillation. In this group of patients, therefore, methoxamine is a better choice because it causes mainly vasoconstriction, which tends to reduce the heart rate. Due to the fact that methoxamine reduces the blood flow to the placenta, the use of vasoconstrictors is contraindicated in obstetric anaesthesia and the treatment of choice is ephedrine.

The other drugs used commonly in anaesthesia for their cardiovascular effects are the anticholinergics. They have been discussed previously and are used in the treatment of low heart rates (bradycardias).

RESPIRATORY DRUGS

All general anaesthetic agents, but especially opioids, cause some degree of respiratory depression and may slow the return of spontaneous ventilation at the end of surgery. This is particularly true in elderly patients and those who have respiratory disease. In some cases, stimulation of ventilation can be produced by the drug *doxapram*. This short acting drug causes stimulation of the respiratory centre in the brain without reversing the analgesia provided by opioids. Its effects only last for 20–30 min, by which time the patient should have breathed out enough vapour for a further dose to be unnecessary. Because of non-specific stimulatory effects, it can, however, cause confusion and tachycardia and this makes it difficult to use in those with hypertension and pre-existing tachycardia.

Other respiratory drugs used in theatre tend to be for the treatment of bronchospasm: salbutamol, ipratropium and aminophylline. *Salbutamol* is a selective β_2 agonist. These are the β-receptors found mainly in the respiratory tract and their stimulation causes relaxation of the muscles in the walls of the bronchi, leading to relief of bronchospasm. The drug may be either administered intravenously, by inhalation, or nebulized. The latter is the commonest method used in theatre, usually in the recovery period. Its side effects include tremor, tachycardia and anxiety. Repeated use and intravenous use are more likely to produce these symptoms and may also lead to a lowering of the serum potassium concentration. The intravenous route is employed intraoperatively.

Ipratropium is an anticholinergic and again causes relaxation of muscles in the bronchi but does this by blocking acetylcholine receptors. It is administered by inhalation and nebulization, again mainly in the post operative period, but it can cause tachycardia and thickening of mucous secreted by the bronchi, making it more difficult for patients to expectorate.

Aminophylline causes bronchial muscle relaxation by blocking the enzyme phosphodiesterase in the muscles. It also causes some degree of respiratory stimulation through central nervous system effects and produces an increase in heart rate and blood pressure, by effects on the cardiovascular system. Aminophylline is given by slow intravenous injection and/or infusion, in order to treat bronchospasm intraoperatively. Its side effects include cardiac arrhythmias, nausea and vomiting and confusion.

SUMMARY

Although there are many drugs available to the anaesthetist, relatively few are in routine use. It is, however, important to know which drugs to use in the emergency situation and this is discussed fully in Chapter 26.

RECOMMENDED READING

British National Formulary.

Calvey TN, Williams NE 1997 Principles and practice of pharmacology for anaesthetists, 3rd edn: Blackwell Scientific, Oxford.

14

THE LOCAL ANAESTHETIC DRUGS: DOES THE IDEAL AGENT EXIST?

A. C. Skinner

Local anaesthetics (LA) are drugs that reversibly block the conduction of nerve impulses along nerve axons. Many drugs have some local anaesthetic properties and some drugs such as phenol, although they are not local anaesthetic agents, are used to block nerves permanently in the treatment of pain due to malignancy. This chapter is only concerned with drugs that are primarily used as local anaesthetics.

USES OF LOCAL ANAESTHETICS

1. As the only anaesthetic for surgery.
2. To supplement a general anaesthetic for surgery.
3. Postoperative pain relief.
4. The treatment of other acute pain, for example in obstetrics.
5. Other (unrelated) indications, for example lignocaine for control of cardiac arrhythmias.

HOW NERVES CONDUCT IMPULSES

Nerve cells consist of a cell body, which undertakes the metabolic activities needed to keep the cell alive, and axons (fibres) which sprout out from the cell and transmit the impulses from the source to the destination of that nerve's signals. Each axon carries a specific signal such as touch, heat, pain or a specific command, usually to part of a muscle or a viscus. The individual nerve axons are collected together into mixed nerves, which consist of sensory and motor nerve fibres. These run from the brain or spinal cord to all parts of the body.

Conduction of impulses along the axons is an electrical phenomenon. In a healthy person the extracellular fluid contains about 140 mmol/l of sodium (Na^+) ions and about 4.0 mmol/l of potassium (K^+) ions. Inside the cells these concentrations are approximately reversed and this means that there is a tendency for Na^+ ions to move into cells and K^+ ions to leak out, because each ion moves down its concentration gradient. This leakage is controlled by the permeability of the cell membrane. There are specialized channels in the membrane for each ion and ions are actively "pumped" against the concentration gradient. This pumping uses energy and expels Na^+ and takes in K^+ ions. The net result of this process, which is known as the Sodium Pump, is that the inside of the cell is about 90 mV negatively charged compared with the outside of the cell. The magnitude of this gradient is called the 'membrane potential'.

A nerve impulse spreads down the axon by reversing the membrane potential, from 90 mV negative inside to about 50 mV positive inside. This process is known as 'depolarization' and is achieved by opening Na^+ ion channels in the membrane and allowing Na^+ ions to flow in, making the inside more positive. The Na^+ channels in any part of the membrane open automatically when the voltage across that membrane falls to about 50 mV negative inside (referred to as the depolarization threshold) causing Na^+ ions to flood in down their concentration gradient, completing depolarization. Because of electrical conduction the depolarized cell membrane affects the adjacent membrane and by lowering the membrane potential to the depolarization threshold, it triggers off Na^+ channel opening in the membrane further down the nerve and thus propagates the impulse. Because membrane that has been depolarized cannot depolarize again for a short time (called the 'refractory period'), the axons effectively only pass impulses one way because the refractory membrane behind the impulse stops the impulse from propagating backwards.

The nerve recovers by opening K^+ channels (also voltage triggered) allowing K^+ ions to escape, taking positive charge out of the cell and reestablishing the resting (-90 mV) membrane potential.

This wave of depolarization spreading across the cell membrane of any excitable tissue is known as an 'action potential'. The pumping of Na^+ out of the cell and K^+ into the cell maintains overall a steady state despite the ion flows caused by the passage of action potentials.

Figure 14.1 shows an action potential passing down a nerve fibre. The voltage changes are shown above with the ionic events in the nerve below.

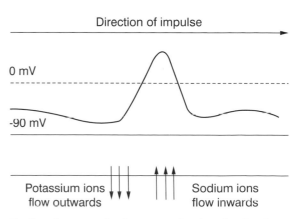

Sodium ions constantly pumped out and potassium ions in to maintain membrane potential

Figure 14.1   An action potential

HOW LOCAL ANAESTHETICS WORK

Local anaesthetics prevent the inward Na^+ ion flow that is triggered by depolarization of the adjacent membrane, probably by binding to the inner end of the sodium channels in the cell membrane. This stops the action potential being propagated. Small axons are blocked at lower concentrations of LA than large axons. Because pain axons are generally smaller than axons supplying the sensation of touch, local anaesthetics are often effective for the pain of surgery but leave the sensation of touch intact. This can be disconcerting if the patient is not warned beforehand.

Larger nerves need more concentrated LA to penetrate them adequately. Because of this, more concentrated LA (say, lignocaine 2% instead of 1%) is used for blocking large nerves than the dilute solution (lignocaine 0.5%) used for infiltration anaesthesia, where the nerves are the smaller terminal branches.

LAs block all types of nerve fibre unselectively and some of their adverse effects are due to blockade of fibres in addition to the fibres that the operator intended to block. These may be quite widespread because many tissues use the action potentials of their cell membranes to control their function. Good examples are

1. Hypotension after subarachnoid block due to blockade of sympathetic nerve fibres.
2. Leg weakness in women having an epidural for childbirth due to blockade of motor fibres.

Neurones in the brain are affected by sufficiently high doses of LA and the electrical activity of the heart depends on similar action potentials in the heart muscle, which can be affected by doses of LA (either deliberately or as a side effect).

GENERAL PROPERTIES OF LOCAL ANAESTHETICS

All LAs will block nerve impulses if they are injected close enough to a nerve in a sufficient dose. Failure to achieve a good block is usually due to an inadequate dose of LA or technical failure on the part of the operator. Some blocks are more reliable than others. For example, subarachnoid (spinal) and epidural blocks are much more reliable than plexus blocks.

LAs in common use today are all chemically 'amide' type compounds. They are absorbed from the site of administration and carried in the bloodstream to the liver where they are deactivated. Older drugs are chemically 'esters' and are metabolized by esterases in the blood.

TOXICITY OF LOCAL ANAESTHETICS

In normal doses LAs are very safe. The potential for toxicity depends on the dose injected, how quickly the drug is absorbed and the site and method of administration. Some sites show more rapid absorption than others and toxicity can be a problem if large doses are used at these sites. The addition of adrenaline to the LA will slow absorption and reduce this problem.

Accidental intravascular injection produces very high blood levels of LA very quickly and thus toxicity can be seen suddenly after small doses. When LA is used it is good practice to aspirate before injecting a large dose in one place to prevent inadvertent intravascular injection.

Toxicity is actually rare if the maximum safe dose is not exceeded and all users of the drug should know this. The common manifestations of toxicity are in the central nervous system and the heart.

CENTRAL NERVOUS SYSTEM TOXICITY

CNS toxicity precedes cardiovascular problems with most LA drugs. Large enough doses of LA would stop conduction of all nerve impulses in the brain but in practice inhibitory neurones are most sensitive to LA and this leaves excitatory effects unopposed. Thus, tremors and restlessness proceed to clonic convulsions resembling epilepsy and may be followed by respiratory failure and cardiovascular collapse. Treatment is with anticonvulsant, such as diazepam, and tracheal intubation and artificial ventilation if this is indicated.

CARDIOVASCULAR SYSTEM TOXICITY

Blood pressure can fall because CNS depression affects the vasomotor centre in the brainstem and there may be a direct effect on arteriolar smooth muscle but cardiac arrhythmias and depression of myocardial contractility are more serious complications. Lignocaine and a compound related to LAs, procainamide, are used to stabilize some abnormal heart rhythms. Other LAs, most notably bupivacaine, can produce arrhythmias at doses that do not cause marked CNS effects and bupivacaine-induced arrhythmias can be very difficult to treat and have caused fatalities. There is no specific treatment but this is the same as the more common causes of cardiac depression, arrhythmias and cardiac arrest. The cardiac effects of bupivacaine can be prolonged, needing resuscitation for a long period.

ALLERGIES

Allergy to modern amide LA is very rare. Patients who are allergic to one are likely to cross react to others.

THE IDEAL LOCAL ANAESTHETIC

LOW TOXICITY

Of the commonly used drugs, prilocaine is probably the least toxic but even prilocaine gets close to its maximum dose for some useful blocks, e.g. axillary plexus blocks. The propensity of bupivacaine to produce cardiac toxicity is particularly hazardous. Other drugs, such as lignocaine and prilocaine, tend to produce CNS toxicity (fitting) at a dose well below that which causes cardiac problems. Since fitting is relatively easy to treat this is a useful safety feature. Ropivacaine, a newer agent, has been specifically developed to be like bupivacaine but with a greater cardiac margin of safety.

Some agents have specific toxicity, such as prilocaine. Large doses can cause haemoglobin to be converted to methaemoglobin, which cannot carry oxygen. Lower overall toxicity would be useful but any new agent will certainly need a similar margin of safety to our current drugs if it is to become widely used.

RAPID, RELIABLE ONSET

This is an obvious requirement but, although lignocaine fulfils this, the other local anaesthetics are not as good from this point of view. Lignocaine is thought by many anaesthetists to diffuse more freely through tissues than the other drugs, resulting in a lower failure rate for blocks. Rapid onset means that the effectiveness (or not) of the block is quickly apparent. Bupivacaine has a slow onset and is thought by many to have a higher failure rate. Missed segments are probably more common in epidural blocks with bupivacaine than lignocaine. Prilocaine seems to be intermediate between lignocaine and bupivacaine.

In addition, the following properties are desirable if the LA is to be used as the sole anaesthetic for surgery.

GOOD MOTOR BLOCK TO PRODUCE MUSCLE RELAXATION

Many surgical procedures need motor blockade for muscular relaxation. Bupivacaine produces noticeably less good, though adequate, abdominal (and other muscular) relaxation than lignocaine.

DURATION OF ACTION LASTING A FEW HOURS

The length of action should be comfortably more than the expected duration of the procedure but not too long so that any adverse effects, e.g. lower limb paralysis after a subarachnoid block or hypotension from sympathetic block, wear off reasonably quickly.

NO SYMPATHETIC FIBRE BLOCKADE

This would avoid the hypotension that is the most troublesome common problem with subarachnoid and epidural blocks. The sympathetic fibres, which are involved in the maintenance of blood pressure by controlling the level of vasoconstriction in the blood vessels, are closely related in the spinal canal to the sensory and motor fibres. Since sympathetic fibres are so easy to block with LA it seems very unlikely that a drug which provides a good block for surgery and no sympathetic fibre block will become available. Lignocaine and bupivacaine are close to the ideal for surgery and the intelligent choice of either one will give good results in most cases. Prilocaine, being less toxic, is used for blocks needing a large dose of LA.

There are further requirements if the LA is to be used for postoperative analgesia.

MINIMAL MOTOR BLOCK, PREFERABLY SELECTIVE PAIN FIBRE BLOCK

Postoperatively motor block is undesirable. Patients like to be able to move their limbs normally, have the full force of their cough and feel in control of their body. Ideally, only pain fibres would be blocked in this context but this seems unlikely to be achievable in practice. Bupivacaine seems to produce less motor block than the other agents but still may cause significant muscle weakness. In an attempt to reduce the motor and sympathetic effects of subarachnoid or epidural blocks, the use of dilute LA combined with opioids and clonidine is becoming popular.

LONG DURATION OF ACTION

In only a few blocks can a catheter be introduced so that the block can be 'topped up'. A drug that lasts for a few days would thus be most advantageous, provided ways of using it without serious side effects (like motor block) could be found. Some very long-acting drugs have been investigated but the LA that can be infiltrated into a surgical wound and provide analgesia for a few days is not likely to be available for clinical use in the near future. Bupivacaine is somewhat unpredictable and has been known to last for up to 36–48 hours after a single administration.

Lack of sympathetic fibre block is also desirable, again to avoid hypotension.

TECHNIQUES OF LOCAL ANAESTHESIA

LOCAL INFILTRATION

The LA is given directly into the operative site. This is technically easy but large areas require many injections and the maximum permitted dose of LA may be reached before adequate analgesia is obtainable.

SINGLE NERVE BLOCKS

Only a few nerves supply the area and LA is injected close to these nerves, producing a large area of anaesthesia with a proportionately small number of injections and a lower dose of LA. Examples are digital nerve blocks for surgery on a finger or femoral nerve block for the pain of a femoral fracture.

PLEXUS BLOCK

The nerves supplying an area of the body run together for part of their course. Nerve fibres from different nerve roots may leave or join the main nerve trunks in the same way as railway lines do as they approach a station. These 'junctions' in the nerve network are known as plexuses and an injection at this site can produce a large area of anaesthesia. Axillary block, for example, is used to provide analgesia for forearm surgery. Plexus blocks often require a high dose of LA at high concentration and a detailed knowledge of anatomy is required if the block is to be effective.

FIELD BLOCK

A combination of nerve blocks and infiltration is known as a field block and is used, for example, to provide pain relief in surgery for inguinal hernia repair.

INTRAVENOUS REGIONAL (BIER'S) BLOCK

A limb is isolated by a tourniquet after draining out some of the blood and dilute LA is introduced into a vein in that limb, from where it gains entry to the nerves via their venous drainage. It is important that the tourniquet is reliable or a toxic dose of LA may leak into the general circulation. In order to minimize ischaemic pain a double cuff tourniquet is often used. The more distal cuff is inflated after the block is effective, after which time the proximal cuff is deflated.

SUBARACHNOID (SPINAL) BLOCK

LA is injected into the cerebrospinal fluid surrounding the lower spinal nerves. Because these nerves supply large areas of the lower body widespread analgesia is obtained with only a low dose of LA.

EPIDURAL BLOCK

LA is injected in between the two membranes covering the spinal cord. A larger dose of LA is needed than for subarachnoid block but a catheter may be used for repeated injections to prolong ('top up') the block. Technically they are more difficult to introduce than subarachnoid block and epidural blocks often require a high dose of LA at a high concentration.

TOPICAL ADMINISTRATION

This involves applying LA to mucous membranes and the conjunctiva and is achieved by spraying the pharynx or larynx, introducing eyedrops or using packs or probes soaked in LA in the nasal cavity. The nose has a very good blood supply and, in patients with allergic rhinitis the use of nasal LA-soaked packs may cause toxic side effects. This is because of the speed at which the LA is absorbed.

DRUGS USED FOR LOCAL ANAESTHESIA

Table 14.1 shows the local anaesthetic drugs in common use. LAs are available in various strengths; generally the more concentrated the LA, the bigger the nerve it will block and the longer it will last. The total dose of any LA is limited by toxicity, primarily in the brain and heart, so the most dilute LA that will suffice should be used.

Some LAs are used with added adrenaline (epinephrine). This slows down absorption from the site of injection, which prolongs the anaesthesia and increases the safe maximum dose. Others are absorbed slowly and the addition of adrenaline makes no worthwhile difference.

Table 14.1 Local anaesthetic drugs in common use						
Drug	Potency	Onset	Duration	Dose in mg/kg		Common trade name in UK
				Plain	Adrenaline	
Lignocaine	1	Rapid	Short	3	7	Xylocaine
Bupivacaine	4	Slow	Long	2	2	Marcain
Prilocaine	1	Slow	Short	4	8	Citanest

LIGNOCAINE

Lignocaine is often used when the operation is to be done purely with LA. It has a rapid onset, lasts between 60 and 120 minutes and produces a high-quality block. This is because it is thought to spread through body tissues freely. The rapid, reliable block and useful duration of action make lignocaine the drug of choice in many circumstances.

PRILOCAINE

This agent has a less rapid onset and is probably less reliable than lignocaine but higher doses are safe as it is rapidly metabolized. For this reason it is the drug of choice for intravenous regional anaesthesia where failure of the tourniquet may cause toxic effects. Large doses can cause haemoglobin to be converted to methaemoglobin that cannot carry oxygen. This can be important in the unfit or anaemic patient. Duration of action and potency are comparable to lignocaine.

BUPIVACAINE

Bupivacaine has a slow onset but lasts considerably longer than lignocaine, up to eight hours in some cases, and is thus used for longer procedures and for postoperative analgesia. It produces less motor block than lignocaine but the reason for this is unclear. It is about four times more potent than lignocaine and is more cardiotoxic than other LAs. It is the only drug commercially available for subarachnoid blocks in the UK.

ROPIVACAINE

This is a new drug that is similar to bupivacaine but less cardiotoxic. The extent to which ropivacaine will come into common use is not clear at the time of writing but it may well replace bupivacaine in the future.

COCAINE

Cocaine is only used for topical anaesthesia of the nose. It is a marked vasoconstrictor and reduces bleeding and shrinks the nasal mucosa. The combination of cocaine and adrenaline was popular for this use but may produce dangerous hypertension. It is controlled under the Medicines Act.

AMETHOCAINE

Amethocaine is used almost exclusively as eyedrops.

CONTRAINDICATIONS TO LOCAL ANAESTHETICS

ALLERGY TO THE LOCAL ANAESTHETIC

Known allergy to a particular LA is the only absolute contraindication to its use.

PATIENT CHOICE

Patients should be able to choose whether surgery is performed solely under LA unless there are specific medical reasons why this should be so. This is also a cultural issue and patients on mainland Europe often expect to have operations under LA.

CONFUSED PATIENTS OR CHILDREN

Patients who are unable to cooperate or children may not be able to understand the need to keep still and they may be frightened. Such patients will benefit from LA techniques as a supplement to postoperative analgesia.

TIME OF PROCEDURE

In practice, many common procedures take too long for LA to be the sole technique and some require an uncomfortable position. Careful use of sedation may help if there is a strong case for using LA.

TYPE OF LOCAL ANAESTHETIC PROCEDURE

There are specific contraindications to most types of regional anaesthetic techniques but the ability to perform the block in that particular patient must always be considered. In addition, the success rate of the procedure must be weighed against the need to succeed and against manageable alternatives.

MEDICAL PROBLEMS

LA techniques should not always be seen as an alternative to general anaesthesia in patients with medical problems. In some cases the medical condition means that LA is not a safe or desirable option. Coagulation problems contraindicate some techniques, such as subarachnoid or epidural blocks, because of bleeding locally. The sympathetic block produced by sub-

arachnoid or epidural blocks precludes their use in patients who are already hypotensive or hypovolaemic or who would tolerate hypotension badly should it develop.

INFECTION

Infection near the site of the injection usually contraindicates LA, either because of spreading the infection or because local infection reduces the effectiveness of LA.

LAs can form a useful part of the anaesthetist's armamentarium. Complex blocks are usually done by anaesthetists rather than surgeons because the blocks have side effects, such as hypotension, which need managing and because treating toxicity, though it is rare, needs the specific skills of an anaesthetist. In addition, the normal need for a skilled practitioner to look after the patient during the operation remains. The surgeon often manages smaller blocks and local infiltration because the risks are then very modest.

15

THE SAFE POSITIONING OF PATIENTS FOR SURGERY

S. Collins & A. Davey

INTRODUCTION

Prior to the introduction of anaesthesia in the 19th century, patients were positioned for surgery on their beds, wooden tables, an operating chair or any hard surface that was available. They were then tied down or held in position by the surgeon's assistants so that surgery could be quickly completed but there was little attention to the rights or dignity of the patient.

Good practice in patient positioning is an essential factor in promoting and safeguarding the well-being of patients in the perioperative period and is achieved through the collaboration of the multidisciplinary health-care team. The acquisition of knowledge and the development of skills, effective communication and team work all contribute to the prevention of complications, avoidance of accidents and the reduction of risks associated with this task. Appropriate and well-designed training programmes play a vital role in this process but clinical practice must also be updated and reviewed regularly in order to maintain currency in the constantly developing fields of anaesthesia and surgery. The resultant quality service, which meets patients' expectations, should be measured against processes such as risk management and clinical audit.

Ideally, preoperative assessment should identify individual needs and potential problems which, recorded in the plan of care and communicated verbally, will focus the team's action plan. Positioning is essentially a team activity but requires an experienced coordinator and this role is most naturally and frequently filled by the anaesthetist. However, if more complicated arrangements such as those involving an operating microscope are indicated, it is usual for the surgeon also to be involved.

Lifting and handling manoeuvres should never be attempted unless there are sufficient personnel present, possessing both the skills and strength required for safe practice.

THE AIMS OF SAFE PATIENT POSITIONING

Warren (1983), and Ignatavicius and Bayne (1991) have described the principal aims that are designed to achieve:

1. Physiological alignment.
2. Minimal interference with circulation.
3. Protection of skeletal and neuromuscular structures.
4. Optimum exposure to operative and anaesthetic sites.
5. Patient comfort and safety.
6. Patient dignity.
7. Stability and security in position.

PHYSIOLOGICAL ALIGNMENT

There are a number of factors that affect the physiological alignment of every individual and these include age, size, gender, general condition, nutritional status and the existence of deformity, disease or injury. This is particularly important if limbs, joints or the spine are involved and the information may be used to modify the way that the patient is positioned, thus reducing risk and increasing patient safety

MINIMAL INTERFERENCE WITH CIRCULATION

It is essential to maintain adequate tissue perfusion at all times. The extremities can be especially at risk in certain positions and stasis or restriction from pressure must be avoided in order to diminish the likelihood of venous thrombosis, potential embolus formation and the potential development of pressure sores.

The use of external pneumatic compression apparatus ('boots') and the adoption of the 'lawn chair' position (this involves slight flexion at knee and hip, thus distributing support more evenly and providing a more 'natural' position) will tend to ameliorate these potential problems. Particular care needs to be exercised with the handling and positioning of patients who have swollen ankles or fragile skin due to existing cardiovascular disease, e.g. varicose eczema and patients receiving corticosteroid therapy. Similarly, special attention is needed for patients whose peripheral circulation is compromised.

In addition, there will be physiological changes as a direct consequence of the final position of the patient. Examples include the Supine Hypotensive Syndrome in pregnant patients and the way ventilation, perfusion and airway pressures vary in the Trendelenburg position. Similarly, patients who have a fixed cardiac output will not tolerate rapid movement into the sitting position and may become hypotensive. This includes patients with valvular heart disease and those who are dehydrated and/or hypovolaemic. A working knowledge of physiology will therefore enable the practitioner not only to predict these changes, but also to compensate for them.

A *pressure sore* is an area of cellular damage occurring in a localized site subjected to unrelieved pressure, e.g.

skin and subcutaneous tissue may be compressed between a bony prominence and a hard surface such as an operating table or piece of equipment. Contributing factors may be intrinsic or extrinsic. Intrinsic factors relate to the condition of the patient and include the state of nutrition and hydration, whilst extrinsic factors include pressure and friction shearing forces. Pressure sores occur when intrinsic and extrinsic factors combine. This is most likely to occur in patients who are elderly, dehydrated or debilitated because the cardiac output is decreased and perfusion is easily compromised. Although this process may begin in theatre it may not become apparent until the patient returns to the ward. It is, however, a very real risk for patients undergoing prolonged surgery and may result in added pain and discomfort for the individual and constitute a drain on the hospital's resources.

Awareness of the risk factors should influence the practice of all those involved with the positioning of patients, thus ensuring that pressure points are recognized and risk is minimized by the use of appropriate aids, e.g. gel or foam pads and the liberal use of gauze padding. Patients may well complain of discomfort resulting from minor pressure areas, such as a catheter mount pressing on the forehead or a sore angle of the mouth because of pressure from an endotracheal tube. In a similar way, minor eye problems due to pressure or rubbing may easily be prevented by suitable protection. Shearing and friction forces may be reduced through the application of recognized moving and handling techniques and the effective use of transfer devices such as rollers and slides.

PROTECTION OF MUSCULOSKELETAL AND NEUROMUSCULAR STRUCTURES

Nerves are extremely vulnerable to damage produced by traction, pressure or untoward joint movements. In 1964, Britt and Gordon discovered that only 30 – 40 minutes in an unfavourable position would be enough to produce nerve damage in an anaesthetized patient. Measures used to protect against potential injury may themselves predispose to damage, e.g. when ankles are supported on foam pads to relieve calf pressure, the unnatural hyperextension of the knee joint may lead to pain from trauma to the ligaments of the knee. Similarly, the normal lumbosacral curvature of the spine may need support with a wedge or pillow, especially if the patient has a history of backache. The above would certainly be unacceptable to an awake patient for any length of time and perhaps this should be used as a good guide to the protective measures advocated for patients who are anaesthetized. Whilst it

is obvious that the restricted joint movements of arthritic patients and the special needs of amputees require additional attention, it should be remembered that positioning aids, e.g. compression from overtight safety straps, may constitute a very real hazard. Constant vigilance from the whole clinical team is therefore most important.

OPTIMUM EXPOSURE TO ANAESTHETIC/OPERATIVE SITE

The setting up of monitoring equipment, anaesthetic induction and the establishment of infusions are usually achieved in the relatively secluded atmosphere of the anaesthetic room prior to entry into the operating theatre, but must take into account the final position of the patient and the operation site. Positioning may be completed in the anaesthetic room or after transfer to theatre.

Transfer to the operating theatre and onto the operating table should be a coordinated, swift and smooth process effected through the interaction of members of the theatre team. Final adjustments to the position are then made, adhering to all protective and preventive protocols and if there is any doubt surgical confirmation should be obtained prior to skin preparation and draping. Anaesthetic access to areas such as the airway or the intravenous route will vary according to the operation site and may involve the use of circuit and intravenous extensions but once the anaesthetist is satisfied with the position of all necessary equipment the operation can proceed.

The position of the diathermy equipment will depend on the site of operation and the use of tourniquets, image intensifiers, microscopes, endoscopy equipment and lasers all demand specific access arrangements.

PATIENT COMFORT AND SAFETY

Almost everything said elsewhere in this chapter could be reiterated here but we will only deal with topics that have not been mentioned before.

Although the majority of patients are anaesthetized there are a significant number of individuals who have their operation performed under local anaesthesia. Under these circumstances it is essential that the patient is aware that their comfort and safety is of prime importance to the theatre team. A member of the team should be allocated solely to look after the patient's well-being and the theatre team should be reminded prior to the patient entering theatre that the procedure is under local anaesthesia, because it is very easy to forget that the patient is conscious.

Temperature regulation is needed to ensure that the patient is comfortable prior to induction of anaesthesia or if the operation is to be performed under local anaesthesia. Of prime importance in patient safety is the maintenance of body temperature and this requires varying levels of intervention depending on such factors as age, general condition, cardiovascular status and length and type of procedure. Thus the neonate, elderly, severely burned and vascularly compromised patients may demand a range of adjustments varying from extra insulation (in the form of additional wrapping or space blankets) to raising the theatre's ambient temperature several degrees. This is fully discussed in Chapter 19.

PATIENT DIGNITY

The maintenance of dignity at this time, when the patient may be most vulnerable, is inextricably bound up with awareness of the role of the practitioner as advocate and with ethical issues centring on patients' rights, choices and beliefs. In addition, there must be an understanding of the needs and requirements of anaesthetic and surgical procedures.

The creation of an environment which supports and respects human values at physical and psychological levels throughout the perioperative episode of care is too complex a matter to be addressed here. Issues, however, include such simple actions as minimizing the exposure of the patient during and after positioning and the attitude of respect for the individual and the acknowledgement of his/her rights and values shown by team members involved in this process. They should also be sensitive to the appropriateness of their speech, interactions and behaviour. Whilst it may seem easy and natural to behave in a suitable manner in the presence of a conscious patient, the anaesthetized patient should not be expected to surrender rights, beliefs and choices along with his/her loss of consciousness.

STABILITY AND SECURITY

The overriding directive for all care professionals is that the patient should come to no harm and the twin objectives of stability and security are vital components of safety during the perioperative period. This is especially relevant during and immediately following positioning on the operating table and during postoperative transport from the operating table to the recovery area.

The effect of position on patient stability is discussed below but may be enhanced by the use of operating table accessories, supports, pillows and straps. Mattresses, pillows or pads from which air may be evacuated offer an effective method of secure fixation.

These positioning aids consist of heavy-duty plastic, airtight bags containing polystyrene granules and air may be sucked out or let in through a valve. When filled with air the appliance is soft and malleable but when air is removed it becomes firm and immobile. Once position is established there is no tendency to slide, with pressure on the skin being evenly distributed. They are especially advantageous for maintaining positions that are difficult to sustain and for lengthy procedures.

TABLES AND MATTRESSES

Preparation of the operating theatre includes selection of the appropriate operating table and accessories from the wide and sophisticated range now available to cater for specific situations. However, certain basic features apply to all and are relevant to safe patient positioning.

The solid steel base or fixed pedestal supports a top, which is divided into four sections, namely the head, upper trunk and lower trunk and leg sections. The head and leg sections may be detachable and interchangeable.

Hydraulic controls or hand-operated levers are used to select and effect the various positions by raising or lowering, tilting laterally or tipping the head or foot end. The full range of table movements should be checked prior to the start of each operating list and any faults identified should be managed according to agreed protocols, including the removal of the operating table from service. Health and Safety at Work legislation requires documented evidence of regular service contracts for all operating tables, thus promoting a proactive approach to risk management.

Before the patient arrives in the operating room it is imperative that an appropriate selection of all ancillary equipment, together with any fixing clamps, is assembled, tested and prepared for use.

The sectional mattresses are manufactured with a sponge base covered in antistatic, non-slip rubber material. The foam should be at least 2 inches thick and smooth rather than ribbed to avoid tissue damage in ischaemic skin conditions. Sections must be completely bonded with all joints sealed and the covering intact in order to minimize the risk of cross-infection and to ensure complete electrical insulation.

SUPINE POSITION

Supine patients lie on their back in a horizontal position. Nearly all patients arrive in theatre and are anaesthetized in this posture and it is the most common position for subsequent surgery. The patient's head is supported on a pillow or head ring and he/she can generally lie comfortably though patients with acute or chronic respiratory disease may experience dyspnoea when lying flat and may need to be raised on pillows into a more comfortable position. Manipulation and access are relatively straightforward. The arms may be positioned by the side of the patient, across the chest or abducted and supported on armboards.

In order to prevent the supine hypotensive syndrome occurring during the operative delivery of pregnant patients, about 20° of right-sided tilt may be added to the supine position, thus removing the pressure of the pregnant uterus from the inferior vena cava.

PHYSIOLOGICAL CHANGES

In the supine position the ventilation:perfusion ratio is greatest in the dependent parts of both lungs.

HAZARDS

Aspiration of stomach contents is a risk in the supine position and precautions, e.g. rapid sequence induction, should always be used if regurgitation is likely.

Nerve damage is usually related to undue pressure or traction during or after the patient is positioned. Brachial plexus damage is usually caused by hyperextension of the arm and the angle between the body and arm should never exceed 90°. The hand is usually pronated, if possible with the head turned towards the extended arm to reduce tension on the nerve roots. It is very easy for the surgeon to abduct the arm while operating and the anaesthetist should constantly be aware of this potential complication.

The brachial plexus and capsules of the shoulder joint are also at risk should the arms be allowed to fall off the table or trolley. Arm restraints should therefore always be in position before the patient is anaesthetized.

The radial nerve, which winds around the humerus, can be easily damaged by pressure from table attachments such as a screen support, while the ulnar nerve, due to its position at the elbow, may be damaged by compression on a mattress edge.

Pressure from inadequately padded catheter mounts and nasal endotracheal tubes may traumatize the supraorbital nerve and the facial nerve is vulnerable to pressure from an excessively tight facemask harness or fixing tape.

The eyes need protection from dehydration and rubbing and from contamination with splashes of lotions, body fluids or aerosols. They may easily be taped to prevent opening but if the operation is on the face protective ointment is better and unless there is a specific indication, an antibiotic-containing ointment should not be used. There is, however, always the possibility of an allergy to the ointment.

It has already been mentioned that care must be taken not to allow prolonged hyperextension of the knee joints. The legs should be uncrossed in order to minimize the occurrence of deep vein thrombosis, the incidence of which may be reduced by the use of heparin or external pneumatic compression.

The sacral and occipital regions must be well padded to guard against the development of pressure areas.

TRENDELENBURG POSITION

Generally, there is a head-down tilt of between 35 and 40° in this position but a more moderate 20° is useful to reduce venous drainage in the legs, thus decreasing blood loss, e.g. varicose vein surgery. The legs remain fully extended and may be 'spread' onto a double armboard to facilitate access to the inner aspect of the legs.

This position takes advantage of gravity by allowing the more mobile parts of bowel to move out of the pelvic cavity, thus improving access for surgery on the pelvic organs. It is therefore the preferred position for many gynaecological procedures. The knees are flexed over the lower break of the operating table and the lower section is angled towards the horizontal position. This prevents the patient slipping towards the head end of the table and a well-secured, non-slip mattress further helps this. Shoulder supports are not recommended due to the vulnerability of the brachial plexus.

PHYSIOLOGICAL CHANGES

Although there are surgical advantages in this position there are definite anaesthetic disadvantages. The level of the carina may be displaced towards the head of the patient and may lead to the endotracheal tube entering the right main bronchus.

Movement of the abdominal contents towards the diaphragm increases the pressure inside the abdomen and decreases the compliance of the lungs. This makes ventilation more difficult and a much greater intrathoracic pressure is needed to produce a similar tidal volume. Morbidly obese patients are an extreme example of this and it may not be possible to adequately ventilate these patients in the head-down position, the preferred position being head-up tilt. Generally speaking if the operation is likely to last a long time or if there is any concern about the patient's respiratory system, muscle relaxation and IPPV should be the preferred anaesthetic technique.

Ventilation:perfusion ratios are best at the apices, which is the reverse of the normal upright posture.

Venous return from the lower limbs is increased in the head-down position and elevation of the legs is the best method of compensating for unexpected hypotension. The haemodynamic effects of this position may present added difficulties in patients with cardiovascular problems or when hypotensive techniques are employed.

HAZARDS

The tendency to downward slippage is the main concern and the adverse cardiovascular changes have been described above.

ANTI (REVERSE) TRENDELENBURG

This position is utilized for neurosurgery and surgery of the head and neck, including thyroidectomy, plastic surgery and middle ear surgery. It decreases bleeding by promoting venous drainage away from the operating site. The sitting position may be regarded as an extreme form of anti-Trendelenburg. If there is a danger that the patient may slip down the operating table the lower half of the table should be moved into the horizontal to prevent this. The arms should be supported either on armboards or by the side of the patient.

PHYSIOLOGICAL CHANGES

Ventilation:perfusion ratios follow roughly the same pattern as the normal sitting patient and the steeper the head-up tilt, the more this is realised. Unfortunately venous return is easily compromised and moderate to severe hypotension may occur in patients who are dehydrated, or hypovolaemic or who have a fixed cardiac output.

Ventilation of the lungs is much easier and slight to moderate head-up tilt is very useful in obese patients, but hyperventilation may further decrease the venous return.

HAZARDS

Perfusion of the brain and vital organs must be maintained. Because the brain is higher than the heart and limbs the perfusion pressure of the brain is lower than that of the recorded blood pressure. This means that severe hypotension may have a significant effect on the blood flow to the brain, possibly leading to ischaemic damage. Hypotension may be minimized by gradually changing the position of the patient. In addition, preloading the circulation is often useful. Parasympathetic blocking agents such as atropine will increase the pulse rate and help to maintain the cardiac output. Unfortunately, they also increase bleeding and should only be used if the advantages outweigh the disadvantage of a very bloody surgical field.

Because the venous pressure is low it is easy for air to be entrained into the circulation. Air embolism is a major problem in neurosurgery performed in the sitting position, especially if the surgery involves the cerebral sinuses. Air entrainment is detected using a Doppler probe placed over the heart.

POSITION FOR KNEE SURGERY

The supine position is established and the lower section of the table is dropped or removed altogether, enabling the knees to be flexed. The knee to be operated on is slightly raised by a pad placed under the thigh. With the introduction of arthroscopic surgery the use of this position has decreased.

POSITIONING FOR THE INTERNAL FIXATION OF HIP FRACTURES

The orthopaedic 'traction' table has a perineal post and adjustable leg extension pieces, both of which pose their own problems and positioning is very much a team approach with emphasis on patient security and stability. These are frequently exacerbated by the frailty of the patient.

The demands of traction and abduction of the affected limb and of access to allow for outer posterior and lateral radiography during the procedure are combined with the very real danger of an unguarded and possibly frail patient's pelvis slipping from the sacral support during positioning, pre- or postoperatively. It is essential that the perineal post is well padded and the sacrum, heels and genitalia require special protection.

The perineal post is positioned toward the unaffected limb and in contact with the symphysis pubis, in order to limit the chances of damage to the pudendal nerve when manipulating the fracture prior to the fixation of the feet within the boots. During positioning it is very easy to damage the skin of the patient by excessive skin traction. The leg extension pieces are then adjusted to provide both the maintained reduction of the fracture and the abduction of the legs, to permit movement of the image intensifier arm. Care should be taken not to abduct the affected limb beyond 20 or 30° so that there is no angulation at the fracture site.

LITHOTOMY POSITION

The name of the position originates from the Greek word for stone, because this was the position used to 'cut for the stone' (bladder) through the perineum. Widely used for gynaecological and genitourinary surgery it can be modified to permit combined access to the abdomen and perineum for laparoscopic and anorectal procedures.

The patient is placed supine on the operating table, after which the knees and hips are flexed, abducted and externally rotated to allow the legs to be placed in slings suspended from vertically padded poles attached to the operating table at hip level. When the legs are safely positioned the lower sections of the table are removed (the foot end may be lowered or removed) and this permits the upper section to slide downwards, thus bringing the patient closer to the operating surgeon.

PHYSIOLOGICAL CHANGES

The physiological changes in this and the other modified lithotomy positions are all variations of the changes that occur in the supine and head-down positions.

HAZARDS

It is important that the presence of arthritis and the range of movement of the hips and knees is known beforehand and any pre-existing back problems should also be identified. Arthritic disease may necessitate that the position of the leg stirrups is modified or that their use is abandoned altogether. The lower limbs must be raised and lowered simultaneously because strains in the sacroiliac, hip and knee joints are a constant threat in even healthy patients. At least two assistants are required to raise or lower the limbs.

If the table has no downward sliding mechanism and the patient must be slid downwards, the cervical spine must be protected from the sudden loss of head support.

The arms should be secured across the patient's chest and supported with padded arm retainers because there is an increased danger of contact with metal or the risk of trapping the fingers if they are kept at the sides. One arm may be extended on an arm board if this required by the anaesthetist. The use of a wedge or pillow to support the lumbosacral curve will reduce the risk of postoperative backache, which can be exacerbated by flexion of the hips.

Stretching of the sciatic nerve may be caused by too upright a position of the thighs, overvigorous rotation of the hip joints or by an assistant leaning on the patient. The peroneal and saphenous nerves may become compressed against the lithotomy poles and are also vulnerable to pressure from the surgical assistant. The poles must therefore be well padded and the theatre staff must be vigilant, especially during long procedures.

Although the lithotomy poles are padded throughout their length it is almost inevitable that there will be a degree of pressure on the long saphenous vein. Careful positioning should minimize this risk but prophylaxis for DVT should also be considered.

LITHOTOMY WITH TRENDELENBURG

Lithotomy with Trendelenburg is commonly used for surgery where access to both the abdomen and vagina is required. The degree of head-down tilt should be sufficient to allow the abdominal organs to fall away from the pelvic cavity. Inflation gas should be allowed to escape completely before levelling the table in order to minimize the postoperative discomfort that results from the gas irritating the diaphragm.

LLOYD DAVIES LITHOTOMY AND TRENDELENBURG

This position is most frequently used in the synchronous combined approach for abdominoperineal resection of rectum, during which two teams of surgeons need simultaneous access to the lower abdomen and perineum. This is achieved by abducting the thighs with only slight flexion of the knees and hips. Lloyd-Davies stirrups support the lower limbs and cradle the calves, holding them in one of a range of available positions made possible by their multi-jointed construction. The limbs, placed in the well-padded calf supports, are held in place by bandages.

THE LATERAL POSITION

As the name implies. the patient lies on the right or left side with the lower limbs flexed and the uppermost arm elevated in an armrest. Unless an evacuatable mattress is available an ischial support, a hip strap, footrests and several pillows are needed to maintain the position. The position is used for renal, pulmonary and some neurosurgical interventions, which tend to be both lengthy and complex procedures, but is also useful for superficial operations on the back.

During renal surgery the table must also be 'broken' over the flank and each section tilted at a 20° angle, thus facilitating the surgeon's access to the extraperitoneal space.

Achievement of the lateral position demands at least three experienced and able assistants to move the patient's chest, pelvis and legs, as well as the anaesthetist who is controlling the head and neck and coordinating the process. Coordination is particularly important and it is essential to decide in which direction the patient is to be turned before commencing the manoeuvre.

PHYSIOLOGICAL CHANGES

The optimum ventilation:perfusion ratio occurs in the lower lung with the upper being less perfused but better ventilated.

HAZARDS

Until patients are fully supported they are potentially unstable and may easily roll to one side, or because they are quite close to the edge of the table, even fall off onto the floor. It is therefore important to ensure that a member of the team stands close to the patient to prevent this happening. A pillow should be placed between the legs in order to prevent the development of pressure areas. The lower ear may also be subjected to pressure or bent back on itself during the positioning process. The head should therefore be placed on a pillow or a well-padded head ring. Cervical spine problems may be exacerbated during rotation of the patient.

If the head support is allowed to 'drop' relative to the position of the upper shoulder, the brachial plexus on this side may be put under strain. The upper arm is usually supported in a cradle-like armrest, which must be well padded because the radial nerve may become compressed against its edge and the lower arm should be positioned in such a way as to minimize venous congestion.

Soft padding should be used under the lower iliac crest so that pressure sores can be prevented and the skin of the uppermost hip must be protected from chafing by the hip strap.

THE PRONE POSITION

Together with the knee-elbow, the face-down or prone position is potentially the most hazardous to set up. It is used for spinal surgery, excision of pilonidal sinuses and where access to the tissues of the back is needed.

Pillows or padded support are essential for the head, chest, pelvis and legs and these should be positioned before the patient is turned. Although only one pillow is usually needed for pelvic support, the number of pillows required under the chest will depend on the size of the patient. The aim of the exercise is to allow the head to remain in a more or less neutral position because this is the most comfortable. Larger (or fatter) patients will therefore need more pillows.

The anaesthetist is always responsible for the care of the head, face and airway and must make sure that the eyes are adequately protected. In addition, it is useful to insert a large mouthpack to absorb any secretions that are produced.

A team of four, under the supervision of the anaesthetist, is required. The team members must possess the skills, strength and knowledge to perform the task and to avoid harm to the patient and to themselves. It is useful to attach the patient to a ventilator before the patient is moved. This frees the anaesthetist for the manoeuvre and ensures that the patient is adequately ventilated. Three of the assistants stand on one side of the table, taking responsibility for the chest and arms, pelvis and lower limbs, while the fourth pushes the patient, firstly into the lateral position and then onto the waiting arms of the three assistants. At the same time the anaesthetist rotates the head ensuring that it is kept in the same position in relation to the rest of the body. In order to facilitate this move, the anaesthetist may first lower the head of the table. The patient is then gently laid on the pillows and the adequacy of the supports confirmed so that the abdomen is relatively free from compression. Access for head and neck surgery may demand that the arms be positioned by the sides, in which case they must then be supported by well-padded arm restraints. Usually, however, they are extended on either side of the patient's head in a natural sleeping position. An armboard fitted under the mattress of the table head section may support the position of the arms.

PHYSIOLOGICAL CHANGES

In this position the anterior portions of the lungs have the better ventilation:perfusion ratios. Pressure on the abdomen may cause venous congestion in the great veins, which in turn may result in increased venous and capillary bleeding.

HAZARDS

There is a danger of damage to the cervical cord through hyperextension of the cervical spine, especially during turning and in patients with cervical arthritis. The radial nerve may be traumatized if the arm is allowed to hang over the edge of the table. In this position the ulnar nerve must be protected from compression by the edge of the mattress.

Excessive and inappropriate movements of the shoulder may lead to dislocation in susceptible individuals. The judicious placement of pillows or pads will protect the anterior superior iliac spines, the knees, feet and toes while chest pillows must allow for lateral displacement of the breasts in the female patient.

THE KNEE-ELBOW OR MOHAMMEDAN PRAYING POSITION

This position is used for spinal surgery and the manoeuvre begins in the same way as described for the prone position. Once in the prone posture, the patient's pelvis is lifted and the legs are moved into the kneeling position. This tends to push the patient up the table towards the anaesthetist and the best way to counteract this movement is for the anaesthetist to use an arm placed in front of the patient's shoulder as a pillar. The foot part of the table is then removed so that the feet, resting on pads, hang over the end of the table. A pillow, secured by a strap, is then put over the calves and the knees are moved as near the edge of the table as possible. Once this has been done, the patient and the

supporting pillows are moved down the table so that the patient rests on the knees. The legs, arms and feet are carefully padded so that they are not touching metal and, finally, the abdomen is again checked to ensure that it is not compressed and the table is adjusted to make the back horizontal.

The physiological changes are generally the same as for the prone position.

HAZARDS

These also are very similar to the prone position but it is important to make sure that the feet are not hyperextended, i.e. they are free to hang over the edge of the table and not touching metal. The knees should be well padded and must not be allowed sink into the gap between the two parts of the mattress.

The knee-chest or Mohammedan praying position has now been largely superseded by a development, which involves the use of a frame supporting the ischial tuberosities, the chest and the head.

SUMMARY

The positioning of patients for surgery is a potentially hazardous procedure, but with good teamwork, a sound knowledge of the patient's pre-existing pathology and an awareness of the anaesthetic and surgical goals it may be accomplished both safely and efficiently.

RECOMMENDED READING

Ignatavicius DD, Bayne MV. Interventions for interoperative clients. Medical/Surgical Nursing, 19, 454–471.

Warren MC. The circulatory nurse. Operating Theatre Nursing, 11, 76–80.

16

PRINCIPLES INVOLVED IN THE MANAGEMENT AND USE OF EQUIPMENT

M. Greenall

INTRODUCTION

The management of equipment in the operating department is a demanding task that should involve both the medical and non-medical members of the theatre team. If operating theatres are to be run in a safe and efficient manner, management structures must include the policies and protocols needed for the day-to-day management of equipment as well as long-term strategies.

Equipment is constantly introduced into hospitals for a variety of reasons, such as new equipment replacing that which is old and worn out, the development of new technology and, of course, the new devices that improve our working lives. Manufacturing companies may promote them as being more user friendly, time saving, cost efficient or safer but the theatre user must become familiar with all equipment and learn how to use it safely and wisely.

The introduction of equipment to a hospital is a complicated process and involves many different groups of people, i.e. the manufacturers, engineers, servicing departments, repair specialists, departments within the hospital and the individual user. It is for this reason that adherence to clearly defined policies, procedures and guidance within the theatre environment is so important. This chapter attempts to show how all these strands can be drawn together in order to provide a safe and efficient theatre service. I will also discuss some of the potential hazards that may occur when equipment is used, with particular reference to the diathermy.

MANAGING THE USE OF EQUIPMENT

WHAT IS MEDICAL EQUIPMENT?

Medical equipment is equipment intended to diagnose, treat or monitor the patient under medical supervision and which makes physical contact with the patient or conveys energy to or receives energy from the patient. The type of protection that equipment provides against electric shock is classified as follows:

- Class 1 equipment relies on protective earthing mechanisms.
- Class 2 equipment relies on sturdy insulation.
- Internally powered equipment is classified separately.

DESIGN OF MEDICAL EQUIPMENT AND THE MANAGEMENT OF RISK

Medical equipment must not only be safe to use but also inherently safe. Although this chapter primarily deals with the management and use of equipment, it is important to have a basic understanding of how medical equipment has evolved in terms of safety. When anaesthetic machines were first introduced, it was not possible to accurately control the concentration of anaesthetic vapour that the patient received and even today many anaesthetic machines are incapable of preventing the delivery of a hypoxic mixture of gases to the patient.

In order to minimize risk and make apparatus produced by different manufacturers interchangeable a series of quality standards were introduced that included the pin-index system, colour coding for gas cylinders and requirements for electrical safety. The International Standard ISO 5358 was first published in 1980. This has now been adopted by many countries or, in the case of the United Kingdom and the United States of America, has been incorporated into the national standard. Most ventilators, anaesthetic machines and monitors conform to the electrical and safety requirements of the International Electrical Commission (IEC) standard IEC 601–1, which is identical to the British Standard BS5724. In broad terms, it ensures that equipment remains safe even if one safety component has failed.

Within anaesthetic practice, the greatest danger to patients arises from hypoxia, over- or underdose of anaesthetic, over- or underventilation, barotrauma, burns and electrocution. All of these have been addressed in new technology by active systems and machine alarms but in the final event, the safety of the machine depends on the user and the way that it is checked before each use. This subject has been discussed in Chapter 10. All electrical equipment must satisfy the requirements of IEC 601–1 and specially trained medical physicists or engineers must test it before it is used on patients.

AN APPROACH TO ELECTRICITY AT WORK REGULATIONS

Portable appliances

All portable electrical appliances are registered, tested and labelled to this effect. An approved contractor will carry out all testing. Employees are made aware of the requirements and are obliged to report any equipment that is not correctly certified, together with any damaged or faulty equipment.

Permanently wired equipment

All work on mains electricity will be undertaken by a qualified and approved contractor, who will operate under a permit to work, which will be issued by the Health and Safety Manager.

All contractors, patients, visitors, and employees that bring portable electrical equipment into the hospital must comply with items above.

THE MEDICAL ENGINEERING DEPARTMENT

The medical engineering department (MED) or, as it is sometimes known, the electrical biomedical engineering department (EBME) is responsible for organizing the maintenance and scheduled servicing of trust equipment as well as the purchasing of new equipment and the loaning of devices from suppliers. In addition, it is often involved in the purchasing negotiations that are ongoing throughout the hospital. Some of the more complicated and specialized medical devices, e.g. autoclaves and CAT scanners, require specialist engineers to service and maintain them and this involves external companies and agencies working closely with the EBME department, sometimes as a joint servicing exercise.

Both surgeons and anaesthetists rely on complex equipment to provide a safe and effective service to the patient. Between 10% and 14% of all accidents in the theatre environment are due to problems with equipment, whether this is due to human error or equipment failure. It is very important to properly manage this risk and regular maintenance that is carried out on time, according to clearly defined protocols, plays a major part. (If patients are injured as a result of a critical incident, the service record of any equipment involved is one of the first things to be scrutinized.) Thus, it can be seen that the coordinating function of this often hard-pressed and underresourced department plays an essential part in patient safety.

ACCEPTANCE PROCEDURE FOR NEW AND LOANED EQUIPMENT

A formalized acceptance protocol is needed to ensure that every item of equipment that enters the hospital is logged and can be controlled by the equipment management system. Characteristically, the procedure takes the form of an initial inspection that includes an exhaustive safety check (including an electrical safety check if this is indicated). The equipment is then given a specific identity number.

Although the exact way that this is done varies between hospitals the number, e.g. TH107, usually consists of two parts. In this example, 'TH' refers to the department, i.e. theatre, and '107' is the unique

equipment identity number within the theatre department. In this way, every item of hospital equipment can be identified and entered into an *asset register*, which includes its purchasing price, current value and its proposed date of replacement.

COMMISSIONING OF EQUIPMENT

While the acceptance procedure is being undertaken, other safety checks are carried out to ensure that there is no damage to the apparatus, e.g. damage in transit leading to the integrity of the appliance being compromised. The piece of equipment is then entered into the *equipment inventory*, which is often the same document as the asset register. It contains a complete record of the service history and maintenance schedules, together with details of any reported faults and repairs. In this way, common faults or frequent breakdowns can be acted upon to ensure that changes can be implemented to improve the in-service life of the equipment.

Commissioning of equipment is normally arranged by the EBME/MED in conjunction with the supplier, if appropriate, and should include:

- A comprehensive function test to ensure that the apparatus is working properly.
- A demonstration of how to operate the device and prepare it for use.

This demonstration should ideally involve the supplier and all relevant personnel. It may be necessary to organize further training sessions to include other staff who may be asked to operate the apparatus. Once again, this is a risk management issue designed to ensure safe operating practice.

MODIFICATION OF EXISTING EQUIPMENT

Equipment may be modified to improve performance or safety and this course of action often follows the publication of a safety action bulletin or hazard warning notice. The manufacturer or the Medical Devices Agency (MDA) issues these notices to warn of possible danger, so that preventive action can be taken at the earliest opportunity. If there is a need to modify equipment during its repair or service, the authorization of the manufacturer should be sought, together with an agreement as to who would be the most appropriate to perform the task. Following any modification to existing or new equipment or after the introduction of new practice techniques, training courses must be organized in order to update all users.

It is important to understand that equipment that is modified by the hospital and subsequently exported to an outside agency is classed as a manufactured product.

The hospital must register with the MDA and must comply with its rules governing such issues. Only approved experts can carry out the work. (This does not only apply to equipment but to prostheses and prescribed drugs and solutions that are made up in hospital pharmacies.)

MEDICAL DEVICES AGENCY

The Medical Devices Agency is responsible for the safety and quality of all medical devices used throughout the UK. There is an enormous range of equipment for which the agency is responsible, from a complex piece of equipment such as a ventilator used in an ITU unit to a syringe used to give medicine to a child.

The success of the MDA is dependent on good communication between manufacturers, doctors, nurses, clinicians and other professional health-care workers who provide relevant information about devices. In this way, safety aspects can be improved constantly, ensuring that quality and safety are maintained at a high standard.

If, within a department, an adverse incident takes place that causes potential injury or harm to patients or staff, the Adverse Incident Centre (AIC) is the first point of contact. First, the incident or the faulty device should be reported to the appropriate department within the MDA. An investigation may have to take place involving the manufacturer, the person who reported the incident and the medical device specialist who was appointed to investigate the incident.

If the case proves to be high risk, urgent or extremely dangerous, a *hazard warning notice* will be published. This will allow appropriate action to be taken immediately to deal with the problem and/or to ensure that all necessary measures are taken to make safe all similar devices.

The *safety notice* is issued in less urgent situations and requires users to be aware of a danger whilst using a device, thus avoiding a repeat of the incident.

A *device bulletin* is issued to inform of general guidelines in the use and management of a device.

Serious problems are fortunately very rare when compared to the number of devices used on a daily basis throughout the UK. This indicates how well the system works but safety often depends on the individuals who are using the equipment, so be clear about your position in maintaining a safe environment.

THE USE OF EQUIPMENT WITHIN THE CLINICAL ENVIRONMENT

DECONTAMINATION OF EQUIPMENT

Equipment must be cleaned and decontaminated prior to its service, repair, inspection or transportation. This is essential in order to protect those individuals who are working with or who may come into contact with that item of equipment. It is the legal right of these workers not to be exposed to any form of risk from infected or contaminated equipment.

The Health and Safety at Work Act (1974) states that:

> a written safety policy should be provided to ensure that procedures carried out by hospital staff, representatives of suppliers, recipients of items that are involved in repair, inspection, and transport are protected and not placed at risk by exposure to contaminated or infected apparatus.

A safe system of working must be implemented so that individuals are able to provide such a service and a responsible person should be nominated to deal with such issues as training, documentation and other necessary legislative requirements. This person is known as the Safety Officer. Ignoring the Act may lead to prosecution.

Legislation dealing with the Control of Substances Hazardous to Health (COSHH) provides further regulations, which apply to both chemical and biological hazards.

The Management of Health and Safety at Work Act (1992) states that there should be cooperation between employers, any contractors and any other staff involved. They should share clear communication in health and safety matters associated with transfer of material or equipment.

There may be occasions when it is not prudent to decontaminate equipment or materials, as may be the case in an investigation into equipment failure or into an incident that causes injury to patients or staff. Decontaminating under these circumstances may alter key factors that are necessary for a complete investigation. However, a few steps may be taken to ensure that the recipient is aware of the state of equipment prior to inspection, including:

- *a warning by label* to inform the user of the hazard prior to opening the package;
- the inner package should not be able to contaminate the outer package;
- the packaging should be strong enough to withstand handling during transport from sender to receiver;

- the provision of information to the recipient about the status of equipment. A Declaration of Contamination Status should travel with the item and this should contain relevant information to inform of contamination. A typical format is illustrated in Figure 16.1.

EQUIPMENT BREAKDOWN OR FAILURE

If an item of equipment breaks down or ceases to function properly, a protocol for removal of faulty equipment must be implemented in order to ensure that neither staff nor patients can be harmed or injured due to the faulty apparatus.

A responsible person must be notified as to the condition of equipment, giving them necessary information as to what happened or how it came to be noticed. The apparatus should be taken out of use and a 'Faulty Equipment' sticker or tag should be attached to the equipment where it can be seen clearly. The appropriate department should then be contacted so that provision can be made to have the equipment repaired or replaced. EBME/MED or the supplier should provide a replacement as soon as possible so

that the smooth running of the department is not compromised. Replacement and service/repair times are usually included in the service agreement with the supplier or EBME/MED and must be realistic. Knowledge of these times is essential so that users of the equipment may reschedule lists or obtain a replacement from an alternative source.

THE MANAGEMENT OF ADVERSE INCIDENTS ASSOCIATED WITH EQUIPMENT

If an incident occurs that involves equipment, an incident form should be completed. If the event caused harm or had the potential to cause harm or injury to personnel or patients, an investigation must be implemented to establish the sequence of events and the possible cause. In the first instance, EBME/MED should be informed and if sufficiently serious, the MDA should be notified, together with the manufacturer of the apparatus and this could lead to the initiation of a hazard warning. It is also important to establish how the apparatus was being used at the

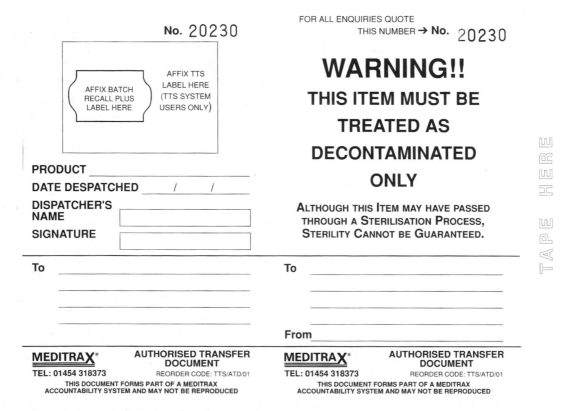

Figure 16.1   Declaration of Contamination Status

time of the incident. (Training may have to be implemented for staff to ensure that operators are not using poor technique.) Sometimes incidents result from failure to follow instructions or to switch on and properly use the built-in alarm systems, both of which may have implications for the trust's insurers.

In the event of a serious incident or fatality occurring within the theatre department, it is essential that the correct procedure is strictly adhered to. The following example is intended as a guide to show how local policies and procedures are used to protect the parties involved.

- The item of equipment must be isolated and immediately withdrawn from service.
- The item should not be tampered with in any way prior to investigation.
- Emergency services may have to be called.
- Any spilled materials should be dealt with appropriately.
- Witness statements should be obtained.
- Opinions as to how the incident occurred should not be voiced.
- Any item of evidence that may have contributed towards the incident should be retained for inspection.
- Maintenance and service records must be made available for inspection.
- If the incident resulted in a fatality, *the body must not be disturbed in any way*, i.e. endotracheal tubes, cannulae, infusions, ECG electrodes, etc. must all be left *in situ*.
- The trust's insurers must be informed.

Following an incident of this nature, both the medical and non-medical staff involved will be under great emotional stress. It is important that they receive full and sympathetic support and this may include formal counselling.

THE ELECTROSURGICAL GENERATOR/DIATHERMY UNIT

Diathermy and the electrosurgical unit are now an integral part of most modern surgical techniques. In the 16th century William Gilbert, a physician to Elizabeth I, conducted experiments that used electricity and magnetism and earned him the title 'the father of electrotherapy'. During the early part of the 19th century a physicist called Becquerel demonstrated the principle of electrocautery, by passing electricity through a needle which subsequently became heated, to produce a controllable source of heat coagulation. However, the development of modern electrosurgical

units that use high-frequency current can be attributed to the work carried out by Darsonoval in 1891. He discovered that frequencies of 20 kHz and greater could be passed through the body without causing an electrical shock, with only heat being generated to the tissues. This principle is used to great effect in electrosurgical units in current use.

All personnel using an electrosurgical unit should be trained and familiar with its working principles. If this is not the case very serious injuries may occur. It is therefore necessary to understand the theory and properties of electricity relevant to electrosurgery.

PROPERTIES OF ELECTRICITY

Current is the flow of electrons between two points during a period of time. The larger the current, the more electrons are moving and flow is expressed in a unit called the ampere (A).

Voltage is the force that pushes the current through the circuit and is measured in volt (v).

Resistance is the restriction to the flow of electrons and is measured in ohm (Ω). As a result of this restriction, heat is produced at the point of the circuit that offers resistance.

A circuit is the pathway that electricity uses to travel from a source of generation to its destination. It must be continuous and will eventually return to earth by the intended circuit or by any other available pathway.

Current density produces the heating effect that is used in electrosurgery. The current flows through the circuit to the patient at the same rate as it is flowing from the patient to the electrosurgical unit. The current, however, is concentrated at the narrow diathermy point and thus the current density is greater here than anywhere else in the circuit (Fig. 16.2). As a result, heat is generated at the tip and it is this heat that cuts tissue or coagulates bleeding points.

The reverse happens at the site of the earth plate. Here, the surface area is very large and thus the current can leak to earth without generating heat. If the patient earth plate becomes loose or detached or its surface area is reduced, the current also becomes concentrated at the site of the plate, resulting in an increase in current density that may lead to a burn at this site. Any compromise to the patient earth system may result in an increase in current density. *Remember! Energy always takes the easiest way out.*

Other sites that may be affected by current density are digits and appendages, such as fingers, toes, the penis and the base of pedicle flaps. The former may result in

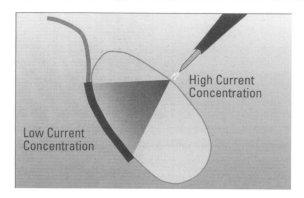

Figure 16.2   Current concentration/density (reproduced from *Electrosurgery Self-Study Guide*, courtesy of Valleylab Inc., Boulder, Colorado)

a burn to the thumb or, if the current density is sufficiently high, coagulate the blood vessels of the digit, resulting in avascular necrosis. Burns may also occur when the current returns to earth by an alternative route other than through the earth plate. Examples include ECG electrode sites through a monitor and if the patient is touching metal.

MONOPOLAR DIATHERMY

This electrosurgical apparatus is the most common form used in the operating department; it is both versatile and effective for most types of surgery (Fig. 16.3). The circuit consists of:

- The electrosurgical generator.
- An active electrode.

- The patient.
- A patient return electrode.

BIPOLAR DIATHERMY

Bipolar diathermy is very useful for smaller procedures that do not require the versatility of monopolar diathermy; neither does it require an earthing plate. It may also be used on digits and extremities.

The circuit comprises:

- An electrosurgical generator.
- A double-lumen lead.
- The patient's tissue.

The double lumen lead carries the current to one of the tips of the forceps and returns it via the other, with the tissue that is between the forceps now forming part of the circuit. Because tissue does offer resistance to current flow, the heat that is generated results in coagulation of the blood vessels (Fig. 16.4).

COAGULATION AND CUTTING WAVEFORMS

Electrosurgical generators are capable of producing different waveforms to achieve different outcomes that are relevant to the type of surgery being performed. Normally this is pure cutting or coagulation but there are other waveform types used during electrosurgery that are helpful to the surgeon. These are known as *blend waveforms* (usually 1, 2, and 3). They are not a mixture of the cut and coagulation waveforms but are interruptions in a waveform cycle to produce different effects; heat produced rapidly causes vaporization of tissue while heat produced slowly causes more of a coagulum (Fig. 16.5).

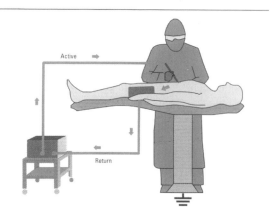

Figure 16.3   Monopolar circuit (reproduced from *Electrosurgery Self-Study Guide*, courtesy of Valleylab Inc., Boulder, Colorado)

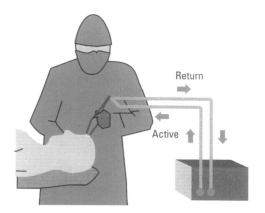

Figure 16.4   Bipolar circuit (reproduced from *Electrosurgery Self-Study Guide*, courtesy of Valleylab Inc., Boulder, Colorado)

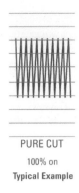

PURE CUT

100% on

Typical Example

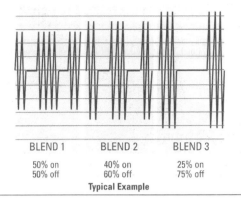

BLEND 1	BLEND 2	BLEND 3
50% on	40% on	25% on
50% off	60% off	75% off

Typical Example

Figure 16.5   (A) Cut waveform. (B) Blended waveforms (reproduced from *Electrosurgery Self-Study Guide*, courtesy of Valleylab Inc., Boulder, Colorado)

RETURN ELECTRODE

The importance of the return electrode is often underestimated and severe burns can result with poor positioning of the return electrode or if good earthing plate contact is not achieved. A suitable site for attachment must always be considered carefully because the earthing plate is part of the circuit and we have already established that any resistance to current flow produces heat. The site selected for the earthing plate must take into account the following considerations.

- The position of the patient on the operating table.
- The need to select a well-vascularized area, close to the operation site.
- Excessive skin will reduce the contact area of the earthing plate.
- Bony prominences may reduce blood flow to the skin, resulting in poor electrical conductivity.

Most of the reported accidents involving electrosurgical units could have been prevented if more attention had been paid to the common causes, including earthing plates, damage to the insulation coatings, 'sharps' injury involving the active electrode and ensuring that the patient is not touching metal. The latter may easily occur during the positioning of the patient on the operating table. Once again, making sure that all theatre staff are trained and familiar with the electrosurgical unit before using it may reduce accidents.

BASIC ELECTRICAL SAFETY

The human body may be thought of as an electrical system, with nerves carrying signals back and forth between the brain and the body organs. The main effects on the body may be neuromuscular (involving sensory and motor nerves and muscle contraction) or due to physical heating of the tissues.

NEUROMUSCULAR EFFECTS

The effects on the body vary greatly, depending on the density, frequency and duration of the current as well as the condition of patient, e.g. dry skin may offer some protection against electrocution. This is illustrated below by considering the effects of different current strengths on the body when 50 Hz (mains power) is passed between the hands.

1 mA	Perception
10 mA	Cannot let go of the electrical contacts
100 mA	Severe pain, interference to heart and chest function
1 A	Ventricular fibrillation and death

HEATING EFFECTS

High currents passing through the body would cause tissue heating, the extent of which depends on the current density and resistance to current flow. Thus, small contact areas and a high skin resistance would cause heating, leading to tissue necrosis. This is in effect the same as that achieved when using the diathermy for coagulation and/or cutting.

MACROSHOCK AND MICROSHOCK

Macroshock refers to shock or electrocution due to a large current passing through the skin, a portion of which may pass through the heart.

Microshock describes the passage of a small electrical current, which is applied in close proximity or directly to the heart.

The frequency band most likely to affect tissues is between 40 and 60 Hz but this is also the frequency of most domestic and industrial power supplies. The route that the current takes through the body will also determine whether or not the heart is affected.

Circuit breakers are used in domestic and industrial power supplies. When the circuit breaker detects the leakage of a small current, e.g. 30 mA, the power supply is interrupted. Unfortunately, this method is not always suitable in the clinical environment because it may interrupt the power supply of equipment on the same circuit. Thus patients connected to electrical equipment are isolated from earth potential using a device known as an isolation transformer.

In summary, electrical safety is of paramount importance in the modern operating theatre environment. Accidents will always occur but the frequency of such events may be minimized by the user being familiar with the equipment and by strict adherence to health and safety protocols.

RECOMMENDED READING

International Electrical Commission 1988 Safety of medical electrical equipment IEC 601-1, 2nd edn. IEC

17

UNDERSTANDING SUTURE MATERIALS

M. H. Scott

INTRODUCTION

Put most simplistically, operative surgery consists of nothing more than cutting the body's tissues and subsequently sewing them back together again. Therefore to the uninitiated it probably seems that the whole issue of suture materials is simple to understand. There are, however, probably few surgical subjects that generate as much heated debate as the 'correct' use of the 'appropriate' suture in a particular clinical situation. All surgeons have their own opinions as to the ideal suture material for each situation but sadly this is a decision that is often based on habit, tradition or whim. Surgeons thus empirically find the suture material which best suits them. Therefore different surgeons will often use quite different materials and dimensions of sutures for the same purpose. With increasing knowledge about the physical properties of different suture materials and the tissue reactions to these materials, it becomes increasingly clear that for a given purpose one suture or type of suture is often far more suitable than others are.

The purpose of this chapter is therefore to guide the reader through the suture options available, whilst outlining some of the reasons why the diffuse variety of sutures and needles needs to exist.

THE HISTORY OF SUTURE MATERIALS

The use of thread for wound closure and for ligature is described in the literature as far back as 2000 BC. Since then a great many materials have been used for these purposes, including dried gut, dried tendon, strips of hide, horsehair, women's hair, bark fibres and textile fibres of various kinds. The Greeks were leaders in the field of medicine and the Romans later adopted their techniques. Galen, in the second century AD, used silk and harp cord for ligatures as well as strands of animal intestine to close the wounds of Roman gladiators. In the 10th century Rhazes is credited with being the first to stitch abdominal wounds with harp strings made from spun strands cut from animal intestines.

Before the introduction of antisepsis the use of sutures and ligatures presented great problems since their application almost invariably resulted in infection. Pus formation and secondary haemorrhage were therefore common complications. The introduction of antisepsis by Lister in 1867 resulted in a considerable improvement in the infection rate. A further important step came with Lister's promotion of the chrome treatment of catgut in order to delay its absorption in

tissues and thus contribute to longer lasting strength of sutures and ligatures. When Claudius introduced sterilization of suture materials using potassium iodide in 1902, the rate of infection was further decreased. As time went by other methods of sterilization were discovered and currently, suture materials are sterilized with ionizing radiation or with ethylene oxide.

Until the 1930s the suture materials used in surgery were predominantly catgut and silk and, to a lesser degree, linen and cotton. Steel wire came into use around 1932 and synthetic fibres were introduced on a large scale during and after World War II, starting with nylon in 1941. Soon after this, a large number of suture materials with various physical and biological properties flooded the market. Generally speaking, the synthetic fibres made their appearances first in the textile market and their use as suture materials came as a secondary offshoot.

MODERN SUTURES

One only has to walk into any modern operating theatre to appreciate the huge number of sutures that are kept as routine stock for operative surgery. With so many sutures currently available, it is essential that the reader understands the differences in the structure and properties of the sutures.

In order to simplify the matter somewhat, sutures can be considered as:

1. absorbable or non-absorbable;
2. synthetic or natural;
3. monofilament or polyfilament.

Figure 17.1 helps to clarify this classification.

ABSORBABLE VERSUS NON-ABSORBABLE SUTURES

Probably the most important distinction between sutures is those that are absorbable and those that are non-absorbable. The commonly used absorbable materials are catgut, polyglycolic acid (Dexon), polyglactic acid (Vicryl), polydioxanone (PDS) and polyglyconate (Maxon). Materials other than these are accordingly non-absorbable. Non-absorbable materials do lose strength after implantation in the tissues but to such a small extent that it is of no practical importance. Compared to other non-absorbable materials, silk loses its strength comparatively quickly when buried in tissues.

Various enzymatic processes break down absorbable materials after implantation in the tissues. They first

		Absorbable	Non-Absorbable
N A T U R A L	Monofilament	Cat Gut – Plain – Chromic	Wire
	Braided		Silk Cotton Linen Wire
S Y N T H E T I C	Monofilament	Polydioxanone (PDS) Polyglyconate (Maxon)	Nylon (Ethilon/Dermalon) Polypropylene (Prolene/Surgilene)
	Braided	Polyglycolic Acid (Dexon) Polyglactic Acid (Vicryl)	Polyester (Ticron/Dacron) Nylon (Nurilon)

Figure 17.1   Suture materials and their characteristics (typical brand names in brackets).

lose strength and then gradually disappear from the tissues. A distinction must be made between the time it takes for the suture material to completely disappear and the time that the material maintains its strength, because it can remain in the tissues long after it has lost

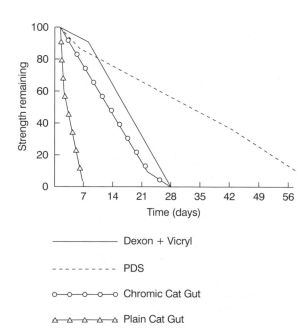

Figure 17.2   Strength of suture materials.

its strength. Although the absorption rate of suture material is of importance in respect of late suture complications, such as suture granuloma and sinus formation, the rate at which the material loses its strength is of greater interest to the surgeon. Generally speaking, the strength of catgut is maintained for little more than a week, that of Dexon and Vicryl for two weeks and PDS and Maxon for considerably longer (see Fig. 17.2).

The strength of catgut declines even more quickly in the presence of infection but this is not generally true of the synthetic absorbable sutures. Absorbable sutures are often used in the skin to avoid the need for removal, typically in children, circumcisions and scrotal operations. Due to the inflammatory response they provoke, absorbable skin sutures generally give a poorer cosmetic result.

Because the non-absorbable sutures retain their strength indefinitely they are used when a repair will take a long time to reach full strength (e.g. abdominal wall closure). Non-absorbable sutures are widely used for skin closure as they often give the best cosmetic results and are most easily and painlessly removed.

NATURAL VERSUS SYNTHETIC MATERIALS

Catgut has been around in some form or another for thousands of years and despite its history, it is still one of the most widely used suture materials. It consists mainly of collagen and is made from the dried small bowel mucosa of sheep or the serosa of cattle intestine. Silk and linen also have a long and distinguished history but their use is declining. Many surgeons believe that silk has the best handling and knotting properties of any material but, unfortunately, the strong inflammatory response it provokes is exceeded only by linen. Silk is mainly used for skin sutures, where its softness means there are no sharp ends to irritate the nearby skin. This is particularly important for operations involving the mouth and the perineum.

In general, natural materials are much cheaper than their synthetic counterparts which, of course, is a matter of importance in underdeveloped countries. The more modern synthetic suture materials are, however, becoming rapidly more popular than the older natural ones. They provoke little or no inflammatory reaction and can be scientifically designed to meet the specific requirements of absorbability, duration of strength and handling.

MONOFILAMENT VERSUS POLYFILAMENT SUTURES

Monofilament materials have an extremely smooth surface and can therefore be pulled through the tissues with minimal friction. This makes them easier to insert and remove than polyfilament or braided materials. Conversely, monofilament materials are stiff, springy and more difficult to knot. Although braided materials have better handling qualities, the interstices between the braids provide a haven for bacteria. This problem is partly overcome by the manufacturers applying surface coatings to the braid.

GAUGE OF SUTURE MATERIAL

The traditional method of describing suture gauge is confusing for the newcomer and derives from the time when sutures were much thicker than those used today. The finest suture then was designated 'gauge 1' with 'gauge 2' and upward applying to heavier sutures. As finer and finer sutures came into use, the scale had to be taken progressively backwards from 1, i.e. gauges O, OO (also known as 2/0), OOO (3/O) and so on. Nowadays the finest suture available is 11/0, which tends to be used for extremely delicate surgery such as in the eye. A more rational metric gauge based on suture diameter is in use but the traditional gauging method is still more widely used and understood.

The gauge of suture chosen for a particular task depends largely on practical experience. This takes into account several of the following factors:

1. Strength of repair required.
2. Type of suture material being used. For a given gauge, the various materials have different strengths; catgut is the weakest.
3. Cosmetic requirements. Multiple fine sutures give a better result than fewer heavier sutures.
4. Delicacy of the tissues. Paediatric tissues require finer sutures than adult tissues.

A simple guide to the use of different sutures in different situations is shown in Figure 17.3.

NEEDLES

For every kind of suture material, there are many different types of needles available. Until approximately 20 years ago suture material had to be threaded onto a needle but the industrial technique of swaging of needles onto suture material now almost entirely obviates the need for threaded needles.

SITE	FUNCTION	MATERIAL	SIZE
SKIN - FACE - LIMB ABDOMEN	WOUND CLOSURE	SILK / NYLON NYLON / PROLENE NYLON / PROLENE	5 / 0 or 6 / 0 3 / 0 or 4 / 0 2 / 0
ABDOMINAL WALL (SHEATH)	CLOSURE	PDS MAXON NYLON	GAUGE 1 GAUGE 1 GAUGE 1
GASTRO INTESTINAL TRACT	ANASTOMOSIS	VICRYL CHROMIC CATGUT PDS / MAXON NURILON	2 / 0 2 / 0 2 / 0 3 / 0
ARTERIES	ANASTOMOSIS	PROLENE	2 / 0 to 7 / 0 DEPENDING ON SIZE OF VESSEL

Figure 17.3 Guide to sutures commonly used in various situations.

Generally speaking, suture needles are either straight or curved. The degree of curvature varies up to 5/8ths of a circle, as does the length of circumference. Needles are supplied in lengths from approximately 4 to 60mm depending on the individual requirements.

SHAPE OF NEEDLE

Straight needles tend to be used for skin suturing or applying sutures to wound drains.

Curved half circle needles are used for most purposes, quarter circle for microvascular anastomoses and three-quarter circle for the hand closure of abdominal walls (see Fig. 17.4).

LENGTH OF NEEDLE

The length of the needle varies according to the required depth of penetration and delicacy of surgery.

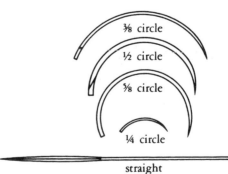

Figure 17.4   Types of suture needles

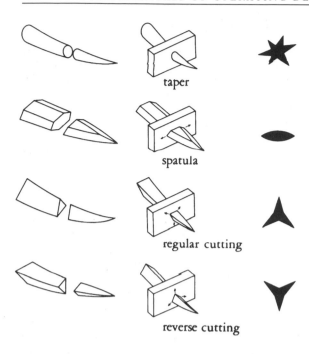

Figure 17.5   Tissue penetration characteristics.

TYPES OF NEEDLE	USAGE
HAND HELD	SKIN CLOSURE
INSTRUMENT HELD	UNIVERSAL
STRAIGHT	SKIN CLOSURE
CURVED 1/2 CIRCLE	MOST PURPOSES
1/4 CIRCLE	FINE VASCULAR PROCEDURES
" J SHAPED "	DIFFICULT CAVITY CLOSURES (FEMORAL HERNIAS)
ROUND BODIED (TAPER)	MOST SOFT TISSUES GUT / FAT / FINE FASCIA
CUTTING	TOUGHER TISSUES (SKIN / SHEATH / BREAST)

Figure 17.6   Usage of different types of needles.

TISSUE PENETRATION CHARACTERISTICS

The cross-sectional shape of the needle varies depending on its required function. Round-bodied needles with pointed tips tend to be used in soft delicate tissues, needles with an angular cross-sectional shape are known as cutting needles and are used for tougher materials (see Fig. 17.5).

Figure 17.6 demonstrates the difference in types of needles and their usage.

PRACTICAL USAGE OF SUTURES

As mentioned at the start of this chapter, all surgeons have their own personal preferences of suture material, size of suture and needle type. In reality, there is no 'right' and 'wrong' suture but it will be apparent that certain suture materials are more suitable for particular applications than others. For example, strong non-absorbable sutures on a large cutting needle are eminently more suitable for abdominal wall closure than a thin, rapidly absorbable, small-needled suture. The converse is true in closing more delicate wounds.

STAPLES AND CLIPS

Some of the traditional duties of sutures and ligatures are now being usurped by the use of mechanically inserted clips and staples. Whilst these are not technically sutures, it seems appropriate to briefly mention them in this chapter.

CLIPS

Simple occlusive-style clips have been developed to take the place of tie ligatures. They can be inserted in conventional surgery or at laparoscopic procedures. They are usually made of stainless steel but are also produced in titanium alloys and from absorbable materials. The clips are either loaded singly into a non-disposable applicating forceps instrument (often known as 'liga' clips) or may be contained in a disposable 'multifire' device. The advantages of these types of clips are that inaccessible structures may be more easily occluded and time can be saved. They may, however, be dislodged after application and therefore manipulation of the clipped tissues immediately after insertion should be kept to a minimum. Patients should be warned when metallic clips are inserted because they may cause problems if patients ever require certain type of X-rays (e.g. magnetic resonance imaging).

STAPLES

The most common surgical use of staples is in skin closure. When this method of closure was first developed the clips were applied singly using non-disposable instruments. Gradually automatic disposable multifire applicators were introduced although initially these were extremely expensive. Nowadays, many companies manufacture disposable clip applicators, which retail for similar prices to skin sutures. Skin staples are quick, easy to insert and remove and leave very cosmetically acceptable scars.

SPECIALIZED STAPLING DEVICES

A number of stapling devices with specialized functions have been developed over the last 15–20 years. Generally speaking, these are manufactured by one of two companies, Ethicon and Autosuture. The specialized staplers fall into three groups.

Linear staplers

Examples of linear staplers include the TL30, TL60 (manufactured by Ethicon) and TA30, TA55 and TA90 (produced by Autosuture).

When fired, these staplers leave two parallel rows of staples. They are usually used to occlude gastrointestinal tract structures (e.g. stomach, small bowel or colon) but can be adapted for use with large vessels and bronchi.

Linear staplers that also cut

TLC55, 75, 90 (Ethicon) and GIA 60, 90 (Autosuture) are examples. These instruments place two double staggered rows of staples in the tissue and in the same operation divide the tissues between these pairs of staggered rows. The instrument was initially employed to form side-to-side intestinal anastomoses with serosal opposition. It is now used for resection as well as for other forms of anastomosis.

Circular cutting staplers

The circular cutting stapler – CDH (Ethicon) and CEEA (Autosuture) – is sometimes known as an end-to-end anastomosis gun. It was first developed in the Soviet Union in the 1950s and, when it first came to this country, was known as 'the Russian gun'. In the early 1960s the instrument was introduced into the United States. Through research and development, primarily by the US Surgical Corporation (Autosuture), the instrument was refined to its current state.

EEA instruments are tubular devices, employed for end-to-end and end-to-side minimally inverting anastomoses. The ends of the bowel to be anastomosed are secured with pursestring sutures about a central rod, the device is tightened, central rings of tissue are stamped out by a circular knife and the staples are applied in an encircling anastomosis. These instruments come with a variety of diameters so that they can be used in different parts of the gastrointestinal tract. This particular type of stapling device has become most popular in oesophageal and rectal anastomoses, with some documented reports of superiority of these anastomoses over their sutured counterparts.

Although some surgeons now prefer to use a stapler for their routine anastomoses because it saves time in the operating theatre, it still represents an expensive way to perform the procedure. Therefore many surgeons still use the conventional methods of anastomosis as described earlier in this chapter.

CONCLUSION

The further development of sutures continues apace. On the whole, these do tend to be synthetic absorbable sutures, which have been developed for specific circumstances.

With a general understanding of the nature of suture materials, it is hoped that the reader will be better equipped to deal with the everyday demands of the surgical profession!

18

FUNDAMENTALS OF PAEDIATRIC SURGERY AND ANAESTHESIA

P. D. Booker

It is easy to appreciate that a newborn baby is markedly dissimilar to the mature adult. Babies are not just small in size but have different body proportions and react to their environment differently, not only compared with adults but also with older children. Many of the fundamental dissimilarities between neonate and adult are understandable when one considers that the newborn has had suddenly to switch from intra- to extrauterine life, and some of the mechanisms whereby this is achieved may persist into early infancy. However, even older infants and children should not be classified as small adults as the growth and development of many organ systems is not in proportion to the change in the child's overall size. This differential anatomical and physiological development leads to ever-changing responses to the environment and to therapy throughout childhood.

DEVELOPMENTAL ANATOMY AND PHYSIOLOGY

THE CENTRAL NERVOUS SYSTEM

The intact skull is less rigid in infants than in adults so that expansion of the fontanelles (spaces that occur at the junction of some of the skull bones) and separation of the bony suture lines can accommodate small increases in the volume of its contents. Fontanelle pressure reflects intracranial pressure (ICP) and has been used to show, for instance, that awake intubation of neonates can lead to large rises in ICP. Infants have a relatively large brain and by two years of age, the brain has reached 80% of its adult mass. Neuronal development is almost complete by 28–30 weeks gestation and term neonates can perceive pain, identify their mother and react to various stimuli with complex behaviour patterns.

THE CARDIOVASCULAR SYSTEM

The neonatal heart has about half the amount of contractile tissue and more supporting tissue than in the adult heart and this results in relatively stiff ventricles which cannot easily increase the amount of blood they pump out with each beat (stroke volume). Thus an adequate heart rate is particularly important in babies because their cardiac output (CO) is so rate dependent. At birth the two ventricles are equal in size but the left ventricle enlarges disproportionately so that by six months of age the adult ratio of ventricular size is reached. The neonatal blood pressure (BP) is governed by the relationship between a high CO and a low systemic vascular resistance (SVR), which is the total resistance produced by the ability of blood vessels to contract on the left side of the circulation. The CO, which is in proportion to metabolic rate, tends to increase in relation to body surface area over the first year of life and then stays approximately the same in relation to size thereafter. Myofibril (heart muscle fibre) size and maturity increase throughout infancy so that by one year of age, the heart is anatomically and physiologically mature. The SVR increases throughout childhood such that the BP gradually increases (see Table 18.1).

The pulmonary vascular resistance (PVR) is the equivalent of the SVR in the pulmonary circulation. In the newborn it is very labile and hypoxia and/or acidosis may result in a dramatic increase in PVR, causing the right ventricular pressure to be greater than the pressure in the left ventricle. Blood is therefore shunted from the right side of the heart to the left and bypasses the lungs, starting a vicious circle of increasing hypoxia. This is much more likely to occur in the neonate as, although the ductus arteriosus and/or foramen ovale close functionally soon after birth, complete anatomical closure may not occur for some weeks. The picture of a cyanosed neonate with an

Table 18.1 Normal physiological parameters						
Age	Height (cm)	Weight (kg)	Heart rate	Blood pressure	Haemoglobin concentration (g/dl)	Respiratory rate
1 month	54	4.5	120	90/50	15–16	35
1 year	76	10	115	94/55	11–12	30
4 years	103	17	100	95/57	12–13	25
8 years	127	25	90	100/60	13–14	20
12 years	148	37	85	108/65	14–15	15

anatomically normal heart and normal lungs is some-times termed "persistent fetal circulation" for obvious reasons. This tendency of immature pulmonary blood vessels to "overreact" in response to various stimuli is related to a relative abundance of smooth muscle in the walls of the smaller arteries. During the first three months of life the size and number of pulmonary arteries increase rapidly and the excessive smooth muscle regresses.

Total blood volume varies considerably during the first week of life depending on the amount of blood drained from the placenta before the cord is clamped. Moreover, an infant's capacity to compensate for changes in circulating blood volume is poor because of less efficient control of capacitance vessels (large systemic veins which act like a reservoir containing varying amounts of the blood volume) and inactive baroreceptors. Blood pressure is therefore an excellent guide to the adequacy of blood replacement during anaesthesia in the very young. Because the hypo-volaemic infant will be unable to maintain an adequate cardiac output, early volume replacement is essential.

THE RESPIRATORY SYSTEM

There are major anatomical differences between the neonate and adult that have important implications with regard to laryngoscopy and intubation. The epiglottis is long and U-shaped in the neonate, becoming relatively smaller and less obtrusive with age. The tip of the laryngoscope blade must elevate the epiglottis before the glottis can be seen: hence the use of a straight blade laryngoscope is recommended for infants and small children. The neonatal larynx is high up in the neck, situated opposite C3–4 and descends during the first three years of life and again at puberty to its final position opposite C6. This laryngeal position dictates that elevation of the head to the "sniffing position" during intubation will not assist in visualization of the glottis in the very young.

The length of the trachea correlates better with weight than age but varies significantly. As the neonatal trachea is only about 4–5 cm long, accurate placement and fixation of the endotracheal tube (ETT), so that its end lies 2–3 cm below the cords, is essential. The narrowest part of the larynx before puberty is not at vocal cord level but at the level of the cricoid cartilage. Here there is a complete ring of cartilage and a small amount of mucosal oedema will reduce the area of the airway substantially. Insertion of an ETT similarly encroaches upon this space and the internal diameter of the tube will determine the resistance to gas flow. To avoid mucosal trauma and yet use the ETT with the largest internal diameter possible, an uncuffed tube

should be used in children younger than 10 years old. This should be of a size to allow a small leak when an airway pressure of 20 cmH$_2$O is applied.

Because neonatal ribs are almost horizontal their movement is an inefficient means of generating negative intrathoracic pressure and ventilation is primarily the result of diaphragmatic rather than inter-costal muscular contraction. The abdominal viscera are bulky and can readily hamper diaphragmatic excursion, especially if the gastrointestinal tract is distended. Thus, if mask ventilation has resulted in gastric distension temporary insertion of an orogastric tube after intubation is recommended. The nasal air passages contribute 30–50% of the total airway resis-tance in infancy and insertion of a nasogastric tube may increase this resistance by up to 50%. Postoperatively, therefore, the smallest possible tube should be used and placed in the smaller of the two nostrils.

The neonate has a very compliant chest wall, which provides only a weak force to maintain air in the lungs at the end of expiration. The small infant tries to prevent airway closure occurring at the end of each breath by maintaining intercostal muscle tone and by having a fast respiratory rate. Thus airway closure and impaired oxygenation readily occur in the anaesthetized infant. Because of this infants usually require controlled venti-lation during anaesthesia and will benefit from high respiratory rates and/or positive end-expiratory pressure (PEEP) to maintain lung volume and prevent airway closure. As growth occurs, the rib cage stiffens so that it becomes better able to oppose the action of the diaphragm. The number of alveoli in the lungs reaches adult levels by eight years of age but the alveoli continue to increase in diameter until adolescence.

DRUG DISTRIBUTION, METABOLISM AND EXCRETION

Body water makes up 75% of the body weight of the term infant compared to 60% in adults. Although initially a greater proportion of water is extracellular rather than intracellular, by about six months of age the volume of the two compartments is similar. Henceforth, the intracellular proportion increases and the extracellular decreases. A large extracellular fluid compartment means that drugs that are distributed throughout this space, such as suxamethonium, are required in larger doses in infants.

The composition of the body also has an influence on drug distribution; neonates have little fat or muscle. Drugs normally distributed to these tissues, such as fentanyl, will have a longer half-life (the time taken for the concentration of the drug to decrease by 50%).

Protein binding of drugs is less in young infants, because decreased hepatic production of proteins such as albumin results in low plasma protein concentrations and more of the administered drug will be free in the plasma to exert a clinical effect. Drug elimination and toxicity may also be affected, as in general it is only the "free" or unbound portion of the drug that can cross from the intravascular space into the tissues.

Detoxification and metabolic breakdown of drugs takes place mainly in the liver. However, some aspects of hepatocellular enzyme activity are poorly developed at term and adult levels are reached only after about 70 days of life. Hence, drugs such as morphine have a considerably longer half-life in young infants than in adults. Toddlers, however, demonstrate a more rapid elimination of some drugs than do adults, reflecting a high hepatic blood flow and enhanced hepatic metabolic activity.

Drugs excreted via the kidney, such as morphine metabolites, are dependent upon adequate glomerular filtration and their elimination will be prolonged in the neonate in whom there is relatively low renal blood flow and limited tubular function. Renal function matures rapidly over the first few months of life and reaches adult levels by one year of age.

HAEMATOLOGICAL FACTORS

The term neonate has a blood volume of about 80 ml/kg and a haemoglobin concentration of $16\pm(2$ g/dl. Most haemoglobin at birth is of the fetal type (HbF) which has a higher affinity for oxygen than does the adult type of haemoglobin (HbA). HbF (see also Chapter 21) combines with more oxygen but releases it less readily to the tissues than does HbA and thus adequate oxygen delivery to the tissues requires a high haemoglobin concentration.

During the first few weeks of life the haemoglobin level decreases, as a result of reduced red blood cell survival time and decreased production, so that by 2–3 months of age the normal haemoglobin concentration is 9–11 g/dl. However, at the same time HbA has largely replaced the HbF content of the blood so that despite this decrease in haemoglobin concentration, oxygen delivery to the tissues has improved.

TEMPERATURE CONTROL

Because infants have a large surface area relative to body weight and lack heat-insulating subcutaneous fat, they tend to lose heat rapidly when placed in a cool environment. The physiological responses to cooling lead to increased oxygen and glucose utilization and result in acidosis, all of which may compromise the sick infant. To eliminate the need for compensatory responses by the infant, sick infants are usually nursed in a high ambient temperature (e.g. 28–32°C, depending on size). During anaesthesia the normal responses of the infant to cold stress are lost and babies' body temperature can drop very quickly. In addition, because normal peripheral vasoconstriction is inhibited, there is redistribution of body heat from the core to the periphery. Measures to minimize heat loss and avoid cold stress are important during anaesthesia and are outlined below.

DEVELOPMENTAL PSYCHOLOGY

Admission to hospital may have profound emotional consequences for children. The type of disturbance depends largely upon the child's age, social and family factors and, of course, their hospital "experience". All staff who come into contact with children in hospital should realize the important role they can play in minimizing psychological trauma.

Infants younger than six months of age are not upset by short-term separation from parents though prolonged separation may impair parent–child bonding. Older infants and preschool children are more likely to be distressed by a hospital stay, principally because of the separation from family and home. Explanations are difficult at this age and these children show the most severe behaviour regression following hospitalization. School-age children are usually less upset at separation and may be more concerned with the surgical procedure and its possible mutilating effect, whilst adolescents fear the loss of control and the possibility of not being able to cope with their illness. Fortunately, the ever-increasing use of day-care facilities has helped enormously in reducing the trauma of elective surgery. Nevertheless, for all children, whatever their age, an empathic and honest approach is generally preferred to a misleading or ambiguous manner.

Nowadays it is routine for at least one parent to accompany their child to the anaesthetic room. As long as the parent is not too upset by the experience their presence usually has a beneficial effect on the young child and renders sedative premedication unnecessary. Similar arguments have been advanced for allowing parents to be present in the recovery area but logistical and local geographical difficulties often make this arrangement a practical problem.

PREOPERATIVE FASTING AND PREMEDICATION

Infants and children should not be subjected to unnecessarily prolonged fasting. Healthy children may safely be given clear fluids up to two hours before induction of anaesthesia, though solid food should be avoided for six hours before surgery. Infants who are breastfed should be fasted for a period equal to the usual interval between feeds.

Premedication is usually unnecessary for infants and children having day-care surgery but some anxious older children may benefit from sedative premedication given orally. Patients in pain should always be given appropriate analgesia.

ANAESTHETIC TECHNIQUE AND EQUIPMENT

Induction of anaesthesia using a non-irritant gaseous anaesthetic agent such as halothane or sevoflurane is more common in paediatric than in adult anaesthetic practice due to occasional difficulty with venous access in unsedated chubby young children. Nevertheless, intravenous thiopentone or propofol remains a common method of inducing anaesthesia in children, particularly since the prior topical application of local anaesthetic preparations such as EMLA or Ametop is so effective. A Rendell-Baker mask, which fits the contours of the face and minimizes dead space, is often recommended for infants and small children but the occasional user may find it easier to achieve a good seal using a mask that incorporates a circular air cushion. The relatively large tongue in infants or adenoid hypertrophy in preschool children may necessitate an oropharyngeal airway.

Once anaesthesia is induced a laryngeal mask rather than a facemask may be used to deliver the gaseous anaesthetic agent. It has the advantage of producing less airway resistance than an endotracheal tube in spontaneously breathing patients. A laryngeal mask is usually easy to insert and is available in a range of sizes, including one for infants. However, due to reasons given above, endotracheal intubation and controlled ventilation is usually preferable in the very young unless the procedure is of short duration.

For infants and small children a straight-bladed laryngoscope, such as a Wisconsin, is used to obtain the best view of the glottis. The head should be at the level of the table and supported in a low head ring but there is no advantage in flexing the neck until the child is greater than six years old, when a small pillow may

improve the intubation angle and view of the glottis. It is important to be aware of conditions such as Down's syndrome that are associated with an unstable cervical spine and in such cases, great care should be taken to limit head movement. Preformed endotracheal tubes are now commonly used in paediatric anaesthetic practice because these lessen the likelihood of tube kinking and enable easier fixation. Nevertheless, use of these tubes should not preclude the careful checking of tube position, particularly the length of tube passed through the vocal cords, as there is a likelihood of accidental right bronchial intubation. As in adults, dentition can prove problematic during laryngoscopy as many children have loose deciduous teeth and it may be safer to remove an extremely wobbly tooth rather than risk its inadvertent aspiration.

The ideal paediatric anaesthetic circuit should be lightweight with low resistance and dead space, adaptable to spontaneous or controlled ventilation and readily humidified and scavenged. No such circuit exists but the T-piece system most nearly meets these conditions. It has the advantage of having no valves and has very low resistance although it is an inefficient circuit to use for spontaneously breathing patients and it is not easily scavenged. Alternatives include the Bain coaxial circuit, which is a modified T-piece system, and the adult type circle absorber semiclosed system, modified for paediatric use by incorporating small diameter tubing.

Humidification of inspired gases during anaesthesia prevents damage to the respiratory tract by dry gases and minimizes heat loss from this route. The principles underlying the humidification of inspired gases are the same as described for adult systems.

Ventilation during anaesthesia may be controlled manually or by a mechanical ventilator. In order to prevent airway closure rapid ventilation with small tidal volumes is advised in the infant, though hyperventilation and consequent respiratory alkalosis should be avoided. It is mandatory to monitor the end-tidal carbon dioxide concentration using capnography whatever method of controlled ventilation is used. Other routine monitoring of children undergoing anaesthesia is similar to that used in adults, except that monitoring for signs of myocardial ischaemia using an electrocardiogram is only rarely indicated.

Prevention of heat loss assumes a high priority when infants are undergoing surgery. The ambient temperature of the operating theatre should be raised to about 25°C and a heating blanket should be placed under the patient. Because the surface area of an infant's head is a large fraction of total body surface area, heat loss from an exposed head can be significant and is best avoided by use of a woollen cap. The use of warmed intravenous fluids and heated humidified gases is also advisable. After excess skin preparation fluid has been removed the surgical area should be covered with an adhesive plastic film such as Opsite. Postoperatively the use of a hot air blanket may be advantageous. Small infants should be returned to their incubators as quickly as possible.

PERIOPERATIVE FLUID THERAPY

Calculation of the volume and type of fluid required must take account of the patient's body temperature, the fluid deficit incurred by preoperative fasting, the maintenance fluid requirement during surgery and extracellular fluid loss secondary to surgical trauma. Intravenous fluid is not usually required for an otherwise healthy child who is expected to be drinking again within 2–3 hours after an operation taking less than one hour. For surgical procedures of longer duration or when postoperative reestablishment of oral fluids may be delayed, peroperative administration of intravenous fluids is indicated.

Maintenance fluid may contain dextrose (e.g. 5% dextrose with 0.45% saline) but other fluids used to replace losses should be free of dextrose. The adequacy of fluid replacement is best judged by continuous monitoring of the relevant cardiovascular indices and urine output although swab weighing may be helpful.

If blood loss greater than 15% of the patient's estimated total blood volume is anticipated a central venous line should be inserted preoperatively. This amount of blood loss usually indicates the need for blood transfusion but the patient's preoperative haemoglobin concentration must also be taken into account. Intravenous fluids are usually continued into the postoperative period until the patient is able to tolerate oral fluids.

DIFFERENCES IN SURGICAL TECHNIQUE AND PATHOLOGY

Basic surgical principles are the same for all age groups but, particularly in the very young, extra care should be taken to prevent excessive blood loss and unnecessary trauma to tissues. Paediatric surgery mainly differs from adult surgery because of the distinctive nature of the pathology encountered in paediatric practice. Degenerative pathology is not seen and little tumour work is undertaken, the vast majority of paediatric surgery being performed to correct congenital abnormalities or to treat the results of trauma or infection.

MANAGEMENT OF POSTOPERATIVE PAIN

New drugs, new ways of using old drugs, new techniques and rediscovered old techniques have allowed major advances in the treatment of pain in infants and children over the past decade. Even more importantly, new validated methods of assessing pain in the very young have been described and are now in common use.

ASSESSMENT OF PAIN

In infants pain is assessed using both physiological parameters such as heart rate and tissue oxygenation and behavioural indices such as facial expression, cry, bodily movements and posture. Older children may be able to use a visual analogue scale such as a five-point series of faces that have different colours and expressions. Whatever the child's age, it is always worthwhile asking both parents and nurses to contribute towards this assessment exercise.

OPIOIDS

Opioids such as morphine remain the mainstay of postoperative pain treatment and, despite their potential problems, are used in all ages including neonates. Nevertheless, using morphine in the very young requires an increased level of monitoring and a ward nurse:patient ratio of at least 1.4. Other techniques, such as patient-controlled analgesia (PCA), that have been well proven in adults are increasingly being used in children of over five years. Similarly, children between one and five years old can be offered a nurse-controlled system of intravenous opioid analgesia (Nurse-Controlled Analgesia).

REGIONAL/LOCAL ANAESTHESIA

It is common practice to perform nerve blocks under general anaesthesia in order to provide up to eight hours of excellent postoperative pain relief. Moreover, bupivacaine (± fentanyl) continuously infused through a catheter, placed after the induction of anaesthesia into the epidural or paravertebral space or next to the brachial plexus, can provide safe and effective analgesia for all age groups for 2–3 days postoperatively. If regional techniques are used the child should be able to understand the significance of any potentially frightening side effects. (To the child a limb that cannot be felt or, more importantly, moved might be equated to a limb that has been amputated.)

NON-STEROIDAL ANTIINFLAMMATORY DRUGS/PARACETAMOL

Paracetamol is a relatively mild analgesic agent, is safe in all age groups and is often used in conjunction with other analgesic techniques or to help with weaning from stronger drugs. Similarly non-steroidal antiinflammatory drugs (NSAIDs) such as diclofenac are commonly given by suppository, inserted at the time of operation, as an adjunct to a local or regional technique. In order to minimize potential legal problems it is important that older children and parents have knowledge of this before the child goes to theatre.

RECOMMENDED READING

Steward DJ. 1995 *Manual of Paediatric Anaesthesia*, 4th Ed.London:Churchill Livingstone

Ashcraft KW.1994 *Atlas of Paediatric Surgery*.London:W.B. Saunders.

19

FUNDAMENTALS OF HYPERTHERMIA AND HYPOTHERMIA

C. S. Ince

HEAT AND THE MEASUREMENT OF TEMPERATURE

Heat is a form of energy and the magnitude of this energy is expressed in units of temperature. Change in temperature occurs when the body loses or gains heat. The energy of a molecule depends on the mass, its speed of movement and the frequency of collision with other molecules or its container. When molecules collide they may transfer some of their energy and, in the same way, energy may be transferred between bodies. If molecules with a different energy level are introduced to an existing system they will influence the energy level within this system. Thus if cold water (low heat energy) is added to hot water (higher heat energy), the new energy level will be more than the cold water but less than the hot and the hot water will be cooled (i.e. it will have less energy). At a temperature of absolute zero (0° Kelvin) a body has no internal energy.

The unit for measuring heat energy is the calorie. This is defined as the amount of heat required to raise the temperature of 1g of a substance through 1°C and is the specific heat capacity or specific heat of that substance. The specific heat of water is 1. The equivalent SI unit (see Appendix) is the joule, which is equivalent to 4.19 calories. Gases at normal pressures have very low specific heats and although easily warmed, their heat content is small and easily dissipated. This means that inhalational burns by hot gases rarely have a serious effect below the larynx, the exception being scalds from superheated steam. Similarly remotely warmed anaesthetic gases are very close to room temperature when they reach the patient.

Energy is taken in or given out when a substance changes its state. The energy level of a gas is greater than that of a liquid, which is greater than a solid. If, therefore, we wish to change a liquid into a gas we must supply energy to the system. Conversely changing a gas to a solid will give out energy. The energy involved during a change of state is known as latent heat and is defined as the amount of heat taken in or given out when a unit mass of a substance changes its state without a change in temperature.(See Table 19.1).

Latent heat of vaporization takes in energy and when air is humidified in the nose or sweat is evaporated from the skin, heat is therefore lost from the body. That is why the administration of humidified inspired air conserves heat (see later). In a similar way large burns and exposed abdominal contents are potent sources of heat loss.

Heat moves from areas of high energy (hot) to lower

Table 19.1 Types of latent heat

Change of state	Type of latent heat	Energy
Solid to liquid	Fusion	Taken in
Liquid to gas	Vaporization	Taken in
Gas to liquid	Condensation	Given out
Liquid to solid	Crystallization	Given out

energy (cooler) areas and the flow ceases when the energy level in both zones is equal. This principle is used in the measurement of temperature for, when the flow of energy between the object to be measured and the thermometer is zero, a true reading of temperature may be obtained.

Fahrenheit developed a mercury in glass thermometer in 1724 using the melting point of ice and body temperature as fixed reference points. Similarly, Celsius used the melting point of ice and the boiling point of water as fixed points and divided the scale into 100 equal parts.

If an 'ideal' gas is cooled it will occupy zero volume at –273.15°C. This temperature is known as absolute zero or 0° Kelvin and is the lower fixed point on the 'ideal gas temperature 'scale'. The upper fixed point is the triple point of water, defined as the temperature at which water exists simultaneously in gaseous, liquid and solid states (0.01°C). The unit of the ideal gas temperature scale is the Kelvin, named after Lord Kelvin who proposed the adoption of this scale.

Although we refer to temperature in °C, etc., temperature intervals are recorded as, say, 36°C (or 36 hundredths up the Celsius scale). The relationship of the various temperature scales is given in Table 19.2.

Temperature may be measured using any physical property of a material, which varies when energy is applied to or removed from that material. Readings may be either a direct observation of that change or may be through the use of an intermediary such as measuring current or resistance changes in an electrical circuit.

Expansion of a liquid in a glass tube is commonly used to measure temperature. The scale depends on its use and the clinical thermometer uses mercury or sometimes alcohol. In order to make it easier to read, there is a constriction just above the bulb, that prevents the mercury from contracting back into the bulb. This permits the thermometer to be read at leisure and remote from the body. Without this constriction the

Table 19.2 Scales of temperature			
Scale	Unit	Lower fixed point	Upper fixed point
Fahrenheit	°F	Melting point of ice (32°F)	Body temperature (98.4°F)
Celsius	°C	Melting point of ice (0°C)	Boiling point of water (100°C)
Ideal gas scale	K	Absolute zero (0°K, −273.15°C	Triple point of water (273.16°K, 0.01°C)

temperature would fall towards that of the immediate environment, i.e. the air temperature, and as the liquid volume decreased, a false reading would be obtained. Gas thermometers measure the expansion of a gas at constant pressure or the increase in pressure at a constant volume but generally they are only used to calibrate other instruments.

In a circuit electrical resistance increases as the temperature increases and this principle is used in resistance wire thermometers. The voltage (V), resistance (R) and current flow (I) will vary according to the formula $I = E/R$. Thus either the change in current, resistance or voltage may be measured. The platinum resistance thermometer forms one arm of the Wheatstone Bridge, which is used to measure the change in resistance (see Chapter 10). The temperature change of the thermometer alters the resistance and this in turn affects the balance of the bridge. The voltage or current change registered may be calibrated to record temperature.

If electrodes are made of two dissimilar metals and each is kept at a different temperature, a current will flow which is in proportion to the temperature difference between the two electrodes and the response is non-linear. This current may be calibrated as temperature and the instrument is known as the thermocouple. Usually one electrode is kept as the reference and the other is used to measure the temperature but thermocouples are mainly used in the laboratory.

The thermistor is a semiconductor that responds to an increase in temperature with a decrease in resistance. Like the resistance thermometer, its response is non-linear but over a range of about 50°C its response is basically of a linear nature. Thermistors have a rapid response time but because they change their resistance properties with age they must be regularly calibrated. Because of their small size they are commonly used clinically, a good example being the oesophageal temperature probe.

SITES OF TEMPERATURE MEASUREMENT

The significance of body temperature measurement depends on the site at which it was measured. Common clinical sites are the mouth, axilla and rectum but strip thermometers that measure skin temperature are becoming popular. Surface temperature is dependent on skin perfusion and thus the skin/core temperature difference is a useful way of assessing vasodilatation, with a small gradient being indicative of good perfusion. Core temperature may be recorded in the oesophagus or rectum but the rectal temperature is slightly lower. The oesophageal temperature should be measured below the bifurcation of the trachea and nasopharyngeal temperature, which reflects the temperature of the brain, is only accurate if the patient is intubated. These limitations are important because gas flow in the trachea and air passing through the nasopharynx may affect the reading.

THE CONTROL OF BODY TEMPERATURE

THE NEED FOR TEMPERATURE CONTROL

The metabolic processes of the body are controlled and mediated by enzymes and because enzymes are proteins composed of amino acids, their optimum activity is temperature dependent. At lower temperatures metabolism is slowed but at higher temperatures, although there may be some initial increase, activity is limited by the gradual disruption of the enzymatic structure, leading to compromised metabolic function and at extremes of temperature severe brain damage or death may occur. Thus, in order to achieve optimum activity the body maintains a core temperature of between 36.5°C and 37.5°C. This varies with the time of the day and the body's activity, although the temperature at the periphery may vary widely. In women there is a slight decrease in temperature

(0.5°C) a few days before menstruation that is maintained until ovulation and is probably due to the low level of progesterone.

Body temperature is a balance between heat gained by metabolism and heat lost to the environment (Table 19.3). Heat is produced by cellular metabolism and from muscle contraction which may be voluntary or involuntary (heart muscle).

Table 19.3 Sources of heat loss and gain	
Heat loss	Heat gain
Skin and sweat	Metabolism
Warm humidified air	Muscle contraction
Urine	Warm environment
Faeces	
Cold environment	

MECHANISMS OF HEAT GAIN AND LOSS

There are three main ways in which the body may gain or lose heat: conduction, convection and radiation. In addition latent heat is responsible for the heat loss resulting from the humidification of dry inspired air or anaesthetic gases and evaporation from open surgical procedures.

Conduction is the transfer of heat by direct molecular transmission from a high energy area to that with a lower energy. By definition the tissues must be in contact with an object at a different temperature, thus establishing a temperature gradient along which the heat energy may pass. Conduction varies with the nature of the conducting substance and is greatest in metals and is more in liquids than gases.

Convection is defined as the process of heat transfer through a fluid (liquid or gas) caused by the movement of molecules from cool regions to warmer regions of lower density. The flow patterns set up cause cooler fluid to replace the warmer which is a potent source of heat loss in accidental hypothermia. In situations where the airflow is increased, heat loss is greater and this accounts for the rapid hypothermia resulting from exposure to cold winds. A similar situation may occur in orthopaedic theatres using laminar flow systems. Convection is decreased by interrupting the airflow and is illustrated by the use of loose-fitting clothing in winter.

Radiation is the emission from a body of electromagnetic particles along an energy gradient and therefore, the greater the skin/environment temperature difference, the greater will be the loss of heat by radiation. The human skin is an excellent radiator and absorber of heat, being most efficient when there is a large surface area with respect to weight, such as in the limbs, and this is the main route of heat loss in a patient. Because of the difference in the surface area:weight ratio, a neonate must generate about twice as much heat/kilogram as an adult in order to maintain a constant body temperature. In addition, a newborn baby is wet and so there is also a large evaporative heat loss. This explains why neonates lose heat so quickly and why they should be nursed in a hot environment with an overhead external source of heat. The child may also be covered in cling film to reduce evaporation, layers of clothing to reduce convection and conduction and tin foil to reduce radiation. These principles also apply to the neonatal operating theatre.

NERVOUS CONTROL OF BODY TEMPERATURE

Reflex temperature control is mediated by the thermal nucleus in the hypothalamus, which also sets the core temperature. Afferent impulses coming from receptors in the brain and the periphery reach this area and the reflex arc is completed by the returning efferent nerves which cause behavioural changes or modify physiological responses (Table 19.4) leading to heat loss or conservation. Because of its large surface area (1.8 square metres in the average adult), the skin plays a vital role in the control of body temperature through sweating and the variation of its blood flow. If the

Table 19.4 Physiological and behavioural responses	
To gain heat	To lose heat
Skin vessels constrict	Skin vessels dilate
Increased thyroid activity	Decreased thyroid activity
Shivering	Sweating
Piloerection	
Use of brown fat (babies)	
Add clothing	Remove clothing
Seek warmth	Seek shade
Drink warm fluids	Drink cold fluids
Increase body activity	Decrease body activity

integrity of the skin in damaged, e.g. in burns, thermoregulation may become severely compromised.

Heat loss by radiation is most effective if there is a large temperature gradient. In a warm environment the body increases the skin/air gradient by sweating, which also cools the skin. Up to four litres of sweat may be produced in a day and this will result in fluid and salt loss if it is not corrected. Vasodilatation within the skin also increases the loss of heat but as the air temperature rises and approaches body temperature, the air/skin gradient decreases and sweating becomes much more important.

In order to reduce the skin/air temperature gradient in a cold environment, metabolism is increased. Blood flow through the skin is also reduced. thereby decreasing heat loss, but as the blood flow through the skin decreases the skin/core temperature gradient increases. The air in contact with the skin is warmed and this is achieved directly by moving close to a heat source or indirectly by means of insulation with loose-fitting clothing. Piloerection is much more important in animals in which the erect hairs restrict air movement and decrease the rate at which warmer air leaves the surface of the body.

Small babies have stores of brown fat, which are under the control of the sympathetic nervous system utilizing the neurotransmitter adrenaline. Because increased blood levels of carbon dioxide may stimulate the release of adrenaline, the maintenance of high normal levels of carbon dioxide during surgery helps to keep this system active.

HYPOTHERMIA

Hypothermia (a lower than normal core temperature) and hyperthermia (a higher than normal core temperature) occur if normal homoeostasis fails or is inadequate, e.g. at the extremes of age and in prolonged anaesthesia. Cold-blooded animals are unable to maintain a constant temperature and thus they tend to equilibrate to the temperature of the environment.

PHYSIOLOGY OF HYPOTHERMIA

Oxygen consumption and metabolic rate are reduced to about 75% of the basal rate at 30°C and 45% at 25°C. The oxygen dissociation curve moves to the left so that there is less oxygen released at the tissues. Because gases are more soluble at lower temperatures and less carbon dioxide is produced, the partial pressure of carbon dioxide falls as the body cools. Thus carbon dioxide is added to the inspired anaesthetic gas to maintain the PCO_2 level during profound

hypothermia. In addition, by increasing the inspired carbon dioxide, the oxygen dissociation curve will tend to revert to normal as hypercarbia moves it to the right.

In spontaneously breathing patients the minute volume gradually reduces and breathing ceases at about 23°C and during hypothermia a respiratory acidosis develops. In patients undergoing intermittent positive pressure ventilation the decreased carbon dioxide production may lead to the occurrence of a respiratory alkalosis. This may be corrected by reducing the minute volume, by decreasing either the rate or the tidal volume of the ventilator.

Because liver function and insulin production are depressed the blood glucose rises. There is a decrease in splanchnic blood flow and drugs that are metabolized in the liver have a prolonged half-life. Blood flow and glomerular filtration fall during hypothermia and urine production ceases at about 20°C.

Hypothermia causes a bradycardia and the heart becomes progressively more irritable as the temperature falls: dysrhythmias are common below 31°C and ventricular fibrillation is likely below 28°C. As the body cools the blood pressure falls. Tissue perfusion is poor below 28°C and this is due partly to an increase in blood viscosity. Slow rewarming of severe accidental hypothermia is essential if ventricular fibrillation is to be avoided. The brain is protected during hypothermia but associated drug overdose may lead to irreversible hypoxia.

CAUSES OF HYPOTHERMIA

Hypothermia may be accidental or intentional. The causes of accidental hypothermia include drugs, alcohol abuse, anaesthesia and myxoedema. Vasodilatation and the decrease in metabolic rate result in rapid heat loss in a cold environment, whether this is the nearest rough shelter, a mountainside or the operating theatre. In addition, anaesthesia prevents shivering and the humidification of dry anaesthetic gases also results in body heat loss.

Hypothermia is common in anaesthetized patients, especially at the extremes of age, and a cool theatre environment is the commonest cause. The risk is greater in hot countries as the theatre temperature tends to be maintained at a lower level to compensate for the excessive air temperatures out of doors. In the Charnley enclosure airflow is much greater than normal and the surgical staff feel hotter in the special gowns. The tendency to have a lower than normal theatre temperature may make the surgeon more comfortable but often adversely affects the patient's well-being.

Failure to think about the possibility of hypothermia is an important factor, particularly during the setting up of the major case in the anaesthetic room where there may be prolonged exposure. The administration of cold blood and fluids add to this problem. Hypothermia may be prevented by the methods outlined in Table 19.5.

Intentional hypothermia allowed operations to be performed on the heart and brain while metabolism was reduced and gave a measure of protection to the vital organs during circulatory interruption. Currently the use of this technique has declined.

In 1950 Bigelow and his colleagues reversibly arrested the circulation in dogs at temperatures of 20–25°C. This technique was first used clinically by Lewis and Tauffic during the repair of an atrial septal defect.

Mild hypothermia (28–35°C) using surface cooling may be induced using surface techniques, e.g. ice packs, cold water blankets and, in emergencies, cold fluid instilled into the stomach. The use of chlorpromazine may prevent shivering. Moderate (21–27°C) and deep (15–20°C) hypothermia are produced using core or bypass cooling. As the temperature falls ventricular fibrillation develops and the electrocardiogram and electroencephalogram become flat.

Table 19.5 Prevention of hypothermia in theatre

Be aware of the possibility

Monitor the patient's temperature

Increase the theatre temperature

Keep the patient well covered

Warm water or warm air mattress

Warm IV fluids including blood

Use of circle system and soda lime absorber

Warm and humidify anaesthetic gases

HYPERTHERMIA

PHYSIOLOGY OF HYPERTHERMIA

During pathogenic infection the fever is partly a response to the pyrogens produced by the infecting agent. The hypothalamus resets the core temperature, making the patient feel cold, and shivering and vasoconstriction occur to bring the temperature to this new higher setting. When the level of pyrogen decreases, the core temperature is reset and sweating and vasodilatation help to decrease the temperature towards normal. The pyrexia may eventually lead to enzyme dysfunction, protein damage, convulsions and death. A similar mechanism is seen in head injury and in the metabolic response to trauma, e.g. major burns.

CAUSES OF HYPERTHERMIA

Hyperthermia is usually caused by infection. In children febrile convulsions are not uncommon and this was probably also the cause of 'ether convulsions'. Children were given atropine as premedication and the heat from the theatre lights, together with the operating drapes, prevented adequate heat loss, thereby increasing body temperature. Sweating was not possible because of the atropine and so the body temperature increased, resulting in febrile convulsions. Complications of neurosurgery or head injury may lead to the resetting of the temperature-regulating mechanisms in the brain. Aspirin overdose is also a cause of pyrexia.

Malignant hyperpyrexia is a very rare and potentially fatal condition, triggered by anaesthetic agents such as halothane and suxamethonium. Its diagnosis and management are discussed in Chapter 26.

RECOMMENDED READING

Mushin WW, Jones PL. 1987 *Physics for the Anaesthetist* 4th Edn, revised. Oxford:Blackwell.

Moyle JTB, Davey A, Ward C, 1992 Ward's Anaesthetic Equipment. WB Saunders.

20

FUNDAMENTALS OF FLUID AND ELECTROLYTE BALANCE DURING SURGERY

R. M. King

DEFINITIONS

BODY FLUIDS

By strict definition, a fluid may be a liquid or a gas but in this context it is taken to be a liquid.

Fluid exists throughout the body but its composition and functions vary greatly (Box 20.1). Developing a clear understanding of what is considered to be a 'body fluid' is important for two reasons. First, if we are able effectively to manage fluid balance it is necessary to understand how the body responds to the physiological insult of surgery and trauma. In this way we may be able to minimize or prevent many of the changes that may lead to significant patient morbidity. Second, because body fluids are a potential source of infection, it is imperative that the health-care professional has a clear idea of what constitutes body fluid as well as possessing a thorough working knowledge of the ways in which infection risks may be reduced.

ELECTROLYTES

When an acid is neutralized by a base, a salt is produced. Thus, hydrochloric acid reacts with sodium hydroxide (the base or alkaline) to form sodium chloride (common salt) and water.

$$HCl + NaOH \leftrightarrow NaCl + H_2O$$

Acids, bases and salts may break down or dissociate into smaller charged particles known as *ions*. Strong acids, bases and salts are completely dissociated (even in the solid state) while weak acids, bases and salts are only partially dissociated. Each ion carries an electrical charge; a positively charged ion is known as a *cation* because it moves to the negative pole or cathode in an electric field, while a negatively charged ion is known as an *anion* because it moves towards the positive pole or anode. Thus, sodium chloride dissociates into positively charged sodium ions and negatively charged chloride ions:

$$NaCl \leftrightarrow Na^+ + Cl^-$$

A chemical such as a salt therefore comprises a cation and an anion. The solution of charged ions has the ability to conduct electricity and this property has resulted in the commonly used term *electrolyte*. The term *electrolyte solution* refers to a fluid that contains a number of free ions but it can also refer to those individual ions, such as potassium and sodium, within that solution. The most important electrolytes found in the human body are shown in Box 20.2

Traditionally the concentration of electrolytes was measured in mg/100 ml. However, this does not help us to understand how the various electrolytes relate to each other because, for example, 1 g of sodium does not combine with 1 g of chloride or replace 1 g of potassium. Concentrations are therefore now measured in terms of milliequivalents. The equivalent weight of a substance is defined as the weight of that substance in grams that will replace or play the part of 1 g of hydrogen. A milliequivalent (mEq) is the equivalent weight expressed in milligrams. Similarly, the *valency* of an atom is defined as the number of hydrogen atoms that the atom will replace or react with. Thus, the equivalent weight is the ionic weight divided by the valency. In order to convert mg/100 ml to mEq/l we must find the number of milligrams in a litre, i.e. multiply by 10 and then divide by the equivalent weight of the substance. Let us look at an example.

Unfortunately, although the concentration of an electrolyte solution is marked on the bag as milliequivalents/litre, it is still common to refer to the concentration in percentage terms. Thus, normal saline (sodium chloride) is often called 0.9% saline. A 0.9% solution contains 0.9 g/100ml or 9 g/l or 9000 mg/l of sodium chloride. Both the sodium ion and the chloride ion have a valency of 1 and thus the equivalent weight is the same as the atomic weight, which is 23 for sodium and 35.5 for chloride. Therefore, a 0.9% solution of sodium chloride contains 9000 divided by 58.5 (23+35.5) which is 153.8 mEq/l.

Intracellular fluid (ICF)	Synovial fluid
Extracellular fluid (ECF)	Cerebrospinal fluid (CSF)
Blood	Digestive juices
Lymph	Synovial fluid
Urine	Pleural fluid

Box 20.1 Examples of body fluids

Anions	Cations
Chloride	Sodium
Bicarbonate	Potassium
Phosphate	Calcium
	Magnesium
	Hydrogen

Box 20.2 Common electrolytes found in the human body

THE PHYSIOLOGY OF FLUID AND ELECTROLYTE BALANCE

DISTRIBUTION OF BODY WATER

In the body there must be a stable physiological environment for the efficient functioning of its many necessary processes. The amount of water and the concentration of electrolytes in the blood and tissues must therefore be maintained within a fairly narrow range. This applies not only to the total amount of water present but also to the way in which it is distributed. The physiological principles relating to osmotic pressure, hydrostatic pressure and the selective permeability of cell and capillary membranes ensure that these fluids are contained in their respective compartments.

An adult body weighing approximately 70 kg contains 42–45 litres of water, making up 60–65% of the total body weight. This figure is closer to 52% in adult females because they have a higher body fat content (fat contains less water than many other body tissues) but infants also have a smaller proportion of intracellular water. The general distribution of this fluid is divided between two major compartments. Fluid that is found within the cell membrane is known as *intracellular fluid* (ICF) and fluid that is not confined within this membrane is called *extracellular fluid* (ECF). ECF is about 12–17 litres and ICF is about 25–35 litres (figures vary between texts). Extracellular fluid can be further subdivided into:

plasma	3 litres
interstitial fluid	12 litres
transcellular fluid	1–3 litres.

Plasma is found within the blood vessels and lymph, interstitial fluid is found between cells and transcellular fluid includes secretions of the gastrointestinal tract, the respiratory system and cerebrospinal fluid. Transcellular fluid is formed by the transport actions of cells. The division or barrier that separates ICF and ECF is the membrane of the cell. Cell membranes are constructed of lipids and proteins and most of the substances found in the body cannot dissolve in lipid membranes. The consequence of this is that the membrane forms an effective barrier to the net movement of many of these substances across the body compartments.

DISTRIBUTION OF ELECTROLYTES WITHIN BODY FLUIDS

The common anions and cations that are present in body fluids are shown in Box 20.2. Many of the body's processes depend on the presence of an electric potential across the cell membrane. Examples include nerve conduction and neuromuscular transmission. In order to achieve this potential, the concentration of sodium and potassium is different inside and outside the cell. There is more potassium and less sodium within the cell and this differential is maintained by means of an active transport process known as the *sodium pump*. Sodium is actively removed from the cell and this process requires energy. (The electrolytic changes that occur during depolarization are reversed using the sodium pump.) Failure of this mechanism results in serious electrolyte imbalance, morbidity and often death.

There is also an internal movement of water and electrolytes. Saliva and intestinal digestive juices are produced within one part of the digestive tract and reabsorbed in another. The total turnover of this water is in the order of 8 litres in 24 hours and explains why severe diarrhoea and vomiting may have such a profound effect on fluid balance.

MAINTENANCE OF NORMAL WATER AND ELECTROLYTE BALANCE

The human body regulates fluids and electrolytes via homeostatic mechanisms. Sensors in the great vessels detect changes in the circulating blood volume, blood pressure and the oncotic pressure of the plasma (see below). Sensory feedback mechanisms that rely heavily on renal function, involving antidiuretic hormone, ADH, (water retention) and aldosterone (retention of sodium, chloride and water together with potassium loss), therefore maintain fluid and electrolyte balance. This is supplemented by sensations such as thirst and results in the conservation or excretion of sodium, potassium, hydrogen ions and water. We do not intend to cover the detailed structure and function of the kidney but seek to put into context the principles involved in the maintenance of water and electrolyte homeostasis.

Water is the largest component of body fluid and is able to pass across the membrane of cells and move between the various body fluid compartments along concentration gradients. The amount of water that moves is dependent on a balance between the forces tending to move it and those that tend to keep it where it is and compensates for any temporary change in osmotic pressure. Thus the concepts of osmosis, osmotic pressure and hydrostatic pressure are major factors in the regulation and distribution of body water.

Osmosis is defined as the movement of water across a selectively permeable membrane from a solution of low solute (solute is the dissolved substance while solvent is the substance that dissolves it) concentration to one that is higher. The action of osmosis drawing water into a confined area will generate pressure, giving rise to the concept of the *osmotic potential* or pressure of a solution. Osmotic pressure is that pressure equal to the pressure required to prevent the movement of water across the membrane. Osmosis is therefore dependent upon the concentration of the solution on either side of the membrane. (Water always passes from the weak solution to the strong solution in an effort to dilute the strong solution and restore equilibrium.)

Oncotic pressure, which is also known as colloid osmotic pressure, is the pressure exerted by the proteins within the plasma and is estimated to be about 3.3 kPa (25 mmHg). It is one of the factors in Starling's hypothesis that is responsible for the movement of water across the capillary membrane and is fully discussed in Chapter 6. Proteins play an important role in osmosis because the boundary between the tissue fluid and the plasma (which has a high concentration of protein) is relatively impermeable to these proteins.

The number of osmoles of solute per kg of solvent is called the *osmolarity* of a solution. Capillary and cell membranes are permeable to water and subsequently all fluid compartments within the human body will effectively have the same osmolarity as plasma. There are also a number of solutes that can pass through cell membranes in order to achieve equilibrium.

Diffusion is the movement of a substance (across a selectively permeable membrane) along a concentration gradient in order to achieve equilibrium. The 'pores' in the membrane of capillaries allow the movement of electrolytes and glucose across the membrane. Large molecules such as proteins cannot readily pass through the membrane and thus remain in their compartments, e.g. proteins in the plasma. This retention of the large protein molecules within the plasma sets up a differential (oncotic pressure) that triggers osmosis. Water moves from the tissue (interstitial space) into the capillary, from a compartment of low protein concentration to a compartment of high protein concentration, i.e. the plasma. The osmotic effect of the plasma proteins and the interstitial fluid pressure both tend to retain water within the capillary while the blood pressure at the arterial end of the capillary tends to cause water to leave the blood vessel (see Fig. 6.2). It is the net effect of these two forces that determines overall whether water will leave or be retained by the capillary.

In Figure 6.2 the capillary blood pressure, arterial (CAP) or venous (CVP), and the tissue oncotic pressure (TOP) tend to push fluid out of the capillary while the oncotic pressure of the plasma proteins (POP) and the interstitial pressure (IP) tend to retain it within the capillary. At the arterial end of the capillary there is a net outflow of fluid equivalent to 9 mmHg (CAP: 32 + TOP: 10 – POP: 25 – IP: 8 = +9 mmHg). Conversely, at the venous end there is a net inflow of fluid equivalent to –11 mmHg (CVP: 14 + TOP: 10 – POP: 25 – IP: 8 = –9 mmHg). Although these figures vary in different texts they illustrate the fact that there is roughly an equal balance between fluid leaving the capillary at the arterial end and returning at the venous end, any excess interstitial fluid being removed by the lymphatic system and then returned to the great veins. If the lymphatic system becomes overloaded the local tissues become waterlogged. This process is known as oedema formation. Thus, any physiological or pathological change to this equilibrium may profoundly affect water and electrolyte balance.

WATER REQUIREMENTS

The previous section described some of the fundamental processes involved in maintaining normal fluid balance, both within the body as a whole and internally throughout the body compartments. This is only possible if the water and electrolytes leaving the body are matched by a similar amount entering it. In Figure 20.1 it can be seen that the actual losses are very variable. Renal function by controlling the volume and composition of the urine output may be thought of as the short-term control and although the average urine output is about 1500 ml/day, it may be as low as 400 ml. The *obligatory water loss,* including the minimum urine output and insensible losses from the skin and lungs, is about 1500 ml/day. Similarly, sweat production varies with the temperature of the environment and with the body temperature and may be up to 15 litres in 24 hours in severe tropical fevers.

The amount of metabolic water produced depends on the level of exercise and the food source that is metabolized. Water intake and the water content of food are obviously very variable. Fluid losses also depend on the surface area of the body and children therefore have relatively greater fluid requirements. In addition, metabolic activity (the *respiratory quotient* or RQ) varies with surface area. It is possible to calculate the average daily fluid requirements and we can use the formula that is generally applicable to children because it takes into account the changing surface area and hence the RQ in relation to weight. A typical formula is as follows:

100 ml/kg body weight/24 hours for the first 10 kg
50 ml/kg body weight/24 hours for the next 10 kg
20 ml/kg body weight/24 hours thereafter.

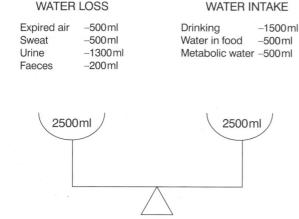

Figure 20.1 Average water balance in an adult

ELECTROLYTE REQUIREMENTS

Normally the salt taken in through food, drink and seasoning (170 mEq) matches the losses through the skin (10 mEq), urine (150 mEq) and faeces (10 mEq). In addition, there is an interchangeable salt pool that involves the plasma (450 mEq), the tissue fluid (1600 mEq) and the rest of the body tissues (1000 mEq). This pool can partially compensate for excessive loss or intake of sodium. An average intake of about 75 mEq/day is needed for normal salt balance.

Potassium is mainly found in the cells, which have a concentration between 100 and 150 mEq/l compared to a plasma concentration of 3.8–5.1 mEq/l. The body contains about 3500 mEq of potassium, the average intake being about 100 mEq/day, but only about half of this intake is needed for normal balance. Potassium moves into the cells when protein is being deposited, during alkalosis and when glucose is metabolized in the presence of insulin. The reverse happens during sodium loss, acidosis and catabolism. Because more potassium is found inside the cell compared with the ECF, compensation for potassium loss tends to be at the expense of the intracellular potassium. Thus the amount of potassium needed to replace the losses will be about twice as much as that calculated from the levels of potassium in the plasma. It has been suggested that a fall of 1 mEq/l in plasma potassium may be equivalent to a 200 mEq loss in total body potassium.

Although only sodium and potassium balances have been specifically mentioned, body levels of bicarbonate, calcium, magnesium and the many trace elements are also important.

MAINTENANCE OF ACID–BASE BALANCE

The number of hydrogen ions present in a solution is measured by means of pH, which is defined as the negative logarithm of the hydrogen ion concentration. Thus, an acid has a pH below 7 and an alkaline has a pH greater than 7. Because enzymes are only able to function within a narrow band of pH, the body must control its pH within these limits. In order to prevent sudden changes in pH, the body has a number of different buffers, substances that are able to absorb hydrogen ions with a minimum change in the pH. Such substances are therefore the short-term controllers of pH within the body and are usually the salts of weak acids and strong bases. Examples in the blood include bicarbonate, phosphate, haemoglobin and the plasma proteins.

The long-term compensation is via the kidney, which excretes the fixed acids, e.g. phosphate and sulphate, and via the lungs that excrete carbon dioxide. Carbon dioxide is a by-product of metabolism and is the principal source of the plasma carbonic acid according to the equation:

$$H_2O + CO_2 \leftrightarrow H_2CO_3 \leftrightarrow H^+ + HCO_3^-$$

The conversion of carbon dioxide into carbonic acid is facilitated by the enzyme carbonic anhydrase. Carbonic acid is transported to the lungs as bicarbonate and this process, known as the *chloride shift*, is described in Chapter 7. Thus change in the rate and depth of respiration will affect the pH of the blood. Changes in pH are affected by electrolyte balance, especially potassium.

ABNORMAL FLUID AND ELECTROLYTE BALANCE

If compensation for changes in water and electrolyte is not possible, the body's physiological processes may be impaired and in extreme cases death may result. It is very uncommon for water and/or electrolyte imbalance to occur in isolation and usually the presentation is of a mixed picture. For the purposes of explanation, however, the effect of the imbalance of water or a single electrolyte in isolation will be described and these will then be illustrated by some clinical examples.

SIMPLE WATER LOSS

Dehydration refers to pure water loss and this term should not really be used in conditions in which water loss is secondary to salt depletion. It is seen in preoperative starvation and in situations in which the patient is unable to drink, e.g. unconsciousness following surgery or trauma, and in conditions where there is excessive water loss such as diabetes insipidus. Although water intake has ceased, insensible loss through the skin and lungs still continues, as does the obligatory urine loss. This is exacerbated after major surgery because the tissue damage leads to increased urea production and potassium load, both of which require a larger volume of urine for excretion.

At first, the concentrations of sodium, potassium and water in the ECF begin to rise, thus increasing the osmotic pressure. Water therefore moves from the cells in an attempt to restore a normal osmotic pressure and urine production is decreased. This is reflected in an increasingly concentrated urine with a higher than normal specific gravity. The end result is a reduced ICF and a slightly reduced ECF. If the depletion is not corrected haemoconcentration, hypovolaemia and eventually hypotension occur, leading to renal failure, coma and death after a loss of about 15% of the body weight. However, these are late changes. Symptoms begin to appear after about 2 litres of water have been lost and if the patient is conscious, they may complain of thirst and a dry mouth. Clinically, in addition to the changes in the plasma electrolyte concentrations, there is a decrease in the elasticity of the skin.

Dehydration is usually classed as mild, moderate or severe and corresponds to about a 4%, 6% and 8% loss of total body weight loss respectively. Treatment is to replace water either orally or by means of 5% dextrose intravenously. In older patients or if there is a history of heart disease, replacement should be managed slowly in order to prevent the development of heart failure.

OVERHYDRATION OR WATER INTOXICATION

Water retention may occur immediately after surgery because of increased production of ADH. If there is coincidental salt depletion, which is treated with water replacement, water intoxication may occur. The osmotic pressure of the ECF falls and water moves from the ECF into the cells, which then increase in size. It is this overhydration of the brain cells that leads to convulsions. This syndrome is especially seen in children and is due to the inappropriate secretion of ADH. Treatment of overhydration is by means of hypertonic saline and/or by encouraging water loss.

HYPONATRAEMIA

Sodium and chloride may not be lost from the body in the same amounts and in fact sodium is by far the most important in terms of osmotic effect. Salt depletion

may occur in Addison's disease, in some renal conditions, in burns, severe sweating and in the loss of intestinal secretions. Clinically, the most common scenario is when salt and water loss is replaced by water alone.

Following a decrease in the concentration of the ECF sodium, the osmotic pressure of the ECF falls and water is lost in an attempt to correct this. Some water moves into the cells but the net effect is a falling plasma volume, presenting as dehydration although the patient does not complain of thirst. The falling plasma volume results in an early decrease in renal function with obvious skin desiccation and a decrease in the intraoccular tension. Symptoms begin to appear after the equivalent of about 4 litres 0.9% saline have been lost and death is as a result of circulatory failure. Treatment is usually with 0.9% saline but in severe cases hypertonic saline may be used.

HYPERNATRAEMIA

Sodium retention occurs postoperatively but may be exacerbated by treating simple dehydration with saline when the amount of sodium excreted by the kidneys is less than the intake. The osmotic pressure of the plasma rises and thus water moves from the cells into the plasma and because of this there may not be a great rise in the plasma sodium concentration. The end result is peripheral and pulmonary oedema with death being due to respiratory failure. Treatment is by restricting the sodium but not the water intake.

WATER AND ELECTROLYTE LOSS

A combination of water and electrolyte loss is the commonest clinical presentation. It occurs when there is inadequate salt and water intake, following severe burns and in ascites, oedema and paralytic ileus. In the last three examples fluid does not actually leave the body but the end result is the same. Symptoms include a combination of the oliguria and thirst of dehydration with the circulatory changes and desiccation of salt loss. Treatment involves the use of 0.9% saline to replace losses.

HYPOKALAEMIA

Low serum potassium or hypokalaemia is a common postoperative occurrence and is often due to failure to manage intravenous fluid therapy appropriately. It is also seen in patients who lose a large amount of intestinal fluid, including diarrhoea, or from fistulae involving the gastrointestinal tract. Large amounts of potassium may be lost in the urine in catabolic patients after major surgery or in the exudate of major burns.

Hypokalaemia is associated with alkalosis and symptoms of hypokalaemia include lethargy, muscle weakness and paralytic ileus. ECG changes include a sagging ST segment, a low or inverted T-wave and cardiac arrhythmias. Serum potassium levels below 1.5 mEq/l are often fatal. Treatment is by oral or intravenous potassium. Because of the effects on the heart, not more than 20 mEq should be given intravenously in any one hour.

HYPERKALAEMIA

Abnormally high serum potassium is called hyperkalaemia. Although it occurs in renal failure, in the context of abnormal fluid balance it is either due to an excessive intake of potassium or because of dehydration. Uncontrolled diabetes results in high potassium levels due to dehydration but in reality there is an overall potassium loss from the body. Levels greater than 7.5 mEq/l may affect the neuromuscular conduction of the heart muscle and ECG changes include an abnormally high T-wave. If the plasma potassium continues to rise, heart failure may occur.

ABNORMAL ACID–BASE BALANCE

There are two components to acid–base balance: a respiratory component and a metabolic component. For the purpose of this discussion, we will use the bicarbonate buffer as an example. Let us again consider the reaction involved in producing bicarbonate.

$$H_2O + CO_2 \leftrightarrow H_2CO_2 \leftrightarrow H^+ + HCO_3^-$$

Because the three stages of this reaction are reversible and in equilibrium with each other, any change in concentration in one stage will automatically affect the others. Thus, if there is an increase in carbon dioxide production or a decrease in its excretion, there will be an increase in the partial pressure of carbon dioxide in the blood and a corresponding increase in the concentration of carbonic acid and hence bicarbonate. The hydrogen ion can be buffered and eventually excreted by the kidney. If there is an increase in carbon dioxide excretion by the lungs resulting in a decrease of its partial pressure, the reverse happens and the level of bicarbonate will fall as the reaction moves to the left. The end result is a small decrease of pH in the former and a small rise in the pH in the latter.

Because both of these situations are the result of change in respiratory function, the former is called *respiratory acidosis* and the latter *respiratory alkalosis*. The lung is unable to compensate for the changes in pH because it is the prime cause of those changes and any long-term compensation is thus through the kidney, leading to a rise in bicarbonate in respiratory acidosis and a fall in bicarbonate in respiratory alkalosis. In other words, respiratory acidosis is compensated with a metabolic alkalosis (see below) while respiratory alkalosis leads to the development of a compensatory metabolic acidosis.

Metabolic acidosis occurs if there is an increase in the hydrogen ion concentration. A typical example is the ketoacidosis that occurs in uncontrolled diabetes mellitus. Because the normal metabolic pathways are unavailable due to a shortage of insulin, there is an increase in the ketoacids. This is partly buffered by the bicarbonate ion and initially only a small fall in pH occurs. The change in pH stimulates respiration and reduces the partial pressure of carbon dioxide in the blood. This in turn produces a compensatory respiratory alkalosis.

A *metabolic alkalosis* occurs if the bicarbonate is increased (excessive use of alkalis in dyspepsia) or if the amount of hydrogen ion is reduced (excessive vomiting). In this case there is a tendency to depress respiration, thus providing a compensatory respiratory acidosis. In both metabolic acidosis and alkalosis long-term compensation is renal unless, of course, the kidney is the cause of the initial problem. Table 20.1 summarizes these blood gas changes. Treatment is generally aimed at the cause but if this is metabolic, it is usual only to half correct the deficit in the first instance, thus allowing the body to manage its own final compensation.

BLOOD LOSS

The management and replacement of blood loss is described in Chapter 21. Failure to replace blood loss adequately results in progressive hypovolaemia. This in turn leads to hypotension, shock and potential renal failure. Anaemia will occur if volume is replaced at the expense of red blood cells. Its significance will depend on the condition of the patient and the degree of anaemia. Usually haemoglobin concentrations greater than 8 g/100 ml blood do not cause a major problem.

Let us now look briefly at some examples of conditions that may lead to fluid and electrolyte imbalance and see how the pathophysiology may help us to understand the processes involved.

PERSISTENT VOMITING

Because the stomach contains a large amount of chloride and hydrogen ions, vomiting leads to dehydration associated with loss of hypochloraemic alkalosis. A typical example is seen in pyloric stenosis.

PERSISTENT INTESTINAL FLUID LOSS

Intestinal obstruction, paralytic ileus or a fistula will result in a mixed water and electrolyte disturbance but the actual type of electrolyte loss will depend on the level of the pathology, e.g. distal to the stomach, potassium and sodium loss will be much more significant.

PREOPERATIVE STARVATION

For practical purposes, preoperative starvation is mainly enforced dehydration. In small children, however, there is also a potential for hypoglycaemia and this is dealt with elsewhere (Chapter 18). Using the formula previously mentioned, a 70 kg adult would require about 2500 ml of fluid/24 hours. Traditionally, patients were starved from midnight until their operation. If surgery were planned for the afternoon the patient would already be short of about 1250 ml of fluid. Nowadays patients scheduled for afternoon surgery are given an early breakfast and generally all patients are allowed to drink water until about two hours before surgery. Obviously this is only guidance and is dependent on the clinical condition of the patient.

ANAESTHESIA AND SURGERY

Of prime importance is the preoperative preparation of the patient. Any major fluid and electrolyte imbalance should have been corrected, if at all possible, before the patient comes to surgery. The surgical team often manages this process but the anaesthetist must be kept closely informed of progress and current blood investigations should be available in theatre. Careful fluid and electrolyte resuscitation enables the patient to be in the best possible condition to face the physiological trauma of surgery but there is often a compromise between the time needed for resuscitation and the urgency of the surgery.

The management of fluid and electrolyte balance in anaesthesia and surgery basically involves the maintenance of blood volume and kidney function. Simply, fluid balance is artificially maintaining fluid homeostasis – what comes out must be replaced! Estimating blood and fluid loss, such as occurs in intestinal obstruction and subsequent replacement therapy, is standard practice in operating theatres but it must also take into account the normal maintenance requirements. During surgery, between 5 and 10 ml/kg/hour of crystalloid will compensate for preoperative dehydration and normal fluid balance but this is in addition to the replacement of abnormal fluid loss.

ANAPHYLACTIC SHOCK

Anaphylactic shock is a good example of what happens when the capillary fails to function as a semipermeable membrane. The normal physiology was described above and illustrated in Figure 6.2. As a result of the allergic response, chemical mediators cause the capillary wall to become much more permeable and protein molecules can now pass out of the capillary and into the interstitial space. They still, however, exert an osmotic effect and the net result is to cause large volumes of fluid to move out of the plasma. This results in rapidly developing hypovolaemia, hypotension and finally cardiac arrest. The patient may become very oedematous as a result of the large fluid shifts. The following example illustrates the magnitude of these changes. If oedema formed subcutaneously to a depth of 1 mm and the body surface area were 1.8 m^{-2}, the total fluid loss would be the surface area multiplied by the depth of oedema fluid. In order to calculate this in ml, we need to multiply the surface

Table 20.1 The interpretation of acid-base disorders	
Blood gas measurement	Interpretation
pH under 7.4	Acidosis
pH over 7.4	Alkalosis
Raised $PaCO_2$ and low pH	Acidosis of respiratory origin
Raised $PaCO_2$ and high pH	Respiratory retention of CO_2 to compensate for metabolic alkalosis
Low $PaCO_2$ and high pH	Alkalosis of respiratory origin
Low $PaCO_2$ and low pH	Respiratory elimination of CO_2 to compensate for metabolic acidosis
Low HCO_3 and low pH	Acidosis of metabolic origin
Low HCO_3 and high pH	Elimination of HCO_3 to compensate for metabolic alkalosis
High HCO_3 and high pH	Alkalosis of metabolic origin
High HCO_3 and low pH	Elimination of H^+ to compensate for respiratory acidosis

area by 10,000 ($1m^{-2}$ = 10,000 ml^{-2}) and divide the depth by 10 (there are10 mm in 1cm). Thus the total fluid loss would be 1.8 x 10,000 x 0.1 = 1800 ml. It is not surprising, therefore, that the speed of onset of anaphylactic shock is so rapid.

Because the main cause is massive fluid loss, the initial treatment is immediate replacement of that loss with any available fluid and oxygen administration. Further management as described in Chapter 26 may then be instituted.

BURNS

Fluid losses from a major burn arise from:

- The burned skin that cannot prevent the uncontrolled evaporation of water from the body surface (up to 140–180g of water/m^{-2}/hour).
- Heat causing capillary damage and a great increase in permeability that leads to oedema formation. This is partly due to lymphatic overload but the lymphatic system also fails to function efficiently.
- Loss of plasma from the skin-denuded surface (2–3 L/24 hours).
- Inhalation of smoke and the products of combustion which have a similar effect on the pulmonary capillaries and increase the overall fluid requirements.
- Failure to maintain normal fluid and electrolyte intake.
- Bleeding from the surgical excision of the burn and from the skin donor sites.

Some of the fluid loss is manifested by oedema, especially if the limbs are affected. In addition, all the fluid and electrolyte changes that occur as a result of the stress response are superimposed on the above.

The overall effect is to lose large amounts of protein-rich fluid and, if untreated, the end result will be dehydration, hypovolaemia, hypotension, renal shutdown and death.

Treatment is aimed at replacing these fluid losses and at the same time providing the normal fluid and electrolyte requirements for the patient. Resuscitation may be with crystalloid, colloid or a combination of both but the development of significant oedema is more likely with crystalloid therapy. This is because the fluid is not completely retained within the circulation but is distributed throughout all the body compartments.

Although the safety of albumin is being questioned, most UK burns units still use it as the mainstay of resuscitation. Treatment is calculated from the time of the burn and is divided into 3 × 4-hour periods, 2 × 6-hour periods and one period of 12 hours. For each period, human albumin solution is given at the rate of 0.5 ml/% burn/kg body weight. In addition, dextrose solution is given at the rate of 1–2 ml/kg body weight/hour. These formulae are only intended as guides and a starting point. Frequently more fluid is needed and repeated blood tests determine the nature and composition of that fluid.

DIAGNOSIS OF ABNORMAL FLUID BALANCE

Before we can attempt to correct the abnormal fluid balance, we must have an idea of how much water and electrolytes the patient needs. As with all clinical diagnosis, this is based on the history of the condition, examination of the patient and special investigations.

HISTORY

From the above discussion it is obvious that important information may be obtained by questioning the patient. The patient's symptoms, the site of fluid loss and the length of time that the patient has been affected will indicate the type and volume of fluid and electrolyte derangement. In addition, a careful review of the fluid balance chart should confirm our suspicions and give a guide as to the severity of the disturbance.

EXAMINATION

The examination partly confirms conclusions from the history but also gives us a more objective view of the problem, e.g. signs of dehydration, hypotension or shock. If the patient appears to be worse than the history suggests it may be that there is some hidden fluid loss such as an intestinal obstruction.

SPECIAL INVESTIGATIONS

Special investigations add a quantitative dimension to the history and examination and provide data on which to base the resuscitation. The actual values are assessed against the normal values for that particular investigation. Thus the amount that the haematocrit has increased will allow an estimate of the volume of fluid required in order to correct the dehydration, taking into account the patient's body weight, while the concentration of electrolytes in the serum will indicate the type of resuscitation fluid required. Calculations to correct any imbalance are based on the assumption that these values were normal before the patient became ill but in some circumstances, e.g. Addison's disease, they also provide a diagnosis. It is important to remember that the electrolyte content of any fluid lost may be measured, including gastric aspirate, intestinal juices and urine.

PRINCIPLES INVOLVED IN THE TREATMENT OF ABNORMAL FLUID BALANCE

Once the above process has been completed it should be possible to identify:

- The normal fluid and electrolyte requirements for maintenance therapy.
- The amount of fluid needed to correct the deficit.
- The amount of sodium, potassium and other substances needed to correct the imbalance.
- A corrective fluid regime based on these assumptions.

The aim is to adjust the imbalance approximately and allow normal body processes to achieve this correction in full. In practice, this exercise may take many hours and regular blood investigations are needed to assess the progress of the resuscitation and the effectiveness of the fluid therapy. As previously stated, there is often a compromise between the urgency of the surgery and the adequacy of resuscitation. Fundamental to this compromise is patient safety and, except in cases of genuine emergency, the patient should have a relatively stable cardiovascular system and be broadly in fluid and electrolyte balance.

INTRAVENOUS INFUSION FLUIDS

The preparation for and the administration of intravenous fluids, including blood products, is a common routine for practitioners but requires the same knowledge, responsibility and consideration as for any other substance given to a patient. Intravenous fluids are often divided into two categories: crystalloids and colloids. A *crystalloid* may be described as an intravenous fluid that will cross a semipermeable membrane, thus allowing movement of electrolytes to correct any imbalance. Examples of crystalloids are saline 0.9% (normal saline), dextrose and Hartmann's solution. A *colloid* is a fluid that will initially remain within the cardiovascular circulation and although useful for replacing blood volume, it is less effective for correcting electrolyte imbalance. Generally, colloids have a higher molecular weight than crystalloids and are more expensive. Colloids include blood products,

hetastarch, gelatin derivatives and the dextrans. Colloids together with blood products and their use will be considered in Chapter 21.

The way that water moves between areas of differing osmotic pressures has already been described but it is also important to know if an intravenous solution will be osmotically active when it is given to the patient. This property may be described as the *tonicity* of the fluid. An *isotonic* solution is one that has the same osmotic pressure as the tissue fluids. It does not attract water from the tissues and neither will water pass from it to the tissues and except by the normal process of filtration. A *hypotonic* solution has a lower osmotic pressure than the tissue fluids and water is therefore drawn from it into the tissues. On the other hand, a *hypertonic* solution has a higher osmotic pressure than that of the tissue fluids and therefore tends to draw water from the tissues. Most of the commonly used IV infusions are isotonic. The use of hypotonic solutions may give rise to pulmonary oedema, whereas hypertonic solutions are useful in neurosurgery for their effect of decreasing the intracranial volume. The more common intravenous fluids will now be described.

5% DEXTROSE

5% dextrose is effectively a means of giving water to the patient without affecting the electrolyte balance (apart from the dilutional effects) or causing haemolysis. The addition of dextrose provides a small amount of energy source (5 g of dextrose sugar/100 ml), which is fully metabolized leaving free water. It is isotonic with plasma, has a pH of 4.55 and is the fluid of choice in patients retaining sodium or at risk from heart failure. Dextrose is also suitable for diluting drugs unless they are acid labile, e.g. the penicillins and amphotericin B.

10% DEXTROSE

10% dextrose contains 10 g of dextrose sugar in each 100 ml of water and is more suitable for patients who need a supply of intravenous calories.

NORMAL SALINE OR 0.9% SALINE

The term 'normal' refers to the fact that it is physiologically normal or isotonic with the plasma. It has a pH of 7.0 and contains 0.9 g of sodium chloride in each 100 ml of water. In order to meet the sodium requirements the average patient needs the equivalent of about 500 ml of 0.9% saline each day. Rapid infusion may raise the blood pressure for a short period but excessive administration increases the salt content of the body, leading to fluid retention and oedema. It should only be used for drug dilution if specifically indicated.

DEXTROSE/SALINE

Dextrose/saline is a mixture of 0.18% saline and 4.3% dextrose. Thus, it contains 0.18 g of sodium chloride and 4.3 g of dextrose in each 100 ml of water. Effectively, this solution is equivalent to giving a patient one part of saline to four parts of dextrose and is a useful way of giving a mixture of salt and water.

HARTMANN'S SOLUTION (RINGER'S LACTATE)

Hartmann's solution, sometimes known as balanced salt solution, is designed to replace extracellular fluid loss and is therefore isotonic and has a composition very similar to that of plasma. It contains 131 mmol/l of sodium, 2 mmol/l of calcium, 112 mmol/l of chloride and 28 mmol/l of lactate. (In the body the lactate is metabolized to bicarbonate.) It is widely used for general fluid replacement but it may precipitate a lactic acid acidosis in the diabetic patient and is therefore best avoided in this condition.

8.4% SODIUM BICARBONATE

This solution contains 8.4 g of sodium bicarbonate in each 100 ml of water. It is used for correcting acute metabolic acidosis, e.g. following cardiac arrest and diabetic acidosis if the body pH falls below 7.1–7.2. In order to prevent rebound alkalosis, it is usually used in amounts of between 50 and 100 ml. It also increases carbon dioxide formation and raises the plasma osmolality.

MANNITOL

Mannitol is an alcohol procured from a plant and is available in 10% or 20% solutions. Because it is osmotically active it causes water to move from the extracellular and intracellular compartments into the cardiovascular circulation. Mannitol is excreted by the kidneys and promotes an osmotic diuresis leading to dehydration of tissues. This has been used to advantage by decreasing the intracranial pressure, e.g. following head injury.

USING THE INTRAVENOUS ROUTE

REASONS FOR USING INTRAVENOUS ROUTE

1. The replacement of fluid, electrolytes, proteins and blood products. (If needed, large volumes of fluid can be administered quickly.).
2. Induction of anaesthesia.
3. To feed patients who are unable to take sufficient oral nutrition for their metabolic needs.
4. As a route for drug administration because drugs reach the site of action more quickly than by any other route and the subsequent action is more certain. Equally, some agents are not absorbed in the alimentary tract. In shock drugs may not be absorbed from the gastrointestinal tract or from the muscles.
5. As a method of altering body chemistry, e.g. diuretics and electrolytes.

SITES FOR CANNULATION

Venous access is usually via a needle or cannula inserted into a vein, either peripherally or centrally. The most common site for cannulation is a peripheral vein, usually the cephalic vein or one of its branches in the upper limb or the dorsal aspect of the hand. It is not unusual, however, to use the lower limb and in small children scalp veins are commonly used. The vein chosen depends on the reason for cannulation, the availability of a suitable vein and, in the case of surgery, the operation site. If possible, the needle or cannula should be away from known arteries and should also avoid joints whenever possible to allow the patient the maximum freedom of movement.

Central venous cannulation is indicated for:

- Central venous pressure (CVP) or pulmonary artery pressure monitoring.
- The use of irritant or vasoactive drugs.
- Unsuccessful peripheral cannulation.
- Long-term fluid administration.

Double or triple-lumen CVP catheters are commonly used in intensive care units. Unfortunately, they only have small lumens and are unsuitable for the rapid administration of fluid and blood products. If rapid transfusion is a possibility an alternative intravenous route should be established.

Common sites for central venous cannulation include the internal and external jugular veins, subclavian, cephalic, and femoral veins.

EQUIPMENT

Before commencing cannulation it is important to make sure that:

- All equipment is in working order.
- All equipment needed is in the work area.
- All equipment is in date and sterile where appropriate.

The equipment needed for an intravenous infusion is essentially the same as for an intravenous injection but a giving set is used instead of a syringe. The various items are listed below.

- Skin disinfectant (antiseptic).
- Local anaesthetic if required.
- Intravenous cannula.
- Fixation for the cannula (strapping, Opsite, etc.).
- Administration set or syringe.
- Fluid or drug.
- Support for the intravenous infusion administration equipment.

Needles and cannulae are used to introduce substances to or remove substances from the body. Although there are relatively few sizes in clinical use, there are many different designs and manufacturers. The final selection will depend on use and value for money. Christopher Wren first described the use of needles for injection in 1659 and this developed via the use of metal tubes and stilettes into the hypodermic cannula and trocar of the 19th century and the modern needles of today. The four main types used in theatre practice are hypodermic needles, intravenous needles, cannulae and epidural and spinal needles.

Hypodermic needles have many uses in the theatre arena varying from single-dose injections to surgical aspiration. The gauge (G) defines the size of a needle or cannula. This classification developed from the wire and cable industry and is based on the number of times the wire is drawn through the draw plate during manufacture. The gauge refers to the external diameter of the needle but the internal diameter may vary depending on the different materials used and the required needle strengths. Colour coding of gauge measurements for hypodermic needles is mandatory in the UK and is illustrated in Table 20.2.

Intravenous needles such as 'butterflies' are commonly made from metal with plastic tubing and plastic winglike supports. Because they are rigid they have the potential of piercing the wall of the vessel in which they are placed when the limb is moved or manipulated. They are usually used for short-term or single-dose access but since the advent of plastic cannulae their use is less common.

The introduction of single-use plastic *cannulae* in the 1970s led to research into the effect that different sizes of cannula had on the flow rate of the fluids passing through them. A British Standard for the size of cannulae was based on this work. Table 20.3 gives an indication of the choice of cannula available for clinical use and a guide to colour coding.

The administration set consists of:

- A piercing needle.
- Filter.
- Drip chamber.
- Tubing.
- Flow regulator.
- An injection port (variable).

The internal diameter of the tubing is 4 mm and, if present, the filter in the drip chamber has a pore size of 170 μm. If an extension is used it will increase the resistance to flow and hence decrease the flow rate. Non-blood administration sets do not have a filter, the float chamber is narrower and it is not possible to increase the flow rate by squeezing the float chamber. They are, however, much cheaper.

A number of different methods are available to control the infusion rate. Gravity-fed infusion sets are the most commonly used. Regulation by a simple plastic roller clamp or similar manually controlled in-line flow regulator mainly depends on the height of the infusion above the patient (gravity) and variation in the patient's venous pressure. Control is inaccurate and fluids are rarely given over the correct period although this is usually of no clinical significance. They are unsatisfactory, however, if accurate control of flow rate is required.

Paediatric infusion sets still ultimately depend on the above but use a screw clamp for easier adjustment and have a graduated burette to give better volume control. Infusion sets for crystalloid administration have a smaller, less variable drop size. In one type the number of drops/minute is equal to the ml/hour delivered. Blood or colloid should not be given using this type of giving set.

Other devices including volumetric pumps, e.g. Ivac, Imed and Valleylab, are more accurate and are alarmed. They are, however, much more expensive. Syringe

Table 20.2 Colour coding of hypodermic needles	
Gauge	Colour
26G	Brown
25G	Orange
23G	Blue
22G	Black
21G	Green
20G	Yellow
19G	Cream

Table 20.3 Flow rates and colour codes for different sizes of cannulae		
Gauge of cannula	Flow rate in ml/minute	Colour code
14G	250–360 ml/min	Orange
16G	130–220 ml/min	Grey
18G	75–120 ml/min	Green
20G	40–80 ml/min	Pink

pumps are the most accurate but should be alarmed for occlusion and overpressure. Care must be taken to ensure that extravascular injection does not occur if the needle becomes dislodged from the vein. If there is a need for rapid infusion it is important to ensure that a large cannula is in situ. Squeezing the float chamber is one way of achieving this but placing a pressure infusion cuff around the collapsible plastic fluid container and inflating it is by far the most efficient method. Securing the needle or cannula adequately is most important, especially in children. The aim should be to give the patient the maximum flexibility of movement but at the same time preserve the integrity of the system. If the giving set tubing is looped near the drip site the possibility of pulling the cannula out of the vein will be minimized.

PREPARATION OF EQUIPMENT

All equipment that is requested by the clinician should be available within the clinical area and its sterility confirmed (if relevant). Intravenous fluids should be checked in the way that drugs are checked and this is summarized below.

- The fluid is in date.
- There is no moisture between the wrapping layers as this may indicate a failure of sterility.
- The fluid is clear.
- The batch number is noted (unfortunately this is rarely done).
- If any additives are to be used, they are compatible and the patient is not allergic to them.
- If the anaesthetist adds any substance to the infusion, a label is attached and signed.

CANNULATION OF THE VEIN

It is important that the intravenous infusion is set up in a sterile manner and that the tubing does not contain any air. Once the size of cannula to be used has been decided, the procedure can begin. **Remember at all times to wear gloves if you are likely to be in contact with body fluids**.

In order to aid cannulation, the limb is gently squeezed proximal to the intended site and gentle slapping of the site usually helps venous filling. Distal veins are usually selected initially, so that if the first attempt is unsuccessful more proximal veins can still be used. The insertion of large-bore cannula often requires a subcutaneous injection of a local anaesthetic agent to reduce the pain of cannulation. In extreme cases, a surgical 'cut-down,' onto a peripheral vein may be necessary.

It is important to tell the patient what is going to happen. The site is cleaned with a suitable agent and the cannula is introduced after first warning the patient. Venous blood should then flush into the cannula. (If the blood looks arterial or the blood is noted to pulsate within the cannula the needle should be removed and the procedure repeated. In this way the chance of intra-arterial injection will be minimized.) The introducer is then removed and either the infusion is connected to the cannula or the cannula is capped prior to intravenous injection. **All sharps must be placed in the appropriate receptacle. Do not put sharps, syringes or glassware on the patient's trolley or pillow**. The cannula may then be fixed carefully in place (taking note of any allergies to the tape used) because poorly secured cannulae will become dislodged by the patient or staff. It is always useful to fix a loop into the infusion tubing so that it does not become accidentally dislodged. Many times this has saved the day when moving patients as it is very easy to leave the infusion still attached to the stand. Finally, the flow clamp should be opened to check that the fluid is flowing properly.

DISPOSAL OF IV INFUSION EQUIPMENT

Great care must be taken when disposing of equipment used in intravascular procedures. All needles, including the piercing end of infusion sets, must be regarded as contaminated sharps and disposed of in designated sharps containers. Used blood bags are potential sources of infection and should be handled with care and disposed of according to departmental policy.

REMOVING CANNULAE AND NEEDLES

Cannulae and needles are often removed in the recovery area and a protocol similar to the one given below should be followed.

1. Tell the patient what is to happen.
2. Remove supporting adhesive tape.
3. Place a swab over the site of entry.
4. Gently press with the swab and at the same time remove the cannula.
5. Apply pressure over the puncture site in order to prevent haematoma formation.
6. Place strapping over the swab to seal the area.

If an arterial cannula is to be removed pressure must be applied to an arterial puncture site for at least five minutes.

COMPLICATIONS OF INTRAVASCULAR CANNULATION

These may be grouped into those resulting from cannulation and using the intravascular route, those specific to central venous access and those relating to intravenous infusion.

Complications following cannulation include haematoma formation, thrombophlebitis, extravascular injection, haemorrhage and infection. Haematomas are more likely to occur following arterial cannulation but are often associated with repeated attempts at cannulation and with poor technique. Thrombophlebitis is an inflammatory process that leads to blockage of the blood vessel with substances such as fibrin. Its occurrence varies with the duration of cannulation, the material from which the cannula is manufactured, the infusion rate (it is less in faster infusions) and the pH and the irritant nature of the drug that is given. Extravascular injection is a common complication but it is only negligent if it is not recognized and dealt with in an appropriate manner. The patient invariably complains of pain on injection or a swelling is observed at the site of the injection or the infusion. Potential tissue and nerve damage may occur if the extravasated drug or fluid is irritant to the tissues. Haemorrhage is most likely if the administration set, the central venous or the arterial line becomes disconnected from the cannula. If this occurs

during arterial monitoring and it is not recognized the outcome may be fatal. Infection is not always the result of poor technique but may be due to cannulation through infected tissue, e.g. burns.

Central venous cannulation is a technique that is easy to learn but may be dangerous if performed badly. There is, however, a complication rate even in the best hands of between 5% and 10%. To some extent complications depend on the site of cannulation but some examples are given below.

- Arterial puncture.
- Haematoma formation.
- Haemorrhage.
- Pneumothorax (1% of subclavian punctures).
- Infection.
- Venous thrombosis.
- Abnormal position of the catheter.
- Hydrothorax.
- Cardiac tamponade.
- Catheter knotting.
- Catheter breaking in the vein.

It should therefore only be used if there is a specific indication. All patients who have had CVP lines inserted prior to an operation should have a chest X-ray to exclude pneumothorax, because if a pneumothorax is present it will expand when anaesthetic gases diffuse into it. This may seriously compromise the patient's respiratory function.

There are a number of complications arising from the use of intravenous infusions. Overinfusion may cause circulatory overload and this may well lead to heart failure. Osmotic imbalance can occur with the excessive use of hypertonic or hypotonic solutions, resulting in cellular dehydration or the formation of oedema (the 'waterlogging' of tissues). Air embolism is caused by air entering the cardiovascular system. This is especially likely when the infusion fluid runs out and air enters the tubing of the administration set. If a new bag of fluid is then connected, the air will be forced into the venous system. Pressure infusors are a major concern because the air will be forced in under pressure when the infusion has run out. Systemic infection may occur if potentially unsterile fluids are used.

CONCLUSION

Properly managed fluid and electrolyte balance is essential if patients are to survive increasingly complex surgery. Attention to detail must include not only the fluid therapy itself but also the techniques used to deliver that fluid therapy.

RECOMMENDED READING

Kox WJ, Gamble J. *Clinical Anaesthesiology. Vol 2, Fluid Resuscitation.* London: Baillière Tindall, 1993.

Taylor TH, Major E, *Hazards and Complications of Anaesthesia. 16 Complications of Fluid Therapy.* London: Churchill Livingstone, 1987.

21

THE PHYSIOLOGY OF BLOOD AND ITS ADMINISTRATION

P. Bolton-Maggs

This chapter will address the special properties of the red blood cells in promoting oxygen carriage, the methods of safe blood and blood component transfusion and consideration of the hazards of these procedures.

THE PHYSIOLOGY OF BLOOD

The vascular system and the blood which flows within it can be regarded as the communication and nutrient highway of the body. Blood consists of a fluid phase, plasma, and cells of the haematopoietic system (e.g. red blood cells, leucocytes and their precursors). Plasma contains numerous elements, chemical messengers and protective proteins, including coagulation factors. The cellular part of the blood consists of red blood cells, which are discussed in more detail below, platelets, which are essential for normal haemostasis, and white blood cells, which are the travelling immune system responsible for host defence.

RED BLOOD CELLS

Haemoglobin is packaged into red blood cells, which normally have a lifespan of 120 days. During this time they probably travel about 300 miles and must be sufficiently deformable to pass repeatedly through the microcirculation where the vessels are less than half the red cell diameter. The special properties of the red cell skeleton (forming a biconcave disc) and metabolic pathways are crucial to these features and any disturbance of these, such as inherited or acquired structural abnormalities (e.g. spherocytosis) or enzyme defects, is likely to adversely affect function and therefore oxygen carrying capacity.

One of the key functions of blood is the transport of oxygen (mainly by the haemoglobin in the red cells) to the tissues and removal of carbon dioxide from them. Red blood cells are produced in the bone marrow, originating from pluripotent stem cells, and are released in a carefully controlled manner so that the production of new red cells (about 2×10^{11} per day) balances the rate of destruction. The rate of production can be increased considerably (up to about eight times the normal rate) and occurs when demand is increased as a consequence of anoxia, haemorrhage, haemolysis or at increased altitudes. Red cell production is controlled by many factors such as the supply of essential constituents and cofactors (including iron, B12 and folate), specific hormones and cytokines, erythropoietin in particular, and others such as growth hormone, thyroxin, corticosteroids and androgens. Erythropoietin is produced mainly in the kidneys, with some produced in the liver, and it enhances red cell production in response to tissue anoxia.

THE PHYSIOLOGY OF HAEMOGLOBIN

Haemoglobin is a unique chemical permitting oxygen exchange. It consists of four polypeptide protein chains—two pairs of globin chains (α and β) – each with a haem group, which lies in a cleft (Fig 21.1). The nature of the globin chains vary with age, in particular before and after birth because of the different physiological requirements of the fetus in utero compared with life outside the womb breathing air. While an adult has mainly haemoglobin A (HbA), the baby at term has predominantly haemoglobin F (HbF). This HbF has a higher oxygen affinity, which is required to permit oxygen exchange in utero across the placenta from the maternal HbA. Haemoglobin production starts to switch from F to A at about 32 weeks gestation, but is not complete until several months after birth. This is important because serious disorders (such as sickle cell disease and β–thalassaemia major) will not be evident clinically at birth. The normal haemoglobins in adult blood are shown in Table 21.1.

THE OXYGEN DISSOCIATION CURVE

The oxygen dissociation curve describes the relationship between the partial pressure of oxygen (pO_2) and the oxygen saturation of the haemoglobin (Fig 21.2). When haemoglobin receives or gives up oxygen molecules the β–globin chains move to accommodate this and permit entry of a substance called 2,3 diphosphoglycerate (2,3-DPG) into the complex in the reduced (or deoxygenated) state. The presence of 2,3-DPG reduces the affinity of the molecule for oxygen. Each haemoglobin molecule contains four chains and therefore four haem groups; these are not all

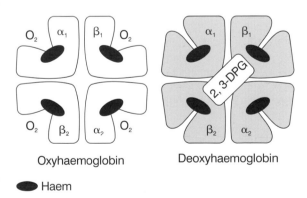

Figure 21.1 Diagrammatic representation of haemoglobin in oxygenated and reduced state, α,β, globin chains of normal adult haemoglobin; 2,3-DPG, 2-3-diphosphoglycerate. (Reproduced with permission of Blackwell Science Publications from Essential Haematology 3E)

Table 21.1 Haemoglobins present in adult blood			
	HbA	HbF	HbA2
Haemoglobin chains	α2 β2	α2 γ2	α2 δ2
Quantity as % present in normal adult	97	0.5–0.8	1.5–3

oxygenated or deoxygenated together, but rather the oxygenation of one will affect the rate of oxygenation of the others – a cooperative effect. When one haem is oxygenated, the attraction for oxygen of the other three haems on the molecule is increased. This characteristic is responsible for the sigmoid shape of the oxygen dissociation curve (Fig 21.2) which means that a large amount of oxygen can be released with a small change in partial pressure of oxygen, as happens physiologically. Arterial blood has a saturation of 95% with a mean arterial oxygen tension of 95 mmHg and venous blood has a saturation of 70% with a mean venous oxygen tension of 70 mmHg. A number of factors can influence this curve and some examples are given below.

1. Lower oxygen affinity (curve shifts to the right – oxygen is given up easily):
   - Increased concentrations of 2,3 DPG.
   - Increased hydrogen ions and carbon dioxide;
   - Anaemia.

- Raised temperature.
- Sickle haemoglobin.
2. Increased oxygen affinity (curve shifts to the left – oxygen is given up less easily:
   - Haemoglobin F.
   - Reduced concentrations of 2,3-DPG (as is the case with transfusion of stored blood and severe septicaemia or acidosis).

WHITE BLOOD CELLS

White blood cells are very important to body defence, but are not a significant part of blood or blood component transfusion at present. In a donor unit of blood the number of neutrophils is inadequate to contribute to the defence system when transfused into a recipient. The presence of white blood cells in donor blood may be deleterious under some circumstances: donor lymphocytes may be viable in a recipient for a prolonged period of time and, if the recipient is immunosuppressed, may attack the host, giving rise to 'graft-versus-host' disease. These white cells can be inactivated by irradiation of the blood prior to transfusion which is therefore indicated for immunosuppressed recipients, e.g. bone marrow transplant patients, babies with congenital immunodeficiency syndromes and some other patients undergoing chemotherapy for malignant diseases. White cells in donor blood are also immunogenic to the recipient, i.e. are likely to provoke an antibody reaction, especially in individuals who are repeatedly transfused. These antibodies develop to tissue type antigens and increase the likelihood both of febrile transfusion reactions (see below) and sensitization to other red cell antigens. Because of these considerations methods of reducing the white blood cells in blood have been introduced. Under certain circumstances a filter can be used at the bedside to remove white cells.

BLOOD AND BLOOD COMPONENT TRANSFUSION

Blood transfusion is the infusion of a blood product from one person (the donor) into another person (the recipient). While transfusion is usually safe and

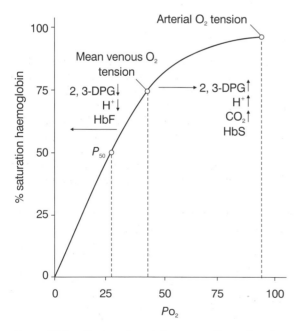

Figure 21.2   Oxygen dissociation curve (Reproduced with permission of Blackwell Science Publications from Essential Haematology 3E)

effective a high standard of practice is required at each step from selection of donors, processing, selection and matching of products through to infusion into the correctly identified recipient in order to avoid dangerous errors. Careful documentation is required at every stage to provide a complete audit trail from donor to recipient.

HISTORY OF BLOOD TRANSFUSION

Although there are accounts of transfusion of blood from animals into man as early as 1667, the first successful transfusion of blood from one person to another is attributed to James Blundell in 1818. He subsequently performed at least 10 transfusions, about half of which were successful. Landsteiner identified ABO antibodies in 1900, leading to the important identification of the ABO blood group system. This was not fully exploited until 1907 when Ottenberg was the first to use compatibility testing (crossmatching). Anticoagulation of blood was essential and, in 1914–15, citrate was introduced which permitted the use of stored blood during the First World War. In subsequent years the anticoagulant solution was refined and reduced in volume and other constituents were added to enhance the quality and the storage life of blood. The advent of plastic bags and tubing from 1949 enabled blood to be separated into components – a major advance in the 1950s.

BLOOD GROUPS AND BLOOD GROUP ANTIBODIES

The surface of the red blood cell is covered by a large number of chemicals that are genetically distinct and which are antigenic, i.e. if transfused into an individual who has not been previously exposed to them, antibodies may develop. More than 300 such antigens have been described but fortunately only a small number are of any clinical significance. There are about 16 major groups of antigens, the most important of which are the ABO and Rhesus (Rh) groups, and all blood donations are typed for these. A number of other antigens, however, can give rise to problems because of the development of antibodies.

Antibodies to blood group antigens may be 'naturally occurring', as with the ABO system, or stimulated by exposure to the antigen, e.g. Rhesus antibodies.

NATURALLY OCCURRING ANTIBODIES

The importance of the ABO system lies in the presence of naturally occurring antibodies. Individuals of one group will develop antibodies to the antigens not present according to Table 21.2. These antibodies are either not present or only present in low titres at birth, but soon increase. They are immunoglobulins (IgM) and usually reactive optimally at 4°C (so-called 'cold') but also react at 37°C. When an individual is transfused with blood of an ABO group to which he possesses naturally occurring antibodies, e.g. group A blood given to a group O individual, the antibody reacts with the red cells causing rapid destruction of the transfused cells (Fig 21.3). This results in a transfusion reaction that may be associated with severe consequences such as renal failure and, at worst, death (10%). Anti-A and anti-B are the most important of these. Because of these antibodies, ABO compatibility is essential for safe blood transfusion.

IMMUNE ANTIBODIES

These are antibodies provoked after an immune challenge, usually a previous blood transfusion or pregnancy because small leaks of blood from the foetal to the maternal circulation are relatively common. The most important antibodies develop in the Rhesus (Rh) system. About 15% of the population are negative for the most important antigen of the Rh system–'D'; 50% of Rh D-negative persons transfused with D-positive blood will develop anti-D antibodies. Immune anti-

Table 21.2 ABO blood groups and corresponding antibodies				
Blood group	Genotype	Red cell antigen	Naturally occurring antibodies	Frequency in the UK (%)
O	OO	O	Anti-A and Anti-B	46
A	AA or AO	A	Anti-B	42
B	BB or BO	B	Anti-A	9
AB	AB	A and B	None	3

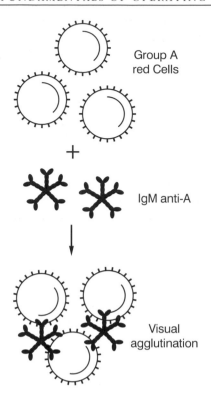

Group A
red Cells

+

IgM anti-A

Visual
agglutination

In ABO blood grouping, Igm antibodies (for example, anti-A) will directly agglutinate red cells carrying the appropriate antigen

Figure 21.3   Reaction of anti-A with a group A-positive red cell. (With permission of BMJ Publishing Group taken from ABC of Transfusion 2E)

bodies are normally immunoglobulins (IgG), react best at 37°C (so-called 'warm') and will cross the placenta with the potential to cause haemolysis in a D-positive fetus. This is known as haemolytic disease of the newborn.

Sensitization against D can be prevented by avoiding transfusion of D-negative individuals with D-positive blood and by giving injections of anti-D to any D-negative woman after the birth of a D-positive infant. The introduction of anti-D prophylaxis in 1969 has greatly reduced the incidence of rhesus haemolytic disease.

It is important to note the Rh system has five antigens – c, C, e, and E as well as D. There is no 'd' antigen – rather 'd' denotes the absence of the antigen known as D. This is in contrast to 'c' and 'e' which, like 'C' and 'E', are antigens and can provoke antibodies. The Rh groups are inherited as two haplotypes (describing the genetic make-up), each of three determinants. An individual who is 'Rh negative' is 'cde/cde', with no 'D'.

The frequency of the common haplotypes (genetic composition) and phenotypes (the outward manifestation of the genetic composition) is given in Table 21.3. It should be noted from these considerations that 'Emergency' Group O Rh Negative blood is not safe for everybody in an emergency and dangerous transfusion reactions may occur.

Other 'irregular' antibodies can develop to antigens other than those of the ABO and Rh systems and are most commonly found in multiply transfused patients, especially those of different racial origin. Before embarking on a regular transfusion programme these patients should have a more extensive red cell typing so that blood for transfusion can be matched against other red cell antigens which are particularly likely to provoke antibodies. In addition, the red cells should be depleted of white cells that make sensitization more likely. This is most easily performed using a bedside inline filter.

TRANSFUSION REACTIONS AND THE 'CROSSMATCH'

Antibodies in the recipient reacting against the donor red cell antigens are the most important. Of much less importance are the donor's antibodies reacting against the recipient's blood. This is partly because the blood tends to be given with most of the plasma removed (as red cell concentrates or various types of 'plasma-reduced' blood) and partly because a relatively small volume is given in relation to the total blood volume of the recipient. These antibodies may be important under some circumstances and all donor blood is screened by the blood transfusion service for the presence of 'irregular' or unexpected antibodies (i.e. other than the ABO antibodies).

The compatibility test (or crossmatch) tests the donor red cells (taken off a special extra line on the donor blood bag) against the serum of the recipient. Two or three different techniques are used in order to detect any unexpected antibody, which might cause an adverse reaction when the blood is transfused. Usually a hospital transfusion laboratory will screen the serum from a potential recipient for such antibodies when a sample is sent for 'group and save' (now usually a 'group and antibody screen'). If no irregular antibodies are detected by this screening the 'crossmatch' is very unlikely to be incompatible. In some countries the group and antibody screen procedure is deemed sufficient so that routine crossmatching is no longer required. In an emergency it is usually safe to issue group-compatible units (i.e. of the same ABO and Rhesus group) if the recipient has

Table 21.3 Rhesus groups			
Abbreviation	CDE nomenclature	Rh D status	Frequency %
R¹r	CDe/cde	Pos	32
rr	cde/cde	Neg	15
R¹R¹	CDe/CDe	Pos	17
R²r	cDE/cde	Pos	13
R¹R²	CDe/cDE	Pos	14
R²R²	cDE/cDE	Pos	4
Others		Pos (mostly)	5

a negative antibody screen. For reasons given above, it is safer to give ABO and Rh group-compatible blood.

In the UK, about 70% of all blood crossmatched is ordered for surgery, but often this is not used. Blood may be returned to stock and re-crossmatched for another patient to reduce wastage. In addition, it is evident that there are considerable variations in practice between teams performing the same surgical procedures (for example, the number of orthopaedic patients transfused after total hip replacement varies from 60% to 93% in different series). In many hospitals 'maximum blood-ordering schedules' (MBOS) have been set in place after discussion with anaesthetists and surgeons (often via a hospital blood transfusion committee) in order to rationalize cross-matching policies. These are not rigid but are designed to improve efficiency and to reduce unnecessary crossmatching and wastage. A schema is illustrated in Figure 21.4.

BLOOD TRANSFUSION PROCEDURE

Blood transfusion must be safe and all the steps in the process should be managed according to strict criteria.

SELECTION OF 'SAFE' BLOOD DONORS

Blood donors are healthy people between the ages of 18 and 65 (17–70 in Scotland) who can donate approx-imately 450 ml usually three or four times a year. Donors are asked not to donate if they are unwell or are in certain high-risk groups with the potential of trans-mitting infection, e.g. IV drug users, homosexuals and individuals who have recently returned from an area where malaria is endemic.

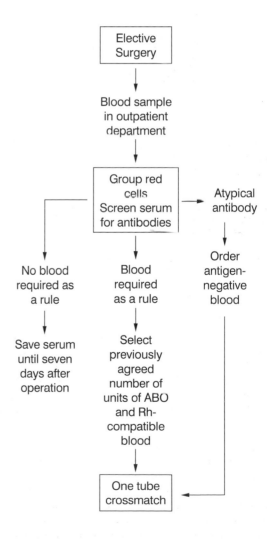

Figure 21.4   Blood ordering policies

SCREENING OF DONATED BLOOD

Donated blood is also tested for potentially transmissible and serious infections. Each donor at every donation is currently tested for evidence of infection with HIV, hepatitis B and C and syphilis. It should be noted that other viruses and infectious organisms, which are not routinely screened for, might be transmitted by transfusion. An important one is cytomegalovirus (CMV). This is of no danger to immunocompetent recipients, but can produce life-threatening illness in immunocompromised recipients (e.g. after organ transplantation or very low birth weight premature babies). CMV-tested blood can be obtained for these patients. Debate is ongoing about other viruses, such as HTLV1, which transmit infection very rarely. HTLV1 can lead to the development of leukaemia after 20 years or so in about 1% of those infected.

Screening for such rare viruses has been deemed not to be cost effective in the UK. Countries where the level of HTLV1 infection in the donor population is much higher (such as Japan where 3–6% of the population is seropositive) have introduced such screening. Recently, in some parts of the USA problems have been encountered with transmission of infections from donors who are immigrants from other countries with a high endemic rate of certain infections, e.g. trypanosomiasis. This kind of risk assessment is ongoing and some tickborne diseases have emerged as potential threats to the blood supply.

PROCESSING AND STORAGE OF BLOOD AT THE BLOOD CENTRE AND HOSPITAL

Currently blood is collected into sterile plastic bags with satellite packs attached. Each bag contains an anti-coagulant solution composed of citrate, phosphate, dextrose and adenine (CPDA). After centrifugation, depending upon the satellite system and requirements, a unit of whole blood is usually separated into component parts (e.g. plasma-reduced blood, plasma and platelet concentrate).

Collected blood must be stored under carefully controlled conditions in a special blood bank refrigerator (with an alarm and temperature chart recorder) to keep the temperature at 4°C (+/- 2°C). Under these conditions the storage life will be 35 days and bacterial growth is minimized. Units of blood must never be stored in a domestic refrigerator on the wards. The temperature in these is not adequately controlled and can vary between +8°C and +10°C at the front to freezing at the rear. Blood that is too warm is a culture medium and freezing leads to lysis of the red cells, with disastrous consequences for the recipient.

CORRECT PROCEDURES FOR IDENTIFICATION OF DONOR AND RECIPIENT, GROUPING AND MATCHING AND FOR BLOOD TRANSFUSION.

When correctly practised, blood transfusion in the UK is very safe. Patients are often anxious about transfusion and the possibility of blood or blood component transfusion should always be discussed with a patient in advance if possible (e.g. prior to elective surgery), preferably with written material available. Patient anxiety often stems from an unrealistic fear of viral transmission, particularly HIV. The risk of this is very low, estimated in the USA at less than one per million components transfused. The risk of hepatitis B transmission is higher, possibly one per 200,000 donations and hepatitis C one per 3000 components transfused prior to hepatitis C screening which was introduced in 1991.

Regrettably, the patient is more 'at risk' from transfusion hazards due to staff mistakes in identification, resulting from failure to observe simple procedures. Each year more than two million units of red cells are transfused in the UK and perhaps four preventable deaths occur, most often due to ABO incompatibility. Deaths are only the tip of the iceberg as only about 1 in 10 ABO-incompatible transfusions is fatal. These occur from two main mistakes of identification: first, the blood samples taken from the potential recipient are wrongly labelled (usually because more than one patient has been bled at a time) and second, because the unit of blood is transfused into the wrong patient. The second error most often occurs in the operating theatre when the patient is unconscious and unable to identify themselves. Mistakes of identification are very rarely made within hospital transfusion laboratories.

Errors undoubtedly occur more often than is realized. A recent study in Glasgow estimated that about 1 in 3300 patients receives incompatible units and the true incidence is likely to be much higher since, due to the frequency of different ABO groups, the 'wrong' blood will be compatible by chance in two-thirds of cases. A national survey of hospital transfusion laboratories responsible for 75% of all units transfused in the UK could identify 111 incidents over two years in which blood was given to the wrong patient.

As a result of these worrying statistics a confidential reporting system was set up at the end of 1996, called the Serious Hazards of Transfusion Reporting System

('SHOT'). A steering group oversees SHOT with wide representation from Royal Colleges and professional bodies. When a major adverse event has been identified, the hospital blood bank or haematology medical staff completes a simple form and sends it to the SHOT office at the Manchester Blood Centre. The adverse events will be analyzed and collated with the intention of making recommendations to further improve transfusion safety.

It should be clear from the above that attention to detail in the practice of blood and blood component transfusion is essential, the following two points being particularly important.

1. When taking samples from a patient for transfusion, the patient must be correctly identified and the procedure carried out as a single uninterrupted operation. The individual who takes the blood must label the tube with the patient's name, date of birth and unique identification number (hospital number). Never prelabel the tubes and never let another person label the tubes for you. The details on the request form must match those on the sample. If the details are incomplete or do not match, the hospital transfusion laboratory will not process your request. Other clearly defined arrangements (i.e. some method of unique numbering of samples) should exist for unidentifiable casualties and major accidents.

2. When a product is to be transfused, two people must independently check that the correct product is being given to the correct patient and both should sign the blood/blood product prescription. At least one of these individuals should be a Registered Health Care Professional.

In addition to the above, it is important that formal records are kept which include the volume of product infused and the duration of the infusion. It is very important that the permanent record includes the unique donation number of every blood component transfused. This is vital if a problem is subsequently identified with a donor (for example, seroconversion to HIV or hepatitis) which necessitates tracking of patients to whom their components have been given. In 1995 hospital blood banks were asked to trace all recipients of donations given in the past from donors who screened positive for hepatitis C when the test was introduced in 1991 (the 'hepatitis C lookback exercise'). This was a mammoth task and although the blood bank may know that a particular product was ordered for a patient, only the record of the donor number at the time of transfusion will confirm that that particular donation was actually given.

Blood should not be removed from the blood bank until it is about to be transfused and it should not be out of the controlled temperature for more than 30 minutes before being set up. Transfusion should last no longer than about four hours, the maximum time from removal of blood from the controlled environment to completion of transfusion being five hours. These limits are set by the transfusion service to reduce the risks of infection. Every hospital should have a written procedure for blood transfusion and an ongoing training programme for all staff involved in order to reduce the risks of error.

Blood Filters

As discussed, the presence of white cells in transfused blood can lead to problems in some recipients. There are two general classes of blood filter available: the microaggregate filter (MAF) which has a mesh of 40 microns and removes microaggregates (consisting of neutrophils, platelets and fibrin strands) and the larger leucocyte-depleting filters which are designed to remove a much higher percentage of white blood cells. The presence of microaggregates may contribute to febrile transfusion reactions and possibly to acute lung injury in the severely ill patient. These MAFs should be considered in multitransfused patients who develop repeated febrile reactions and perhaps in the intensive care setting, although evidence for benefit is not clear. The true leucocyte-depleting filter should only be used for certain patients, usually under the care of haematologists, as mentioned elsewhere in the text.

BLOOD PRODUCTS FOR TRANSFUSION

RED BLOOD CELLS

Red blood cells are available in various volumes and concentrations, which are shown in Table 21.4. It is important to be aware of the differences as 'one unit' of blood can vary considerably in volume. The amount of whole blood issued to hospitals has decreased steadily over the last few years, partly due to pressure for components, and clinicians are encouraged to use the plasma-reduced red cells whenever possible.

FRESH FROZEN PLASMA

Fresh frozen plasma (FFP) is prepared from whole units of blood by centrifugation and separation of the plasma within six hours of blood donation. The units of FFP contain 150–300 ml of plasma and are stored at –30°C with a shelf life of one year. This product is only

Table 21.4 Red cell components

Component	Haematocrit	Volume in bag	Main indication	Precautions
Whole blood+	35–45%	510 ml	Acute severe blood loss	Haemostatic failure if more than twice the blood volume is replaced in a short period of time – monitor platelet count and coagulation tests
Packed red cells	Variable – 55–75%	About 200 ml	Chronic anaemic	Patients on regular transfusion regimes should generally have leucodepleted blood (with suitable inline bedside filters)
Red cells in optimal additive solutions* – SAGM blood	Variable – 50–70%	About 350 ml	Chronic anaemia or any top-up transfusions (including neonates). Often appropriate for use in surgery	Not suitable for exchange transfusions or large volume transfusion to neonates

* Optimal additive solutions are added to resuspend red cells after the plasma has been removed. A commonly used one contains saline, adenine, glucose and mannitol – SAGM. The cells are relatively packed, but easy to transfuse because removal of plasma proteins reduces the viscosity.

+ Fresh whole blood is not generally available. Blood is not released by the blood transfusion service unless it has been fully grouped and screened which is usually when it is more than 24 hours old. In the massively transfused bleeding patient a combination of red cells with platelet concentrates with fresh frozen plasma (as determined by coagulation testing) will be equally effective.

indicated for replacement of coagulation factors when abnormalities of coagulation testing have been documented, for example in patients with disseminated intravascular coagulation (DTC) or liver disease when the defects are multifactorial, and it should not be used for volume replacement alone. The starting dose is 10–15 ml/kg and it must be group compatible, i.e. not contain antibodies which will lyse the recipient's red cells.

Standard locally prepared FFP is not virally inactivated and is therefore not as safe as other fluids such as saline, gelatin or human albumin solutions that can be used for volume replacement (see below). Because of concerns about viral transmission FFP which has been virally inactivated (lipid-enveloped viruses only) by solvent detergent treatment has been produced and is commercially available. This process will not eliminate the non-lipid enveloped viruses such as hepatitis A and parvovirus. This product is more expensive to produce and may not be cost-effective to introduce on a large scale.

CRYOPRECIPITATE

Cryoprecipitate is made by thawing FFP at 4°C and collecting the precipitate that forms at this temperature. This fraction (usual volume 10–20 ml) is then stored frozen at -30°C with a shelf life of one year. It is rich in factor VIIIc, Von Willebrand factor and fibrinogen. In the 1960s and 1970s this product was the mainstay of treatment for haemophilia A and Von Willebrand's disease until about 1986. Currently, heat-treated, plasma-derived or genetically engineered factor concentrates are the treatment of choice for these inherited bleeding disorders.

Cryoprecipitate has limited use and is only indicated for the treatment of DIC when there is bleeding and the fibrinogen concentration has fallen to less than 0.8–1.0 g/L. It may also be of benefit in the microvascular bleeding syndrome associated with massive transfusion. In an adult this may require a dose of 15 bags containing a total of 3–4G of fibrinogen. In children one bag per 6 kg/body weight will raise the fibrinogen by 100 mg/dl.

HUMAN ALBUMIN SOLUTIONS (HAS)

HAS have been available for more than 40 years, with a very safe track record. They are sterilized by filtration and heat treatment and there have been no known instances of viral transmission. There are two products: HAS 4.5%, which is used as a plasma expander, and HAS 20%, which has a much more limited use in some hypoproteinaemic patients. HAS

4.5% is probably used more often than really necessary for volume replacement. It is a very expensive option, as illustrated in Figure 21.5. There is now considerable evidence showing that the cheaper crystalloid solutions are effective for primary resuscitation in trauma and haemorrhage. In addition, albumin offers no particular advantage over the other colloid solutions, which are cheaper.

PLATELETS

Whole donor units of blood do not usefully contribute to the recipient platelet pool. Platelets do not remain viable under the normal storage conditions for red cells (4°C). They can be separated from whole donor units at the blood transfusion centre and left suspended in a small volume of fresh plasma (usually up to 50 ml). These platelet concentrates are stored at 22°C in plastic bags that permit gas exchange, are kept moving in an agitator and have a shelf life of 3–5 days. Each donor unit should have at least 55×10^9 platelets and an adult 'dose' would normally be 5–6 units. Platelet concentrates may also be obtained directly by procedures which remove platelets and return the red cells and most of the plasma to the donor, thus reducing the total number of donors per adult 'dose' and hence the risk of viral transmission. These concentrates contain a variable number of white cells which can be removed by a platelet filter, either in preparation or at the bedside in patients who are likely to need repeated infusions

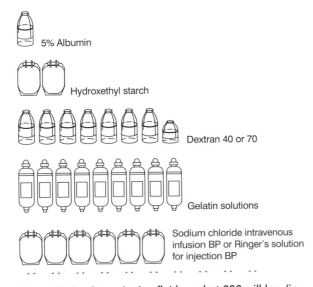

5% Albumin

Hydroxethyl starch

Dextran 40 or 70

Gelatin solutions

Sodium chloride intravenous infusion BP or Ringer's solution for injection BP

Figure 21.5   Resuscitation fluids – what £30 will buy (in 1992) (500 ml units)

(e.g. adults with acute leukaemia or those undergoing bone marrow transplantation).

ARTIFICIAL COLLOIDS

Artificial colloids are of three main groups: dextrans, gelatin solutions and hydroxyethyl starch.

DEXTRANS

Dextran 70 and dextran 40 (lower molecular weight) are complex polymers of D-glucopyranose. Both are effective plasma expanders, the former more than the latter. Dextran 40 is excreted via the kidney and has a shorter half-life in the circulation than dextran 70. The disadvantages include allergic reactions, interference with red cell grouping and crossmatching tests, if blood samples are taken after infusion, and interference with haemostasis which is obviously undesirable in the bleeding patient.

GELATIN SOLUTIONS

These are of variable molecular weight, derived from animal collagen, and show intermediate effectiveness for plasma expansion (less effective than albumin, better than crystalloid solutions). These have become popular in the UK and Europe.

HYDROXYETHYL STARCH SOLUTIONS (HES)

These more recently introduced substances are of precise molecular weight, derived from maize starch and remain in the circulation as long as human albumin solutions. They are excreted in the urine and some is metabolized in body tissues by amylases.

The choice between these various products often depends more upon the personal preference of the medical attendants than on any scientific evidence.

ADVERSE EFFECTS OF BLOOD TRANSFUSION

For convenience these may be divided into 'immediate' or 'delayed' reactions. All patients receiving a transfusion of blood or blood products should be monitored during the infusion to detect any adverse events. If any occur, the infusion should be stopped and appropriate investigations and remedial action taken.

IMMEDIATE REACTIONS

Immediate severe haemolysis due to ABO incompatibility is the most serious but fortunately rare (0.02% of transfusions). The infusion of group A red cells into a group O donor is the most dangerous scenario. The IgM antibodies cause intravascular destruction of the red cells (Figure 21.6) and, in the most severe form, may be evident after only 5–10 ml of blood have been infused. The patient may complain of chills, loin or back pain, dyspnoea or chest pain and may show flushing, tachycardia and hypotension. The damaged red blood cells may trigger the coagulation system, leading to DIC. Many of these symptoms and signs will be masked in the anaesthetized patient. Later, the patient may develop haemoglobinuria or renal failure and death may ensue.

In very rare circumstances the blood may be infected as some strains of Gram-negative bacteria (e.g. Pseudomonas species) proliferate preferentially at the cold storage temperatures and use citrate as an energy source, leading to coagulation of the blood. Shock and hypotension may occur due to endotoxin or septicaemia when infused. The outcome is often fatal. This is one reason why each unit of blood should be inspected before being transfused. Infected units usually show evidence of haemolysis or partial coagulation. Platelet concentrates may also become infected because of their higher storage temperature, most commonly with staphylococcal species, but fatal infections with Salmonella and E. coli have been reported. It is therefore essential to obtain blood cultures in any patient who develops fever during transfusions.

Anaphylaxis may develop due to plasma components. This can also occur with infusion of fresh frozen plasma or cryoprecipitate and may be due to anti-IgA antibodies. A significant number of the general population (one in 700 in the UK) have isolated IgA deficiency and may therefore be sensitized by previous transfusion.

Febrile reactions to transfusions are extremely common (occurring in 5–10% of transfusions) and are due to cytokine release from recipient neutrophils and macrophages triggered by antibodies to white blood cells. These occur most often in previously transfused individuals or women who have had previous pregnancies. The reactions should be documented and investigated. If repeated severe reactions occur, the patient should be given blood depleted of white cells, e.g. by bedside filtration with an appropriate filter.

Urticaria (itchy skin weals) may occur related to allergy to various plasma components. It is usually treated with antihistamines.

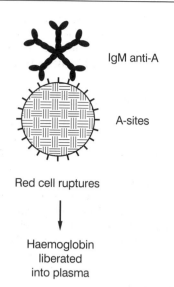

IgM anti-A

A-sites

Red cell ruptures

Haemoglobin liberated into plasma

IgM anti-A on binding to two adjacent A sites activates the whole of the complement pathway (C1-9). C8, 9 make holes in red cell membrane.

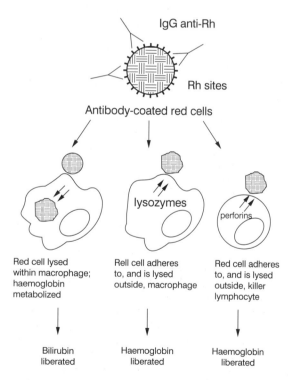

IgG anti-Rh

Rh sites

Antibody-coated red cells

lysozymes

perforins

Red cell lysed within macrophage; haemoglobin metabolized

Rell cell adheres to, and is lysed outside, macrophage

Red cell adheres to, and is lysed outside, killer lymphocyte

Bilirubin liberated

Haemoglobin liberated

Haemoglobin liberated

IgG anti-Rh does not activate complement. Red cell coated with antibody adheres to a macrophage or a killer lymphocyte and is either ingested and lysed or lysed at the cell surface.

Figure 21.6   Mechanisms of red cell destruction by antibodies.

Fluid overload is possible so careful attention should be paid to the volume of blood and blood products infused and also to the rate. All this information should be clearly documented in the patient's case record.

DELAYED REACTIONS

Delayed haemolysis of transfused cells occurs in about 0.2% of transfusions. Such a reaction is rarely fatal and is usually due to IgG antibodies, which lead to extravascular destruction over several days (Figure 21.6). The responsible antibodies are most often from the Rhesus system. The haemoglobin concentration falls over 3–10 days and jaundice may develop, together with a fever. The antiglobulin test will be positive, indicating the presence of an antibody on the red cells. In a mild case the reaction may be missed. Any patient who has had a blood transfusion should be carefully observed over the following 10 days.

Post-transfusion purpura is a rare (<0.01% of transfusions) but potentially life-threatening complication. Individuals negative for particular platelet surface antigens can develop antibodies over 2–14 days post-transfusion if previously sensitized. There is an abrupt onset of purpura and bleeding as the patient's own platelets are consumed by the antibody (the reasons for this are not fully understood). Treatment is with intravenous immunoglobulin or plasma exchange.

Transmission of viral or other infections may become manifest weeks, months or years later. HIV infection has been a very serious problem to haemophiliacs in particular because of the large number of plasma donations pooled to make a single batch of factor VIII concentrate. Since HIV testing was introduced in 1985 there has been only a single British instance of HIV transmission from a donor who was in the 'window' period, i.e. was infected and viraemic but not antibody positive. The tests have been improved in recent years, reducing the window period from 45 to 21 days using HIV antibody tests. The window period can be further reduced to four days but there has to be a balance between the increased costs associated with these tests and the probability of picking up an otherwise missed infection. Although the risk of these infections has been much reduced, as discussed above, there is still a chance of unexpected infection and therefore no blood or blood product should be infused without a clear clinical indication, which has been recorded in the patient notes. Malaria is occasionally transmitted (four reported cases between 1977 and 1986) and the danger is of missing the diagnosis in a febrile, recently transfused patient who has never been out of the country.

MASSIVE TRANSFUSION

When a patient has acute and severe blood loss a considerable proportion of the circulating blood volume may be lost. Massive transfusion is usually taken to mean replacement of more than the patient's total blood volume in less than 24 hours (approximately 70 ml/kg in an adult, 80 ml/kg in an infant). This is most commonly related to trauma, obstetric emergencies or complicated surgery. In addition to the coagulation disturbances that can result, some of these patients will have preexisting coagulopathies (liver disease, shock with DIC), predisposing them to excessive blood loss. Hospitals should have written protocols for the management of obstetric bleeding and gastrointestinal haemorrhage. The priorities in management are given below.

MAINTENANCE OF AN ADEQUATE CIRCULATING VOLUME

Because of the large volumes of fluid required, two large-bore venous cannulae (e.g. 14 gauge) should be introduced. In the short term, a loss of up to 20% of the blood volume (the first litre in an adult) can be achieved by rapid infusion of crystalloid solutions. The maintenance of an acceptable urine output, as measured by an indwelling urinary catheter, is a good guide to the success of the resuscitation.

SURGICAL CONTROL OF THE BLEEDING

It is important that senior medical help is readily available because the Confidential Enquiry into Postoperative Deaths (CEPOD) has identified massive bleeding as a major cause of avoidable perioperative mortality.

MAINTENANCE OF ADEQUATE OXYGEN CARRIAGE

Red cells contain the haemoglobin necessary for the transport of oxygen to the tissues. The haemoglobin concentration or the haematocrit (the proportion of red blood cells in a whole blood sample) is used to determine the need for red cell transfusion. It is most difficult to overtransfuse a patient in the acute phase of massive blood loss. A microcentrifuge in the theatre suite provides a rapid assessment of haematocrit.

WATCH THE COAGULATION PROFILE

Additional blood products such as platelet concentrates, FFP and/or cryoprecipitate should be given according to laboratory results. There is no place for 'formula' replacement of coagulation factors, platelets or electrolytes. It is therefore important to alert the hospital transfusion department as soon as possible and to send adequate initial and repeat samples for estimations of haematocrit, platelet count, crossmatch and coagulation profiles. The hospital should have an agreed protocol in place for obtaining red cell products in an acute emergency. (Is the level of urgency such that the patient should receive group O Rhesus-negative blood?) Often there is enough time to obtain group-compatible units as these should be available within 5–10 minutes if the patient's blood group is already known.

Rapid, large-volume blood transfusion can lead to other complications. If the rate of infusion is more than 50 ml/kg/hour (or more than 500 ml per 10 minutes) a blood warmer should be used to minimize hypothermia. The patient should be monitored for hyperkalaemia (increased serum potassium), acidosis and hypocalcaemia (decreased serum calcium) although the latter is rarely a problem and formula replacement of calcium may be dangerous.

Bleeding problems may be exacerbated by the development of microvascular bleeding manifested as bleeding from mucous membranes, catheter and venepuncture sites, oozing from raw surfaces and petechiae and larger expanding bruises. The most important factor is thrombocytopaenia (platelets often less than 50×10^9/l) due both to dilution by transfusion and increased consumption. Management is with platelet concentrates (e.g. one donor unit/10kg body weight). Other coagulation factors are rarely depleted significantly and should be monitored by regular coagulation profiles. FFP is indicated when the prothrombin time is more than five seconds prolonged and cryoprecipitate given when the fibrinogen falls below 1g/l.

AUTOLOGOUS TRANSFUSION

In recent years, largely because of the impact of HIV transmission, patients prefer not to have donated blood transfusions. The safest blood to have is one's own and there has been increased interest in harvesting the patient's own blood in advance of an elective procedure, with reinfusion at the time of surgery if required. This is a good arrangement for surgery in fit patients who are likely to require 2–4 units, for example for total hip replacement or hysterectomy. Units can be collected weekly, up to four, and screened in the same way as normal units before storage in the standard way.

The logistics of setting up a regular autologous programme may be difficult and although desirable, such units of blood are more 'expensive' to produce than standard donated units to the extent that some transfusion specialists do not consider it to be cost-effective. A recent publication from the USA indicated that the most frequent reason for blood transfusion after a hysterectomy was anaemia caused by autologous blood donation preoperatively. It may be argued that patients should always have the autologous blood returned even though they do not clinically require it.

An alternative way of avoiding transfusion is to salvage the blood shed at the time of surgery and reinfuse it. This is suitable for surgery where the site is bacteriologically clean and free from tumour. Several machines are now available (e.g. Haemonetics Cell Saver systems). The blood is sucked into anticoagulant solution and filtered prior to reinfusion. In some systems the blood is washed and resuspended before reinfusion. The most advanced machines can process about one unit of packed red cells every three minutes which makes them suitable for major surgery with considerable saving of donated blood.

BLOOD SUBSTITUTES

Obtaining blood for transfusion and giving it safely involves several steps and potential hazards, as illustrated above. Not surprisingly, there has been a long-standing and continuing interest in alternative oxygen-carrying solutions that could be safely mass-produced as required, for example, for armies. Despite years of research, the ideal has not yet been achieved but progress has been made and some agents have been used in clinical trials, particularly in Jehovah's Witnesses.

Early studies were made with haemoglobin in solution but toxicity proved to be a major problem. Several products are in existence and animal experiments continue with these. An alternative approach is to use perfluorocarbon solutions that dissolve more oxygen. There was a strong drive to develop all these products in the early 1980s when HIV was first identified in the human blood supply. One product, Fluosol, has been extensively used in Jehovah's Witnesses in Japan. However, in severely anaemic patients there was no survival benefit so this product was not licensed. Research is continuing with second-generation products and it is likely that we shall hear more of these blood substitutes in the future.

RECOMMENDED READING

Contreras M. 1992 *ABC of Transfusion*, 2nd edn. London:BMJ Publishing.

Hoffbrand AV, Pettit JE. 1993 *Essential Haematology*, 3rd edn. Oxford:Blackwell.

McClelland DBL. 1995 *Optimal Use of Donor Blood* Edinburgh:Scottish Office, Clinical Resource and Audit Group.

McCelland DBL. 1996 *Handbook of Transfusion Medicine*, 2nd edn. London:HMSO.

Roberts B. for the British Committee for Standards in Haematology. 1991 *Standard Haematology Practice*. Oxford: Blackwell.

22

FUNDAMENTALS OF PAIN RELIEF

V. Nelson

WHAT IS PAIN?

Pain is a protective mechanism to limit tissue damage. If a person touches a hot object the sensory systems alert them to pain and potential danger so the hand is pulled away, thus preventing further burns. This has evolutionary significance in preserving the human species from harm and explains why we have a nervous system that is very responsive to pain.

Pain is more than a simple reflex reaction however, it is an "unpleasant sensory and emotional experience associated with actual or potential tissue damage". This definition of pain from the International Society for the Study of Pain alludes to suffering as a component of pain.

Pain leads to a series of responses in the autonomic nervous system and the endocrine systems that are aimed at maintaining cardiac output after injury. The pulse rate increases and capillary beds constrict in less essential organs so that blood pressure rises and blood flow to the heart and brain is maintained. Blood clotting is enhanced. Mobilization of blood sugar and increased energy production also occur. All these responses prepare the animal to protect its territory against aggressors or to run from them. This is the "fight or flight" response.

The rise in heart rate resulting from this autonomic response may lead to arrhythmias and cardiac ischaemia in susceptible individuals. Similarly, hypertension increases the risk of haemorrhage and stroke. Pain from an abdominal surgical incision or from fractured ribs causes shallow breathing and poor coughing with the risk of hypoxia and sputum retention (Figure 22.1).

Thus, relief of pain is important for humanitarian reasons and may also reduce the adverse effects of the stress response, which follows surgery.

PAIN ASSESSMENT

Pain is a unique, highly subjective experience and its objective measurement is difficult. Many factors influence the interpretation of a given painful stimulus: fear and anxiety make pain worse and previous experience of pain and cultural differences also affect pain perception. Despite the difficulties, it is important to assess pain in order to determine the effectiveness of the analgesics given. The simplest pain assessment utilizes descriptive categories. The patient is asked to assess their pain as:

No pain   = 0
Mild pain   = 1
Moderate pain = 2
Severe pain   = 3

A standard stimulus such as a laparotomy incision may be rated as "severe" pain by one patient and "moderate" pain by another but both should be reduced if an effective analgesic is given, i.e. the "severe" becomes "moderate" and the "moderate" becomes "mild".

Many more sophisticated pain scales have been devised, such as the continuous "visual analogue scale" (VAS) of 0–10. The patient is asked to mark on a line the point they feel best fits their pain at that moment.

0 _____ 10

NO PAIN   MOST SEVERE PAIN IMAGINABLE

0 represents "no pain", 10 represents the "most severe pain imaginable". This scale allows a greater spread of pain measurements so subtle differences between the effectiveness of different analgesics can be measured.

These techniques can be modified for children with the "FACES" pain-scoring system (Figure 22.2). Here

Response to pain	Advantages	Disadvantages
Tachycardia	Maintains cardiac output	Arrhythmias Cardiac ischaemia
Vasoconstriction	Maintains circulation	Hypertension. Stroke. Heart failure Increased risk of haemorrhage
Heightened awareness	Alert to other dangers	Anxiety and fear
Increased platelet activation	Enhanced haemostasis	Risk of deep vein thrombosis
Substrate mobilization	Enhanced energy production	Hyperglycaemia. Protein breakdown Negative nitrogen balance
Immobilization	Promotes healing	Diaphragmatic splinting. Pneumonia. Sputum retention

Figure 22.1   Summary of the results of pain

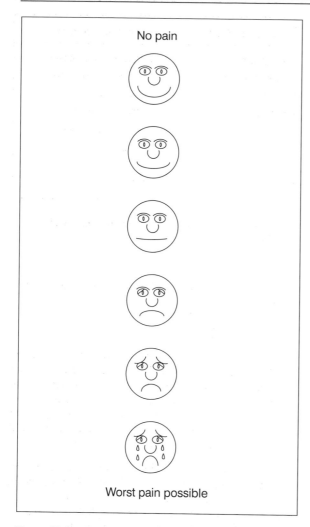

No pain

Worst pain possible

Figure 22.2   Faces pain score.

the child is asked to point to the face that best fits the way they feel. Many hospitals now incorporate a routine pain score measurement on their patient observation charts.

THE IDEAL ANALGESIC

Pharmaceutical companies are constantly researching new drugs. Their aim is to separate analgesia from unwanted side effects. Certain properties of an analgesic are especially desirable.

1. *Rapid onset of action:* the drug can then be titrated to effect.
2. *Easy to administer:* the drug should be stable in solution.

3. *Non-cumulative:* the drug should not accumulate even in the presence of liver or kidney failure.
4. *Cardiovascularly stable.*
5. *No respiratory depression.*
6. *No associated nausea and vomiting.*
7. *No tolerance:* increasing doses should not be necessary to produce the same analgesic effect.
8. *No addiction:* no addictive properties and withdrawal side effects.

Many drugs have been introduced clinically in the belief that they achieve these aims but most fall by the wayside because they have faults. The gold standard is still morphine and, in comparison, most new drugs are less potent analgesics and have increased side effects such as nausea and vomiting.

CLASSIFICATION OF PAIN

The World Health Organization have classified analgesics into three categories: those suitable for mild pain, for moderate pain or for severe pain.

MANAGEMENT OF MILD PAIN

Analgesics such as paracetamol, aspirin and non-steroidal anti-inflammatory drugs (NSAIDs) fall into this category. These drugs are most often used for symptomatic relief of low-intensity pain such as minor surgery, headaches, muscular pains and arthritis. They are not addictive but the recommended dosage must not be exceeded. Overdosage can have serious consequences; for example, paracetamol overdosage is associated with profound liver failure.

These analgesics are effective for mild pain and also have a role as adjuvants to opioids in the management of severe pain. Their mechanism of action is different and therefore additive to the analgesic action of the opioids. Indeed, studies suggest the concomitant dose of morphine can be reduced by up to a third if a NSAID is given as well.

A vast range of NSAIDs is available. Ibuprofen can be purchased over the counter at pharmacies. It is one of the weaker NSAIDs in terms of analgesic action but it is also safer in terms of side effects. Other oral preparations include diclofenac, ketorolac and naproxen. Diclofenac is also available as a deep intramuscular preparation and as a suppository, while ketorolac is available as an intravenous formulation.

MECHANISM OF ACTION OF NSAIDs

When tissue injury occurs there is a localized release of inflammatory mediators, including prostaglandins. Prostaglandins are responsible for the red flare and swelling which occurs around a wound. Aspirin and NSAIDs inhibit the release of inflammatory mediators by blocking an enzyme (prostaglandin synthetase) which is necessary for prostaglandin formation. Prostaglandins also act within the central nervous system to amplify the pain signals that are transmitted along the spinal cord and NSAIDs block this amplification. Although not an anti-inflammatory drug, paracetamol is also thought to act by blocking this central effect.

ADVERSE EFFECTS OF NSAIDs

Prostaglandins occur in most body tissues. Imbalance in their production is responsible for the adverse effects of NSAIDs, which include gastrointestinal problems, bleeding and exacerbation of asthma. New NSAIDs have been developed with the claim of reduced prostaglandin-related side effects.

MANAGEMENT OF MODERATE PAIN

Suitable analgesics include codeine, dihydrocodeine, dextropropoxyphene and tramadol.

Codeine has a similar chemical formula to morphine and about 10% of a dose of codeine is metabolized to morphine within the body. It is probably this that accounts for its analgesic action.

There are many preparations that are based on these drugs in combination with paracetamol. For example, co-codamol is codeine and paracetamol, codydramol is dihydrocodeine and paracetamol. When the dose of the first constituent is kept low, paracetamol is the main constituent and the compound drug should be regarded as a mild analgesic only. With higher dose preparations all the narcotic-related side effects such as nausea, constipation and even respiratory depression can occur.

MANAGEMENT OF SEVERE PAIN

Opioids are the mainstay for relief of severe pain. They act as opiate receptors, which are found throughout the body but in higher concentrations within the central nervous system. Morphine, a derivative of the opium poppy, is the most widely used. Figure 22.3 shows

Desirable effects	Undesirable effects
Analgesia	Respiratory depression
Relief of anxiety	Nausea and vomiting
Sedation	Constipation
Euphoria	Sphincter spasm
	Cough suppression
	Itching
	Tolerance
	Addiction

Figure 22.3 Principal pharmacological effects of opioids.

some of the desirable and undesirable effects of this group of drugs.

MORPHINE

Morphine is the standard against which other opioid analgesics are compared. It is familiar, effective and cheap, being most valuable for the treatment of continuous, dull pain rather than intermittent or sharp pain. It is useful for acute abdominal pain, major trauma, postoperative pain, myocardial infarction and the pain associated with malignant disease.

Morphine is frequently administered intravenously in the perioperative period. Peak analgesic effect is achieved 15–20 minutes after the intravenous injection. The delay is because morphine must penetrate the fatty membranes that surround the central nervous system to produce analgesia. The dosage of morphine required varies tremendously between individuals so it is best titrated to effect. Given intramuscularly, the peak effect of morphine is achieved one hour after administration. The duration of action is four hours but peak analgesia will wane well before this time.

Morphine is active orally although double the dose is required to produce the same effect as when it is given parenterally. Slow-release oral morphine preparations (MST, Oromorph SR) are widely used for pain control in patients with cancer.

As well as the opioid side effects already discussed, morphine can cause a fall in blood pressure, especially if the patient is hypovolaemic. It may also cause an urticarial reaction with redness and hives at the injection site or wheeze in asthmatics, both because of associated histamine release.

PETHIDINE

Pethidine is a man-made opioid. The main pharmacological effects resemble morphine but the drug is less potent. Pethidine produces prompt but shorter acting analgesia when compared to morphine. It is used for analgesia in labour and in the newborn is associated with less respiratory depression than morphine (probably because its action is weaker).

FENTANYL

Fentanyl is another opioid that is structurally related to pethidine. It is more rapid in onset than morphine and has a peak effect after 5–6 minutes as it penetrates the fatty membranes of the central nervous system more readily than morphine. Although a single dose is short acting, repeated doses and infusions become cumulative. Fentanyl is used as a potent analgesic intraoperatively. It is also useful for blunting the circulatory response to stimulation such as laryngoscopy. Its side effects are typical of the opioid analgesics and it causes profound respiratory depression. This can be used to advantage in patients who are being ventilated intraoperatively or in intensive care, as it will suppress the tendency to cough or "fight the ventilator".

OTHER STRONG OPIOIDS

Many drugs have been developed in the hope of producing a painkiller with the analgesic properties of morphine but without side effects. (Figure 22.4). Some of these drugs are swift in onset and relatively short acting so that their main use is as an intraoperative analgesic similar to fentanyl, e.g. alfentanil and remifentanil. Other analgesics have been developed as alternatives to morphine for postoperative analgesia. All these drugs can cause serious respiratory depression.

PARTIAL AGONIST AND MIXED AGONIST-ANTAGONIST OPIOIDS

All the opioid drugs for severe pain described so far have purely "agonist" effects at opiate receptors. This means that they have only positive effects when

Drug	Advantages	Disadvantages	Clinical issues
Alfentanil	Very rapid acting. Short duration	Potent respiratory depression	Intraoperative analgesia. Blunts circulatory response to stimulation
Cyclimorph	Combination of morphine and the antiemetic cyclizine	Cyclizine limits use to 8-hourly	Postoperative analgesic
Diacetylmorphine	Very potent. Produces euphoria	Abuse potential	Strong analgesic for cancer pain or for myocardial infarction
Fentanyl	Rapid acting. Short duration in single dose	Potent respiratory depression. Cumulative in repeat dosage	Intraoperative analgesia. Blunts circulatory response to stimulation
Methadone	Absorbed orally. Long acting	Hard to titrate	Prevention of abstinence reactions in drug addicts
Morphine	Familiar. Cheap	Respiratory depression, Histamine release	Relief of severe pain whatever the cause
Papaveretum	Morphine with codeine and an antispasmodic	Contraindicated in pregnancy	Postoperative analgesia
Pethidine	Slightly faster onset than morphine. Less histamine release	Shorter acting than morphine	Analgesia in labour Asthmatics
Phenoperidine	Rapid acting. Potent	Short duration	Adjuvant to general anaesthesia or to ventilation in ICU
Remifentanil	Rapid onset and rapid offset	Potent respiratory depression	As an intraoperative infusion

Figure 22.4   The strong Analgesics

binding to the opiate receptors, stimulating pain relief and euphoria. Other classes of opioids can have a mixed positive and negative effect. Because of this they are generally not quite as good analgesics but they may have less abuse potential or less respiratory depression associated with their use. These drugs are known as mixed agonist-antagonist opioids. Examples are buprenorphine, pentazocine, nalbuphine and meptazinol.

OPIOID ANTAGONISTS

Severe, life-threatening respiratory depression can occur with any opioid analgesic. Oxygen can be given to counteract hypoxia and maintain oxygen saturation during respiratory depression. This will not combat the accumulation of carbon dioxide that is occurring during hypoventilation and ventilation must be maintained artificially or a specific opioid antagonist should be given.

NALOXONE

Naloxone is the opioid antagonist used clinically and should always be available when opioids are used. The response is rapid and specific, occurring within two minutes of a bolus dose of 400 micrograms (one ampoule). Unfortunately, naloxone also reverses analgesia. Repeat doses may be necessary, especially as the duration of action of naloxone is about an hour, considerably less than the duration of action of most opioids. Renarcotization is a real risk and if naloxone has been used the patient must be observed closely and not prematurely removed from the recovery room.

ROUTES OF ADMINISTRATION OF OPIOIDS

INTRAVENOUS

Direct intravenous injection of an opioid such as morphine is a rapid and highly effective way of administering a painkiller (Figure 22.5). After a bolus intravenous dose of morphine there is a rapid rise to effective analgesic concentrations in the plasma followed by a slow fall-off as the drug is redistributed and eliminated from the body. To avoid this fall-off and prevent recurrence of pain, it is necessary to maintain the effective analgesic plasma concentration with further doses of the opioid. In an ideal world, just enough opioid given as a continuous infusion would be used to achieve this (Figure 22.6).

In practice, it is very hard to predict what infusion rate is necessary as patients vary enormously in their

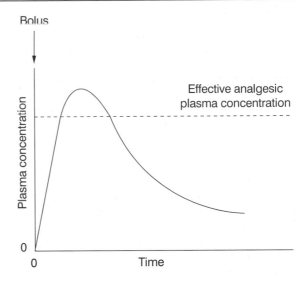

Figure 22.5   Plasma level of opioid after a single intravenous bolus.

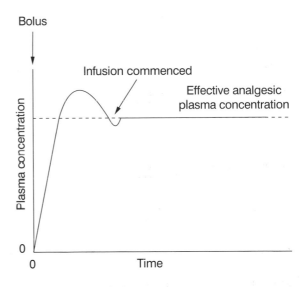

Figure 22.6   Plasma level of opioid after intravenous loading bolus plus infusion (ideal).

effective analgesic plasma concentration and the rate at which they eliminate drugs (Figure 22.7).

If the infusion rate chosen is too high it will give the line "A" in Figure 22.7 where the plasma concentration of the drug is steadily rising, leading to increased side effects and potentially dangerous respiratory depression. If the infusion rate chosen is too low it will give line "B" where the plasma concentration of the drug is steadily falling so that the patient complains of increasing pain. Frequent adjustments have to be made

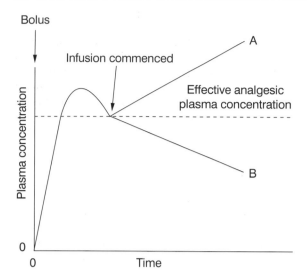

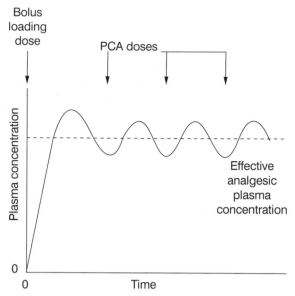

Figure 22.7   Plasma level of opioid after intravenous loading bolus plus infusion (reality).

Figure 22.8   Plasma level of opioid with PCA.

to fixed rate infusions for them to be safe and effective. If a bolus 'loading' dose of an analgesic is given intravenously followed by small frequent bolus doses whenever pain returns, the plasma drug level will stay close to the effective analgesic concentration. (Figure 22.8). This is the principle behind patient-controlled analgesia (PCA).

PCA machines allow the patient to administer a small 'top-up' dose of opioid every few minutes as needed as the machines have a reservoir of drug (commonly morphine). Some of the more sophisticated devices can be programmed to give the initial loading dose from this reservoir too. Further small doses are then given via an intravenous cannula whenever the patient activates the device by pressing a button. As a safety feature the patient cannot activate the device successfully until the previous dose has had time to start working, i.e. usually at least five minutes later. This is known as the 'lockout' period.

Larger PCA devices run off both mains and battery and have a variety of programme options. Some PCA devices can be programmed with different lockout times, and are suitable to be used with a range of drugs. Figure 22.9 shows the Abbott Pain Management Provider pump.

Other PCAs are very simple disposable devices with fixed settings. However, the basic principles are similar. The Baxter 'watch' PCA infuser (Figure 22.10) is a simple disposable PCA device. It is light-weight and pressure driven with a fixed lockout time.

PCAs have become increasingly popular due to improved patient satisfaction when compared with

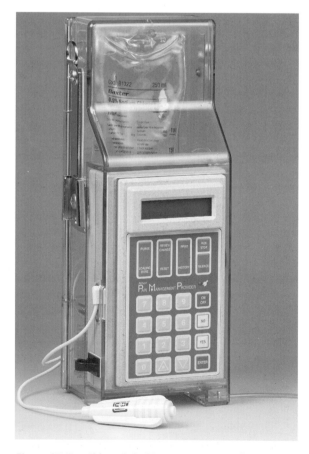

Figure 22.9   Abbott Pain Management Provider pump.

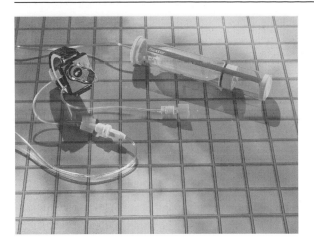

Figure 22.10   Baxter 'Watch' PCA infuser.

traditional intramuscular analgesic injections.

INTRAMUSCULAR

The intramuscular route is a traditional way of administering analgesia for control of postoperative pain. An intramuscular injection starts to work within 30 minutes and reaches peak effect after one hour and thus, compared to the intravenous route, has a slower onset time.

Repeated intramuscular injections give a wider swing in plasma levels than small intravenous doses (Figure 22.11). However, the route is easy to administer even

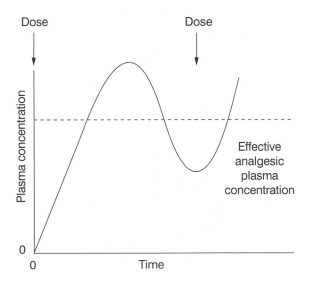

Figure 22.11   Plasma level of opioid after intramuscular injection

when venous access is difficult.

If analgesia is given liberally for pain, the intramuscular route can be highly effective. This is not the case in the shocked patient because the vasoconstriction response to shock means that muscles are poorly perfused; absorption of the drug into the bloodstream will therefore be patchy and slow. When adequate perfusion returns, absorption of the analgesic will occur rapidly, risking overdose.

SUBCUTANEOUS

Although absorption is slower and less predictable than by the intravenous route, the subcutaneous route can be valuable when venous access is a problem. Small cannulae can be placed subcutaneously and taped in position to avoid multiple injections.

ORAL

Many opioids, including morphine and pethidine, are active if taken orally. The dose required is greater than if the intravenous or intramuscular route is used. This is because a smaller proportion of the drug reaches the systemic bloodstream: some is metabolized in the liver first.

Drugs given orally will take longer to work than when given intravenously or intramuscularly but this is an ideal route of administration when pain is long term and predictable, such as the pain associated with cancer.

SUBLINGUAL

Certain opioids are affected by the stomach acidity so that they are ineffective if swallowed. Buprenorphine can be absorbed through mucous membranes, however, and may be given as a sublingual preparation to be dissolved under the tongue.

TRANSDERMAL

Fentanyl is available in slow-release patches applied topically. Analgesia is slow in onset but each patch will last three days. The main use for this technique is in cancer pain where it avoids the need to take frequent medication orally, especially if there are problems in swallowing.

EPIDURAL AND INTRATHECAL

The spinal cord is the dual carriageway of the nervous system. Pain messages are sent up to the brain along it and pain response messages are carried back. A high concentration of opiate receptors lies along the spinal cord and, like traffic lights, they affect the flow of pain messages to and from the brain. By depositing opioids close to their site of action at these receptors, pain perception can be modified. This is the basis of the use of epidural (extradural) and intrathecal opioids and morphine, diamorphine and fentanyl are the most commonly used drugs.

COMPLICATIONS OF OPIOIDS

Whichever route of administration is selected, the same opioid-related side effects can be seen (Figure 22.3).

RESPIRATORY DEPRESSION

The most feared complication is respiratory depression although this is usually reversible with naloxone. Late-onset respiratory depression is a particular problem with epidural and intrathecal opioids as it can occur up to 24 hours after the last dose has been given. Patients receiving opioids by these routes need close observation.

ADDICTION

Although feared, this complication is rare if opioids are used for relief of genuine pain rather than for recreational purposes.

NAUSEA AND VOMITING

This is a common and unpleasant complication with sickness affecting around one-third of postoperative patients overall and up to 90% of patients after certain forms of surgery such as gynaecological procedures. Prolonged bouts of retching increase pain and can contribute to both medical and surgical problems, such as aspiration of gastric contents or wound breakdown.

ANTIEMETICS

PROCHLORPERAZINE (STEMETIL)

This drug may be given intramuscularly, orally, buccally or per rectum. It is the most commonly used antiemetic and is frequently prescribed "as required" when opioids are given.

DROPERIDOL

Droperidol can be given intravenously, intramuscularly or orally. It is more sedating than prochlorperazine. Because it can be used intravenously, it is easy for the anaesthetist to administer. It is compatible with morphine solutions and can be combined with morphine in a single syringe for PCA usage.

METOCLOPRAMIDE (MAXOLON)

A relatively short-acting antiemetic which may be administered by the intravenous, intramuscular or oral routes. Although compatible with morphine solutions, metoclopramide seems less effective than droperidol when used in a PCA. It is also less sedating.

CYCLIZINE

Another sedative antiemetic, cyclizine is an antihistamine. It can be administered separately or in combination with morphine as the drug Cyclimorph.

HYOSCINE

Short acting when given orally or parenterally, hyoscine is also available as a slow-release skin patch.

5HT ANTAGONISTS

This group of drugs, which includes ondansetron, was developed to treat the intense nausea associated with many forms of chemotherapy. 5HT antagonists are also effective in postoperative nausea and vomiting. Because of the cost, they are often used as a second-line treatment when a cheaper antiemetic has failed to control symptoms.

ENTONOX

Entonox is a combination of nitrous oxide and oxygen in a 50:50 mixture and is a useful adjuvant to the analgesic armamentarium. It comes in a premixed cylinder and can be self-administered via a demand valve. Analgesia starts within 30 seconds of inhalation and reaches a peak within two minutes. The offset of action is equally swift as the gas is rapidly eliminated from the lungs when the patient breathes air. It is especially useful to cover short bursts of predictable pain such as during contractions in labour, for changes of surgical dressings or for application of orthopaedic splints to limb fractures.

Entonox can be a potent analgesic if used optimally and is generally safe in short-term usage. It must be avoided in patients who have trapped air within the body such as an undrained pneumothorax. (Nitrous oxide displaces nitrogen by diffusion in a ratio of 35 parts of nitrous oxide in for each part of nitrogen moving out so there will be a rapid increase in pressure within the trapped air.) Long-term continuous usage of entonox for analgesia is not feasible because of an association between nitrous oxide and bone marrow depression.

LOCAL ANAESTHETIC BLOCKS

A suitable local anaesthetic block is an excellent way of providing analgesia, either as the sole anaesthetic, in conjunction with sedation or with light general anaesthesia.

Almost every nerve in the body can be blocked by local anaesthetic when applied with expertise and patience. The most commonly used blocks will be described in more detail (see also Chapter 14).

SPINAL (INTRATHECAL) ANALGESIA

Injection of local anaesthetic into cerebrospinal fluid (CSF) produces temporary blockade of the sensory, motor and autonomic nerves that come into contact with the anaesthetic solution. The sensory block gives the desired analgesia but the associated motor block causes weakness or paralysis while the autonomic block causes vasodilatation of blood vessels within the distribution of the block. Because of this vasodilatation, blood pressure may fall and vasoconstrictor drugs must be readily available to counteract this effect of spinal blockade.

The vertebral level of the injection influences the rate of spread of the block, as does the amount of local anaesthetic injected and the position of the patient. Injection is usually made below the second lumbar vertebra as this is the level at which the spinal cord terminates and there should be less risk of nerve damage from the needle below this level. Fine-bore needles are used, those of "pencil point" configuration and the smallest gauge being the least likely to cause postspinal headache. This is a complication caused by persistent CSF leakage through the hole in the dura (Figure 22.12) made by the spinal needle.

Heavy bupivacaine 0.5% is the most commonly used local anaesthetic. "Heavy" refers to the addition of glucose that makes the solution denser than CSF. Heavy bupivacaine spreads in a very predictable fashion.

EPIDURAL (EXTRADURAL) ANALGESIA

A spinal block requires positioning of the needle through the dural membrane so that the local anaesthetic mixes with CSF. The epidural technique involves positioning of the needle outside the dural membrane in the fat-filled epidural space through which nerves pass after leaving the spinal cord (Figure 22.12).

To establish an epidural blockade, a Tuohy needle of 16 or 17 gauge is used. This is larger than a spinal needle. The epidural space is identified by loss of resistance to a syringe filled with saline or air. When the needle passes through the elastic membranes of the spinal ligaments and into the epidural space, there is a characteristic "give". Either a bolus dose of local anaesthetic is then injected or a plastic catheter is fed through the Tuohy needle into the epidural space in order to permit a continuous infusion technique.

The spinal level at which the epidural is performed will affect the dermatomal height of the resultant block. Lumbar block is performed more commonly than thoracic block and the epidural space is widest (0.5 cm) at this level. Should the Tuohy needle accidentally be inserted too deeply and a tear made in the dura, the subsequent CSF leakage can result in an unpleasant headache.

CAUDAL (EXTRADURAL SACRAL) ANALGESIA

There is an anatomical gap at the base of the sacrum where the fifth sacral vertebra has no spinous process. This gap, known as the sacral hiatus, is utilized in the caudal technique as a low approach to the epidural space (Figure 22.12). Local anaesthetic is injected through the sacrococcygeal membrane, which covers the sacral hiatus, into the epidural space. Larger volumes of local anaesthetic are required at this level to produce an effective block, e.g. 20 ml in the adult patient.

Both intrathecal and epidural techniques require strict asepsis to prevent meningitis or abscess formation. Infection of the overlying skin is a contraindication to these blocks.

BRACHIAL PLEXUS BLOCK

The brachial plexus is formed by fusion of C5, C6, C7, C8 and T1 nerve roots. It can be blocked high in its course down from the cervical vertebrae (interscalene approach), behind the clavicle where it lies on the first rib (supraclavicular approach) or in the axilla (axillary approach).

In the axilla the plexus of nerves surround the axillary artery which is the landmark for this nerve block (Figure 22.13). The patient's arm is abducted to 90° and the needle introduced adjacent to the arterial pulse. Marked pulsation of the needle indicates that the tip lies in the correct fascial compartment, close to the artery.

BIER'S BLOCK (INTRAVENOUS REGIONAL ANALGESIA)

Local anaesthetic can be injected into the venous system to achieve analgesia. After elevation to exsanguinate the limb, a tourniquet is inflated to 50 mmHg

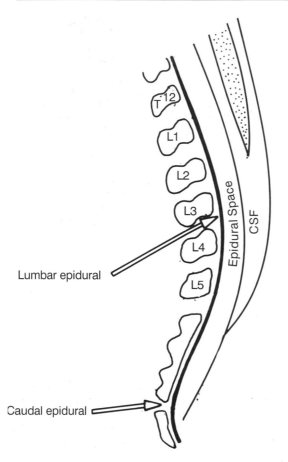

Figure 22.12   Spinal anatomy

above systolic pressure. Local anaesthetic, usually prilocaine, is injected into a vein below the tourniquet. This diffuses out into the tissues and analgesia results. This technique is limited by duration of surgery as the tourniquet becomes uncomfortable after about 40 minutes and tourniquet release would be followed by return of sensation. Tourniquet pain may be minimized by the use of a double tourniquet cuff. The more proximal cuff is inflated prior to injecting the local anaesthetic and, once the block is effective, the more distal cuff is inflated and the former released. This means that the tourniquet is effectively inflated over anaesthetized tissues.

WRIST BLOCK

Partial or complete wrist block is a valuable technique for minor surgery.

The ulnar nerve supplies the medial side of the hand and can be blocked at the wrist immediately to the ulnar side of the ulnar artery.

The median nerve supplies the lateral side of the palmar aspect of the hand. This nerve is located at the midpoint of the wrist between the flexor carpi radialis tendon and the palmaris longus tendon.

The radial nerve supplies most of the dorsum of the hand and it can be blocked by infiltrating in an arc subcutaneously around the radial border of the wrist.

The anatomy is illustrated in Figure 22.14.

DIGITAL NERVE BLOCK

If an injection is made at either side of the base of the digit both palmar and dorsal digital nerves can be anaesthetized. Adrenaline must never be used in the local anaesthetic solution as gangrene could result. This is because the arteries are "end arteries" and do not form connections with other neighbouring arteries. Vasoconstriction therefore cuts off the blood supply to the digit.

INTERCOSTAL NERVE BLOCK

The upper six intercostal nerves innervate the chest wall while the lower six intercostal nerves run down to innervate part of the abdominal wall. An intercostal nerve block can be used to ease the pain of fractured ribs or to reduce postoperative abdominal pain.

Each intercostal nerve runs directly below its respective rib and can be blocked by local anaesthetic placed immediately below the rib.

INGUINAL FIELD BLOCK

This is a useful technique to provide analgesia for inguinal hernia repair.

Three nerves supply the inguinal area: the iliohypogastric, the ilioinguinal and the genitofemoral. Infiltration must cover all three nerves for an effective block (Figure 22.15).

The anterior superior iliac spine is identified and local anaesthetic is infiltrated in an arc from a point 3 cm medial to this. The pubic tubercle is then identified and local anaesthetic is again infiltrated in an arc.

PENILE BLOCK

The dorsal nerves of the penis travel beneath the pubic bone, one on either side of the midline. Good analgesia for circumcision can be obtained by infiltrating each dorsal nerve at the root of the penis. Adrenaline must not be used, as the arteries of the penis are end arteries just like the digital arteries.

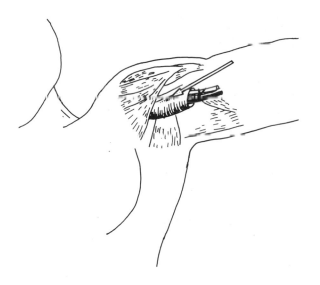

Figure 22.13   Axillary plexus block.

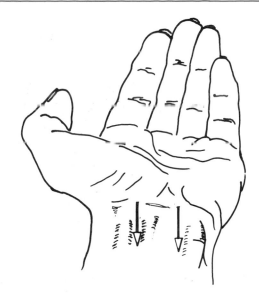

Figure 22.14   Wrist block

FEMORAL NERVE BLOCK

Femoral nerve block can greatly reduce pain from a femoral fracture, in both adults and children. The nerve is easily blocked just below the inguinal ligament, immediately lateral to the femoral artery.

3-IN-1 BLOCK (INGUINAL PERIVASCULAR BLOCK)

Because of local anaesthetic spread, injection of a large volume of local anaesthetic into the region of the femoral nerve may also block the obturator and external femoral cutaneous nerves.

SCIATIC NERVE BLOCK

The sciatic nerve supplies sensation to the back of the thigh and most of the lower leg. Sciatic nerve blocks are useful for fractures below the knee. This block may be achieved in two ways.

In the posterior approach the nerve can be blocked in the buttock. The surface marking for the block is 5 cm below the midpoint of a line joining the greater trochanter of the femur and posterior superior iliac spine.

Using the anterior approach, the sciatic nerve can be blocked, avoiding the need to move the patient if they have a tibial fracture. The nerve here lies between the ischial tuberosity and the greater trochanter.

ANKLE BLOCK

Several small nerves must be blocked at the ankle to produce analgesia in the foot. Subcutaneous infiltration around a large part of the ankle is necessary to cover all these nerves. Nevertheless, this is a useful analgesic technique when combined with light general anaesthesia.

WOUND INFILTRATION

Infiltration of the wound with local anaesthetic at the time of surgical closure is a simple but effective means of decreasing postoperative pain.

PAIN CLINICS AND THE MANAGEMENT OF CHRONIC PAIN

Chronic pain is defined as pain that persists beyond the time period normally expected after an injury. Many factors are implicated in chronic pain, revolving around abnormalities within the central nervous system. It is acknowledged that, just like acute pain, psychological factors are very important and these must also be addressed.

Pain clinics sprang up in the 1950s, initially as "nerve block" clinics. These were usually run by anaesthetists because of their expertise in nerve blocks gained in the operating theatre. Today, the pain clinic is multidisciplinary. In conjunction with physical techniques, considerable input from physiotherapists, psychologists and rehabilitative medicine specialists aids recovery of the chronic pain sufferer.

Nowadays there is much more emphasis on teaching the chronic pain patient coping strategies and rehabilitating them into society. However, physical treatments are still used and the more common ones are described below.

RADIOFREQUENCY LESIONING

Radiofrequency lesioning is a method for destroying nerves through heat. A high-frequency current is passed down a thermocouple probe positioned against the nerve. By careful selection of temperature and duration, pain nerves can be destroyed whilst normal sensation is left relatively intact.

This is a useful technique when cancer pain affects one side of the body only. Lesioning of a part of the spinal cord associated with pain transmission is known as cordotomy. Debilitating facial pain known as trigeminal neuralgia can also be treated by radiofrequency lesioning and low back pain sufferers may sometimes be helped by radiofrequency lesioning of nerves to facet joints.

CRYOTHERAPY

The cryoprobe is a method of freezing nervous tissue. Carbon dioxide or nitrous oxide is forced out of the probe tip at high pressure. The gas expands and the subsequent temperature drop means heat is drawn out of the tissues adjacent to the cryoprobe tip. If the tip is placed close to a nerve it will freeze the nervous tissue. Freezing temporarily prevents conduction along a nerve, often for a couple of months.

CHEMICAL NEUROLYSIS

Nerves that can be blocked by local anaesthetics can be more permanently destroyed with phenol or alcohol injections. Unfortunately, many nerves have motor function as well as sensory innervation and the benefits of semipermanent numbness must be weighed against drawbacks such as motor weakness or incompetence of bladder or bowel sphincters causing incontinence. Blockade of the lumbar sympathetic system of nerves (which control blood vessel tone in the lower half of the body) with phenol can improve the blood supply to the skin of the legs and aid ulcer healing. Similarly, coeliac plexus blockade by alcohol injection is a valuable technique in relieving pain associated with cancer of the pancreas.

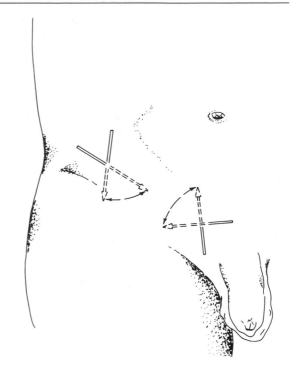

Figure 22.15   Inguinal field block.

INTRAVENOUS SYMPATHETIC BLOCK

Abnormalities within the sympathetic nervous system can cause chronic pain. When this occurs in a limb, injection of the drug guanethidine into the limb may have a beneficial effect through its sympathetic blocking action. Because of the undesirable systemic effects of guanethidine (mainly causing hypotension), it is given under tourniquet using the same technique as the Bier's block.

LOCAL ANAESTHETICS

Various nerve blocks can be performed with local anaesthetic, either to diagnose the source of the pain or as a treatment. In the latter case the local anaesthetic is often combined with a steroid, which reduces any swelling around the nerve which could be contributing to the pain.

STIMULATION TECHNIQUES

These techniques are particularly useful in musculoskeletal pain.

Acupuncture

The traditional Chinese art of inserting tiny needles at special points on the body has been regarded with some scepticism in scientifically based Western medicine. Research has confirmed that acupuncture increases the level of naturally occurring pain modulators (endorphins) within the body, giving a physical basis for its effects.

Sterile stainless steel or aluminium needles of around 30 gauge are inserted at points determined by the cause of the pain. They may then be manipulated by hand or by electrical stimulation.

Acupuncture is remarkably free from complications and in skilled hands it has been shown to be more effective than placebo treatments.

Transcutaneous electrical nerve stimulation

Transcutaneous electrical nerve stimulation (TENS) is simply the application of current from a battery-operated device between two surface electrodes stuck to the skin. This produces a tingling sensation in the area being treated. When sensory nerve pathways are activated by TENS pain-sensing pathways are partially blocked because they utilize some of the same synapses within the central nervous system.

Although not a panacea, TENS therapy may be an effective adjuvant to other methods of pain control. Because it can be self-administered the patient can also regain some independence.

RECOMMENDED READING

British National Formulary. London: BMA and the Royal Pharmaceutical Society of Great Britain.

Sinatra RS, Hard AH, Ginsberg B, Prebble LM. 1992 *Acute Pain: Mechanisms and Management*. St Louis: Mosby Yearbook.

Wildsmith JAW, Armitage EN. 1993 *Principles and Practice of Regional Anaesthesia*. Edinburgh: Churchill Livingstone.

23

FUNDAMENTALS OF DRESSINGS AND DRAINS IN RELATION TO WOUND HEALING

A. Davey & R. M. King

INTRODUCTION

The process of wound healing plays a vital part in the ability of the patient to maintain homeostasis and recover from surgery. An understanding of the principles of wound healing has direct relevance to the choice and use of both dressings and drains. The principles outlined in this chapter apply equally to surgical incisions and minimally invasive techniques, such as cannulation. Essentially, injury may be caused by trauma, outside agents or deliberately, as in surgical incision or puncturing the skin during cannulation.

WHAT IS WOUND HEALING?

Healing is an automatic, self-regulating, natural process that has enabled man to survive disease and trauma. Throughout the ages there have always been healers who through magic, mystery or medicine have sought to speed up this process but generally it is true to say that man healed in spite of them. However, the growth of modern scientific knowledge and technological development within the last 200 years has brought us a health environment in which few wounds are beyond repair and in which most heal quickly and completely.

Healing can be defined as the restoration of the structure and function of diseased or damaged tissues. This process begins as soon as the injury occurs. The body's tissues vary tremendously in their constitution and this variation, together with the type and severity of the wound, is reflected in the way in which that tissue will heal. Thus superficial wounds will regenerate readily and quickly whereas wounds affecting the deeper layers of connective tissue will take longer to repair. Damage to bone, which contains large amounts of inorganic calcium, will heal at an even slower rate.

THE PHYSIOLOGY OF WOUND HEALING

Wounds can be divided into two main types:

1. Closed wounds where no overt tissue loss occurs.
2. Open wounds where there is tissue loss due to excision, trauma, burns or necrosis.

Where there is tissue loss its replacement may be achieved in two ways. First, there may be *regeneration* of identical tissues from undamaged cells in the area, thus replicating both structure and function. Second, where no undamaged cells remain, repair is achieved with *granulation tissue*. Granulation tissue is of a fibrous inelastic nature and fills in the defect adequately; it restores neither structure nor function but eventually leaves a raised and uneven scar.

A wound has been defined as 'an interruption to the continuity of the external and/or internal surface of the body, which may be due to accidental injury, pressure, or disease processes'. Healing in this context is the intrinsic process the human body initiates to repair the wound. This inevitably involves a number of the body systems collaborating to maintain homeostasis, including the cardiovascular, nervous and immune systems. Regardless of how the wound was produced, the physiological response is similar and may be considered to occur in three phases: inflammation, proliferation and maturation, all of which are interrelated and merge into each other.

INFLAMMATION

The initial response is to control blood loss and prevent access to the body of potentially pathogenic organisms. Local vasoconstriction and the establishment of a fibrin clot achieve *haemostasis* but this may result in low oxygen levels and the development of acidosis in the tissue. It is likely that these factors are important in the stimulation of the inflammatory process and often occur between 10 and 30 minutes following the injury. Following any type of wound injury, a complex cascade of biochemical responses by chemical messengers such as bradykinin, histamine, prostaglandins and serotonin stimulates teams of cells, which assist in the inflammatory response. These chemicals cause the capillaries to dilate and increase their permeability, thus allowing cells and fluid access to the wound site once haemostasis has been achieved. The result is the development of heat, redness and swelling, which are the obvious signs of inflammation. Swelling is often accompanied by pain because the nerve endings within the affected tissues are stimulated.

As the circulation to the wound slows *leucocytes* mass on the dilated blood vessel walls. They carry useful substances to the site, which are released when they break down. Phagocytic white blood cells or *macrophages* invade the wound to destroy, ingest and remove dead and foreign tissue. Their numbers increase throughout this phase and they may be considered as part of a cleaning process that prepares the wound bed for further repair. An exudate is also produced and is a factor in nourishing cells and removing necrotic tissue and foreign material. The exudate contains digestive enzymes, antibodies and growth factors, which assist in providing the optimum conditions for wound healing. (If infection becomes established this exudate will also contain the remains of dead phagocytes and bacteria. Its appearance and smell will depend on the infecting organism and it is now known as pus.) The choice of wound dressing is important at this stage as any dressing needs to offer support and a moist environment at the appropriate temperature.

The inflammatory phase is reasonably short, about 4–6 days, and is initiated immediately following injury. Any prolongation of this phase by irritation, infection or damage through untoward movement will prevent the healing process moving to the next cycle.

In summary, therefore, the initial stages of wound healing are haemostasis (where necessary), cleaning and the creation of a warm, moist environment for the subsequent stages of tissue repair and growth. It is important that practitioners are aware of these essential components so that those factors that may potentially hinder the healing process can be minimized. These include disruption of the wound by irritation or movement of the dressing, the presence of foreign material and reducing the temperature of the tissue by cold cleaning agents.

PROLIFERATION

The second phase is the Proliferative Phase, encompassing the processes of granulation, contraction and epithelialization. Damaged or lost tissue needs to be replaced and this is achieved by growth, which is essentially what the proliferative phase is about.

Initially, there is growth of new blood vessels, including capillaries, and they are responsible for giving granulation tissue its bright red granular appearance. The development of an efficient blood supply is essential in order to ensure a good supply of nutrients and oxygen to the tissues so that wound healing may take place as soon as possible. During this phase fibroblasts move into the wound and multiply rapidly. They manufacture a strong connective tissue called collagen that forms fibrous strands, repeatedly bridging the wound to provide a supporting matrix, which is essential for wound strength and which will eventually form the scar.

Fibroblasts only perform well when amply supplied with nutrients and oxygen that are carried to the tissue by the developing blood supply. If substances such as vitamin C and ferrous iron are lacking, collagen production will be reduced if not halted completely. The collagen tends to cause the wound to contract and this decreases the size of the wound surface, thus reducing the space that the granulation tissue has to fill. Inflammation of the surrounding tissue decreases during this period, which begins at about 48 hours posttrauma and can last from four to 20 days.

Once the wound has developed healthy granulation tissue and has begun to contract, the next stage of epithelialization can take place. This is essentially the migration of epithelial cells across the surface of the wound, preferably within a moist environment because it has been shown that the process is 50% faster in moist environments than in dry conditions. The internal structures are thus provided with a waterproof cover by the growth of epithelial cells over the vascular bed. In order for this to occur effectively, the wound should be free from debris, eschar and blood clots. The epithelial seal prevents fluid loss and the entry of bacteria but is still a delicate tissue layer and easily traumatized. This is one of the important aspects of wound healing of which the practitioner must be aware so that the most suitable type of initial wound dressing may be provided. The practitioner must also understand that mild mechanical stress at this time may cause renewed bleeding, thus returning the healing process back to the inflammatory phase.

In summary, the proliferative or reparative phase fills in the defect caused by the wound, reduces its size and covers the area with epithelial cells.

MATURATION

The last phase of the healing process, which is maturation, generally commences at about 20 days following the injury and may continue for up to a year. The previous proliferative phase has filled the wound with granulation tissue and covered it with epithelium, thus re-establishing the integrity of the skin. During this stage the tensile strength and the functional characteristics of the injured area are improved by extensive remodelling of the new tissue through the destruction of the earlier randomly placed bridges of collagen. The new tissue lies along natural folds and stress lines creating more useful networks. Two weeks after epithelialization the wound will have regained 30– 50% of its original tensile strength but further improvement takes many months. The redness of the wound now fades, leaving a whitish, flat, hairline scar. In a minority of patients this phase becomes exaggerated and the scar becomes hypertrophic and keloid in nature. Although surgical wounds should achieve about 80% of their original tensile strength, chronic wounds only reach about 70% of this.

TYPES OF WOUND HEALING

All wounds heal in one of three ways:

1. First intention or primary union.
2. Second intention or granulation.
3. Third intention or secondary suture.

FIRST INTENTION OR PRIMARY UNION

This is the usual way in which surgical incisions heal. The clean, cut edges are approximated so that the normal processes of inflammation, capillary growth and collagen synthesis can proceed without delay in order to produce a consolidated hairline scar. Healing by primary intention tends to be simply a reconstitution of the existing vascular network. A desirable result depends upon the control of bleeding, the limitation of tissue damage, the careful insertion of appropriate sutures (see Chapter 17) and the prevention of infection.

Because all surgical instruments should be sterile, infection should usually only be introduced by poor technique during surgery or on the wards at the time of dressing changes. Bleeding may be controlled either by the tying of blood vessels with suture material or by the use of diathermy. Because diathermy in effect destroys the tissue by burning it, excessive use will produce a focus of dead tissue that will slow down the healing process and may act as a nidus for infection.

The muscle and subcutaneous tissue layers are brought together by accurate suturing but skin edges should not be under tension but merely approximated by the skin closure material (sutures or clips). Drains help to prevent the development of collections of blood or serum but the anaesthetist also has a part to play by allowing the patient to recover smoothly from the anaesthetic. In this way an increase in venous pressure, which may lead to further bleeding, is minimized. Usually, appropriate dressings are used to cover and protect the incision but wounds on exposed areas, such as the face, may be left open and possibly covered with a thin layer of antibiotic ointment.

SECOND INTENTION OR GRANULATION

In these wounds there is either skin loss or loss of tissue or else the wound edges have been allowed to gape. The developing granulation tissue, consisting of immature fibrous tissue and capillary buds, gradually fills the wound from the side and bottom of the cavity. Wound healing by secondary intention, such as a pressure sore, requires the development of new blood vessels and is referred to as *angiogenesis* (*angio* = blood vessels, *genesis* = new). There is a risk that exuberant superficial granulations will develop and these must be controlled. (This is especially seen in burns and these excessive granulations should be removed before skin grafts are applied.) In due course the granulation tissue becomes converted into tissue that is fibrous in nature. During this process, marked contractions or 'puckering' of the scar are produced. The epithelium then slowly grows in from the edges.

THIRD INTENTION OR SECONDARY SUTURE

This is where primary closure of the wound is delayed, usually because of the presence of infection. This results in a wider scar than is associated with primary closure.

FACTORS INFLUENCING THE HEALING OF WOUNDS

If optimum conditions for wound healing are not maintained, the wound may take longer to heal or may fail to heal effectively. At best, this will cause unacceptable scarring but at worst it may result in the death of the patient, e.g. from infection. Internal wound breakdown or dehiscence following surgery, e.g. laparotomy, leads to the development of an incisional hernia.

The factors that affect the ability of a wound to heal are often considered in two categories: those related to the condition of the patient (Intrinsic factors) and those due to outside influences (Extrinsic factors).

INTRINSIC FACTORS

These factors are generally related to body functions and it may be difficult to exert any immediate and direct influence over them. Nevertheless, they need to be considered in the overall plan of care. The general health of the patient does have an effect on the way that the body responds to physical insults and its homeostatic mechanisms, particularly those associated with wound healing.

The *age* of the patient is important, partly because the older the patient is, the more likely it is that the patient will have been treated for degenerative disease, and partly because of changes in the structure of the skin. The elderly patient has more fragile skin with less efficient collagen tissue. Thus wound healing will be slower and less effective.

Circulatory disease influences the amount of oxygen available for normal tissue activity, either because of cardiac failure or because of pathology affecting the vessels that supply the injured tissue. Poor blood supply leads to the development of pressure sores and explains why established pressure sores may take so long to heal. It is also the reason for repeated amputation in patients who have severe peripheral vascular disease.

Anaemia from whatever cause will influence the capacity of the blood to carry oxygen but it will need to be quite severe to influence the healing process.

A normal *immune function* is required for the inflammatory phase of wound healing. A compromised immune system will slow down the cleansing of the wound bed and reduce the body's ability to fight invading pathogens. This may occur in patients with leukaemia or in those treated with immunosuppressive and cytotoxic agents, e.g. chemotherapy for malignancy or following organ transplantation. Corticosteroids also reduce the ability of wounds to heal and make skin much more fragile.

Body weight may affect the delivery and availability of oxygen to the tissues. Obesity, for example, can be a deterrent to healing because adipose tissue is poorly vascularized, thus increasing the likelihood of wound breakdown. This is in addition to the decreased respiratory function and poor mobility. Underweight people may well have problems associated with poor diet or malnutrition, resulting in deficiencies in the body stores of vitamins and minerals and a diminished ability to fight infection.

In *diabetic patients* there is a delayed cellular response to injury, reduced cellular function at the injury site and a defect in collagen production and wound strength. The microvascular circulation is compromised and not only delays wound healing but tends to lead to the progressive amputation of a limb. Thus if amputation is needed it is often more radical than first anticipated.

EXTRINSIC FACTORS

Treatment will be more effective if these extrinsic factors are identified and their effects reduced. The presence of any *foreign material and/or dead tissue* will have a detrimental effect on the wound-healing process, delaying the initiation of the proliferative phase and potentially increasing the infection risk. Thus it is important in the case of trauma that surgical toilet is complete before the patient leaves theatre.

The use of some *chemicals* for wound cleansing may have a detrimental effect by killing healthy cells. Consideration must also be given to the temperature of any agent used to cleanse the wound, particularly as a wound may take some hours to return to ideal temperature after it has been cooled.

Excessive exposure to moisture such as sweat and urine may result in softening of the skin tissue, known as *maceration*, and may lead to a breakdown around the wound. This breakdown of the wound edges has the potential of increasing the size of the wound and encouraging infection. Consideration of the type of dressing to be used will play an important role in reducing this complication. In addition, the optimum temperature for the growth of human cells and therefore wound healing is 37°C. Any factors that adversely affect the temperature of the wound during the healing process will delay the overall process and this should also be borne in mind when choosing a dressing.

Pressure, shearing and frictional forces are all potential *mechanical stresses* that can disrupt a healing wound and the practitioner should bear this in mind when the patient is moved and manipulated. A good example is to note where skin grafts have been placed before a patient is turned onto the side. In this way shearing and frictional forces will not disturb the graft and a further unnecessary visit to theatre may be avoided.

Infection will delay the healing process, particularly in the inflammatory phase, and is often recognized by the classic signs of redness, swelling, heat and pain, together with a discharge accompanied by an elevated temperature. *Radiation therapy* is detrimental to the normal growth and reproduction of cells and also directly affects wound healing.

Each wound is as unique as the patient who owns it and the considerations above demonstrate the numerous factors that contribute to its individual problems and its own set of factors that affect the healing process. Theatre staff have a major role to play in the initial stages of wound healing but they do need to be aware of the relationship that the stage has to the healing process as a whole.

CLASSIFICATION OF DRAINS

FUNCTIONS AND CHOICE OF A DRAIN

A drain is a mechanism that allows fluid to flow from a body space, usually to the outside of the body. Examples include pus, body fluids, blood and cerebrospinal fluid (internal drainage). Effectively, drains reduce the build-up of fluids within the body, thereby reducing the risk of infection and decreasing the size of the cavity. Subcutaneous wound drains also prevent the formation of haematomata, which may lift skin flaps from the subcutaneous tissues and compromise the vascular supply to the flap. Drains are also useful in the management of fluid balance.

The selection of a drain is ultimately the role of the surgeon but in order to anticipate and take part in any team decision, the practitioner should have a sound working knowledge of the properties and uses of the various types of drain. These properties and requirements are listed in a number of relevant texts and are summarized below.

The surgical drain must be:

- Available sterile before insertion.
- Practicable for the scrub practitioner to establish a vacuum.
- Non-irritant to the patient.
- Easy for the surgeon to insert.
- Accessible and convenient for the ward staff to change the drainage container.
- Easy to read to allow accurate monitoring of the drained fluid.
- Of a size and weight that is convenient for the patient to transport.

The design should reduce the potential contact with body fluids for both patients and staff and have some indicator as to the integrity of the vacuum. Potential problems of wound drainage include the risk of infection, accidental removal from the operative site and blocking of the drainage system. The practitioner needs to be familiar with the range and application of drains that are available within their clinical environment, with particular reference to the manufacturer's directions.

Wound drains are generally classified as active or passive.

ACTIVE DRAINS

Most active drains rely on the principle of suction being created by a vacuum within a closed container attached to the actual drain. The subatmospheric pressure achieved in the system draws fluids away from the site or cavity via tubing leading into the container. Traditionally glass bottles with rubber seals were used but now a concertina-style plastic container is the norm. These concertina types of active suction are available in a number of sizes dependent on their use and the expected fluid loss. Examples include the Redon System 600™, Redivac™, Mini-vac™ and Uno-vac™. An alternative is to generate the vacuum by means of a low-pressure suction device.

PASSIVE DRAINS

Passive drains allow the fluids to flow freely into the drainage container utilizing either gravity or capillary action. If these drains are used consideration must be given to the siting of the drain and the potential position and movement of the patient. Although most drainage systems utilize a container, this is not always the case. If superficial tissues require drainage it is sometimes sufficient to use a sliver of plastic or rubber. This acts as a conduit for the fluid to drain by means of capillary action and the fluid is collected in a bulky absorbent dressing.

UNDERWATER DRAINAGE

More correctly referred to as Water Seal Drainage, this system must fulfil a dual purpose. Whilst allowing air, pus, blood or any other fluid to drain from the pleural cavity, it must also prevent the return of either air or fluid to the pleural space, thereby destroying the negative pressure on which inflation of the lung depends.

The drain consists of three items:

1. A chest drainage tube that is placed at the apex of the lung to drain air and at its base for fluid drainage. The chest drainage tube must be of sufficient length to allow the patient to move and turn and to avoid the risk of 'suckback' on deep inhalation.
2. A drainage bottle, which *must* be placed at a level lower than the chest. It has an inlet for the drain, the end of which is led below the level of the normal saline 'seal' in the bottle. This bottle also has an outlet or vent portal in its cap.
3. A one-way valve mechanism provided by the water seal or by a flap valve. Thus, air and fluid, which escape from the pleural cavity aided by gravity and the positive pressure that breathing produces, cannot return.

As long as the bottle is kept lower than the patient, air cannot enter the pleural cavity and nor can fluid flow up the tube. Whenever any untoward patient movement is imminent and the drainage bottle may be raised above chest height, clamping of the drainage tube will prevent fluid entering the lung. This can be dangerous because once the tube is clamped, neither gas nor fluid can escape from the patient's chest. Whilst a short period of clamping is not detrimental, if it is prolonged there is a chance that the dangerous condition of *tension pneumothorax* may develop. Gas enters the pleural cavity but because it cannot escape, the intrapleural pressure increases. This compresses the lungs and later the pericardium to such an extent that the mediastinal space is compromised and respiratory and cardiac function may be fatally threatened. (This is one of the major life-threatening emergencies and is dealt with in Chapter 26.)

A Water-Seal Drainage System is illustrated in Figure 23.1.

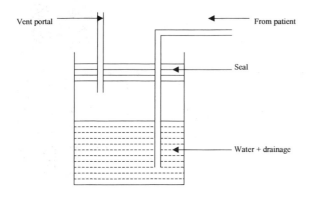

Figure 23.1   A water seal drainage system.

WOUND DRESSINGS

FUNCTION OF WOUND DRESSINGS

The function of wound dressings is to create and maintain an appropriate environment in which wound healing may occur. The properties of the ideal wound dressing are listed below:

- Protection from microorganisms.
- Protection from friction and dehydration.
- Provision of some thermal insulation.
- Maintenance of a high humidity at the wound – dressing interface.
- Allows gaseous exchange.
- Absorption of excess blood, exudate and toxic compounds.
- Provision of some degree of compression, which may assist in the prevention of haematoma.
- Reduces patient interference with the wound.
- Removable without causing trauma at dressing changes.

A wound dressing should also be comfortable for the patient so that there is minimal awareness of the dressing and protection from the pulling of the sutures/staples on clothing and bedding. It should also stay securely in place during movement. Dressings must also be absorbent if there is likely to be oozing from the wound. This may be blood, serum or other body fluids. Finally, a dressing will hide the wound from the patient and other individuals who may be distressed by seeing the site of the operation or injury.

However effective a dressing is, it will be of no use if the patient is allergic to it. Thus prior to anaesthesia and surgery all patients must be asked about any allergies to materials that may be used before, during and after the procedure. This also applies to the fixation materials used by the anaesthetist to secure the airway and cannulation sites.

TYPES OF WOUND DRESSING

Because of its physiological properties the best dressing for any wound is the skin of the individual patient but in most cases this is neither practical nor desirable. The appropriate dressing will be dependent on the site, size and type of the wound and the consideration of a dressing for covering a cannulation site or spinal puncture is just as important as it is for an obvious surgical incision.

The range of wound dressings available is vast but, given the criteria outlined above, the final choice is often influenced by surgical preference and financial restraints. Traditionally, gauze (an open cotton weave) was used as a wound dressing but had a number of disadvantages. It was difficult to keep in position but, of greater importance, although it was absorbent it tended to dry out. This led to a hard dressing that was often difficult and painful to remove and needed frequent changing.

Most modern materials provide a moister environment at the wound surface, enhancing healing and allowing any exudate to stay in contact with the wound surface. They do not tend to adhere to the wound and examples include Melolin™, Telfa™ and Tulle™ dressings. It is, however, necessary to secure them by means of a bandage or adhesive strapping. Partially permeable film dressings usually comprise a clear polyurethane film coated with an adhesive. Adhesive material also surrounds the actual dressing and this is used to fix the dressing onto normal skin. For this reason they are often referred to as island dressings and examples include Bioclusive™, Opsite™, Tegaderm™ and Transite™.

Application of the dressing should be undertaken by the surgeon or scrubbed practitioner whilst the sterile field is viable. Before this, the wound site should be cleaned with an appropriate cleansing solution, preferably at a suitable temperature, and then wiped dry with a sterile swab. It is important not to rub or scrub the actual wound site because this may disrupt the repair. Once the dressing has been applied the drapes can be removed. Finally, the dressing should be fixed securely in place so that it is not possible to remove it accidentally. This consideration also applies to the fixation of drains.

24

THE RECOVERY OF PATIENTS FROM ANAESTHESIA AND SURGERY

M. Maguire

THE ROLE OF THE RECOVERY ROOM

In a relatively short period of time, operating departments have progressed from providing very little postoperative care to having specially designed recovery rooms. Similarly, in the past, staff were not specifically trained for the role but now there is an increasing trend for permanent staff to possess relevant postbasic qualifications. Recovery staff are trained to observe and monitor patients closely during this early postsurgical period and to take prompt and appropriate action to prevent and/or treat postanaesthetic or postoperative complications. The Royal Colleges of Anaesthesia and Surgery insist on a fully functional recovery area whenever patients are in theatre. Failure to achieve this requirement may well result in the withdrawal of training approval for doctors and nonmedical professionals.

The purpose of the recovery room is to provide a calm, quiet environment, where patients are allowed and assisted to recover from the effects of general, regional or local anaesthesia and surgery. At the end of the recovery period they will be ready to be safely transferred to a surgical ward, where relatively less supervision is required. How long patients remain in the recovery room is unpredictable but it must be at least until they are physiologically and surgically stable. The average length of stay may be 30 minutes to one hour but even comparatively minor operations may result in prolonged recovery periods of several hours because of anaesthetic or surgical problems, which may be due to the type of surgery or anaesthesia or the patient's preexisting condition.

These problems may be predictable or unexpected and patients recovering from surgery therefore have many different needs. It is for this reason that some hospitals have a high dependency unit (HDU) attached to the theatre suite. Patients may be kept in the HDU for several hours (and may also be mechanically ventilated) under expert supervision until they are fit to return to the surgical ward. In this way overnight or short-term admissions to the hospital intensive care unit may be reduced.

The recovery room is designed with several bays or bed spaces, all of which are arranged and prepared in a similar way. Whilst recovery rooms are organized according to local practice or guidelines some of the equipment is essential and must be available in each bay or located nearby. A standard layout ensures that the staff are able to find equipment, the most important of which is specified below.

AIRWAY MANAGEMENT EQUIPMENT

- Oxygen supply – preferably with twin outlets
- Mapleson C circuit such as a Waters Circuit or a self-inflating reservoir bag with a non-return valve
- Facemasks to deliver a variety of oxygen concentrations
- Airways – oropharyngeal and nasopharyngeal
- Emergency intubation equipment including a full range of endotracheal tubes
- A fully equipped anaesthetic machine in case a patient needs to be anaesthetized
- A piped suction supply which is backed up by a mechanical suction machine
- Suction tubing and a selection of soft suction catheters and rigid Yankeur catheters

MONITORS, ETC

- Pulse oximeter
- Non-invasive blood pressure monitor
- Sphygmomanometer and stethoscope
- ECG monitor
- Facilities for invasive monitoring
- Thermometer and temperature probe
- Blood glucose monitor
- Availability of gas monitoring
- Availability of a nerve stimulator

TRANSFUSION EQUIPMENT

- Syringes and needles
- Intravenous cannulae in a variety of sizes
- Intravenous infusion sets
- Intravenous fluid, both crystalloid and colloid
- Alcohol wipes
- Tourniquets

DRUGS

- Analgesics and their antagonists
- Cardiovascular drugs
- Respiratory system drugs
- Muscle relaxants and their antagonists
- Sedatives and their antagonists

MISCELLANEOUS

- Vomit bowls/receivers and tissues
- Gloves
- Various dressings and bandages, etc.
- A selection of urinary catheters and drainage bags
- Underwater seal drains
- Recovery charts

Some of the potential problems encountered in the recovery area are also discussed elsewhere. No apology is made for this duplication as repetition is used to emphasize the recognition and importance of the management of these situations. By far the most important function of the recovery staff is to prevent patient hypoxia. The majority of litigious postoperative claims relate to the effects of hypoxia and settlements in excess of £1,000,000 are by no means unknown.

HYPOXIA

THE CAUSES AND PHYSIOLOGY OF HYPOXIA

The function of the cardiorespiratory system is to provide oxygen and nutrients to the tissues and to remove waste products such as carbon dioxide. Failure of any part of this system may result in hypoxia and the fundamental task of the recovery personnel is to ensure that these systems are not compromised. In order to achieve adequate tissue oxygenation, therefore, there has to be:

- Adequate inspiratory effort.
- An acceptable inspired partial pressure of oxygen depending on the condition of the patient (oxygen therapy).
- An unobstructed airway.
- Adequate pulmonary function.
- Acceptable gaseous exchange between the lungs and the blood.
- Adequate oxygen-carrying capacity in the blood.
- Sufficient cardiac output to carry the blood to the tissues.

SIGNS AND SYMPTOMS OF HYPOXIA

Before the invention of the oximeter it was difficult to diagnose mild hypoxia. Indeed, the warning sign was the development of cyanosis, which needed the presence of at least 5 g% of unsaturated haemoglobin to be obvious. A falling oxygen saturation as shown by oximetry is now one of the early indicators.

Thus, restlessness, agitation, hypertension, tachycardia, cyanosis and a falling SpO_2 all point to a hypoxic episode. If this is unrecognized or left untreated, the patient may become unconscious or suffer convulsions. The development of bradycardia, hypotension and finally cardiac arrest must be seen as terminal signs due to hypoxic brain damage. At first, this may be reversible but there is less time from hypoxic cardiac arrest to permanent brain damage than is the case following primary cardiac arrest. If the heart stops due to a cardiac cause, e.g. myocardial infarction, the blood is more or less fully saturated with oxygen at the time of the arrest. In the case of respiratory cardiac arrest the heart stops because it and the brainstem are deprived of oxygen and the oxygen level in the blood supplying the brain is therefore already dangerously low. Immediate action by the recovery practitioner is the only thing separating the patient from permanent brain damage.

Each of the above causes of hypoxia will now be discussed with reference to the function of the recovery practitioner. It is important to appreciate that in most cases hypoxia will not be reversed if the cause is not corrected, no matter how much oxygen is administered to the patient.

The use of oximeters has introduced real-time monitoring, which has greatly improved the continuing care patients receive in recovery departments. However, oximeters are not always foolproof and there is never a substitute for careful observation of patients who are at risk. The saturation monitor may not indicate a drop in SpO_2 for a little while after an obstruction has developed and intervention is preferable before this decrease becomes noticeable. The prevention of cyanosis and hypoxia is always a better aim than their treatment.

Oximeters need good tissue perfusion if the recorded oxygen saturation is to be reliable and vasoconstriction due to hypovolaemia or hypothermia may produce apparently lower readings. This matter is discussed more fully elsewhere.

MAINTENANCE AND PROTECTION OF THE AIRWAY

Airway management is the cornerstone of effective postanaesthetic management and compromise of the airway is the commonest and potentially most dangerous source of complications in the early postoperative period. For this reason it will be discussed first. The 'ABC' of any resuscitation programme corresponds to Airway, Breathing and Circulation. Airway is not the same as breathing and it is common for a patient to have an obstructed airway but still to be making respiratory efforts. A patent airway is a vital prerequisite for any form of resuscitation.

AIRWAY ASSESSMENT

The confirmation of an unobstructed airway is the first priority of recovery personnel when the patient is brought into their care but they must also ascertain that the patient is able to protect their own airway. It is therefore important to ensure that there is an effective cough reflex to avoid the inhalation of stomach contents, blood or secretions.

Even though the airway may not be obstructed, it does not necessarily mean that the patient is breathing. Observation of the facemask misting and clearing as the patient breathes in and out signifies that moist air is being exhaled, but if this is absent it may indicate either an obstructed airway or respiratory depression.

Similarly, observation of the rise and fall of the chest and the patient's colour, listening for breath sounds and the monitoring of oxygen saturation all help in the assessment of a patient's respiratory function, but are not in themselves diagnostic of the cause of a particular problem.

AIRWAY OBSTRUCTION

A sound wave is a slight local pressure disturbance, which travels in a gas, liquid or solid at a speed close to the average velocity of the molecules. In air this is normally about 330 metres/second but sound travels faster in liquids and solids because they are less compressible than a gas. Flow in a gas or liquid through a tube may either be laminar or turbulent. In the former, the molecules flow in a series of layers, with the slowest rate towards the outside of the tube. This is the most efficient type of airflow and the flow rate depends on the length of the tube, the fourth power of its radius and the viscosity of the fluid. This is the type of airflow that occurs in normal breathing and it is quiet and without excessive respiratory effort.

Airway obstruction may be total or partial and the signs and symptoms reflect the changes in physiology. If there is a partial obstruction to the fluid flow or the surface of the tube is not smooth or the tube bends or kinks, the laminar pattern becomes disturbed and the flow becomes turbulent. The flow rate now depends on the density of the fluid and not its viscosity. This is the case in partial airway obstruction and it is the molecular turbulence as the air passes the obstruction that produces the snoring noise of stertorous breathing, which is characteristic of this condition.

The presence of any noise is thus indicative of some form of obstruction or narrowing of the airway. The absence of noise can therefore be an indication of either perfectly adequate breathing or complete airway obstruction: mistaking the latter for the former could have potentially disastrous consequences.

If inspiration or expiration is ineffective the partial pressure of oxygen in the blood falls while that of carbon dioxide rises. The chemoreceptors in the medulla oblongata detect the rise in carbon dioxide tension and send signals to the diaphragm and intercostal muscles to work harder. The resultant respiratory movements are usually abnormal, with the chest and abdomen rising and falling in a "see-saw" fashion rather than in synchrony. In addition, the accessory muscles of respiration begin to function in order to increase the respiratory effort further. These muscles join the shoulder girdle and neck vertebrae to the chest wall and also give the appearance of excessively laboured respiration. Tracheal tug is also a useful sign of obstruction.

By far the commonest cause of airway obstruction is the tongue falling back against the posterior pharyngeal wall. The tongue is most likely to block the airway if the patient is lying supine and therefore, if possible, the patient should be turned on their side. Tilting the head back using a "chin tilt" or lifting the mandible forward using a "jaw thrust" is likely to help bring the tongue forward and away from the posterior wall of the pharynx. This support may be required for some time until the patient regains consciousness.

The same effect may be achieved by inserting a Guedel type oropharyngeal airway or a nasopharyngeal airway. It should be remembered, however, that when an artificial airway is in place, support for the chin or the jaw may still be required and insertion of airways, especially by those unskilled in their use, may also cause complications, e.g. trauma or bleeding. If the airway is not removed in time the patient may bite on it, potentially damaging teeth and soft tissues or possibly precipitating laryngeal spasm and vomiting. It is for this reason that many anaesthetists remove laryngeal masks and endotracheal tubes before the patient is handed over to the recovery staff. Indeed, some may argue that this is a prerequisite of good anaesthetic practice.

The integrity of the mandible, tongue and related muscles plays an important part in maintaining a patent airway. Following radical surgery of the tongue and mandible, this integrity may be compromised and the result is airway obstruction. Most anaesthetics for this type of surgery involve the use of a tracheostomy or nasal endotracheal tube. After breathing has been restored the nasal tube may be withdrawn from the larynx but left in the pharynx. This acts as an airway and is only removed when the airway is stable. An alternative is protecting the airway using a soft latex nasopharyngeal airway. This may be left in place after the patient regains consciousness.

Another cause of the obstructed airway is liquid matter such as blood, vomit, mucus or saliva. Breath sounds produced are of a gurgling nature and the conscious patient will be in some distress. The theatre trolley or bed must be tilted head down so that gravity can aid the drainage of this material and any remaining fluid is removed by pharyngeal suction. The use of suction following throat or mouth surgery must be carried out with great care in order to prevent further trauma to operation sites, which may be producing clots. This is particularly important in post-tonsillectomy bleeding. By tilting the trolley, most of the blood will drain into the mouth and only suction of the buccal cavity will be necessary. Inappropriate or excessive use of suction to pharyngeal and laryngeal areas may lead to laryngeal spasm and/or trauma and oedema. If a patient does not yet have a return of adequate muscle tone or is unable to cough effectively they are at risk of aspiration and should be placed in the same position as described above as a prophylactic measure.

When aspiration is suspected, chest X-ray and chest physiotherapy are indicated together with the possible use of prophylactic antibiotics. This is discussed in detail in Chapter 26.

Laryngeal spasm occurs if the vocal cords are irritated by foreign material or trauma or as a result of a sensitivity reaction to a drug in much the same way as bronchospasm may be precipitated in patients with asthma or chronic airway disease. Whereas bronchospasm is characterized by an expiratory wheeze, laryngeal spasm is manifested by an inspiratory stridor (a crowing noise heard during inspiration).

Laryngeal spasm is often noticed either during induction of anaesthesia or just after extubation when the patient is waking up. During the induction process, deepening anaesthesia may control laryngospasm but if the patient is waking up laryngospasm can be a most frightening experience. Because the airway is partially obstructed, the patient with laryngeal spasm is potentially both hypoxic and hypercarbic and the respiratory centre responds by stimulating an ever-increasing respiratory effort. There is a need to take large gasps of air but this paradoxically leads to further narrowing of the glottis and further hypoxia, which in turn leads to more frantic respiratory efforts. Inspiration becomes noisier as the turbulent airflow increases and this also increases the work of breathing. A downward spiral of less and less effective breathing, more panic and increasing hypoxia develops.

Foreign material is frequently suspected as a cause of laryngeal spasm, especially following nose, throat or mouth surgery, and results from bleeding into the upper airway. Any obvious material may be removed by suction but care should be taken that trauma does not aggravate the problem. In practice, however, a small amount of secretion lodged on the vocal cords is enough to precipitate laryngospasm and although this cannot be removed by suction, a forceful cough by the patient is often effective.

The practice of snapping the inflation port from the endotracheal tube in order to deflate the endotracheal cuff should be avoided because when this is done the cuff either deflates very slowly or fails to deflate at all. The passage of an inflated or partially deflated cuff withdrawn through the vocal cords may traumatize them and precipitate laryngeal spasm.

Treatment involves the correction of any hypoxia and then the treatment of the cause. Oxygen is given via a 'Water's Circuit' (or similar) with the valve partly closed and with light positive pressure applied to the reservoir bag in order to aid inspiration and help to keep the airway open. Patients are reassured by explaining that what they are experiencing is temporary and they are advised to try not to gasp but to take small breaths. A high percentage of inspired oxygen together with reassurance of the patient is usually enough to reduce the feeling of panic and break the vicious circle.

If the laryngeal spasm does not respond to this treatment, the anaesthetist is informed and often a small dose of anxiolytic will relax the patient sufficiently to help relieve the problem. Prior to the introduction of midazolam, the drug of choice was diazemuls but the former is better because it has a shorter duration of action.

In severe cases the use of suxamethonium to paralyse the patient and allow hand ventilation to correct the hypoxia may be necessary. Although some anaesthetists would also reintubate, others would not in case the extubation again resulted in trauma and subsequent spasm. However, if there were a danger of aspiration intubation would be mandatory.

When the laryngeal spasm has eased the patient should be placed in a sitting position (sometimes this is the preferred position from the start), given oxygen by facemask and observed closely for at least half an hour in case of recurrence.

Foreign bodies may pose a threat to the airway, particularly in the unconscious patient. Teeth, tooth caps/crowns and the overlooked throat pack are all capable of causing obstruction and recovery staff should be aware of the possibility of their presence. If a foreign body is suspected visualization with a laryngoscope may ascertain if the upper airway is clear and Magill's forceps can be used to retrieve the item. If the blockage is lower a fibreoptic laryngoscope or bronchoscope may be necessary and medical assistance required. It is important to understand that any instrument introduced into the upper airway over the tongue may cause a gagging reflex and even precipitate vomiting. Thus advice should be sought prior to the intervention unless there is a serious threat to life.

External pressure on the trachea may also cause airway obstruction. This may be due to haematoma or soft tissue swelling following neck surgery.

Haematomas require urgent surgical intervention. The clot must be evacuated and the bleeding point found and ligated as soon as possible. Sitting the patient up to facilitate drainage and sometimes the administration of an antiinflammatory drug is the best way to treat the resulting soft tissue swelling and oedema.

If complete obstruction is feared, it may be necessary to intubate and ventilate until the swelling subsides. In major head and neck surgery this may be done prophylactically but the patient should be transferred to a high-dependency unit or an ICU. Alternatively, a temporary tracheostomy may be performed to ensure there is a patent airway until the swelling has subsided. During thyroid or parathyroid surgery there is a slight risk of damage to the recurrent laryngeal nerves as these run very close to and behind the thyroid gland. Bilateral resection or damage to these nerves would result in paralysis of the vocal cords and a potentially life-threatening airway obstruction. This is a rare complication but after thyroid surgery and before the patient leaves the operating theatre, movement of the vocal cords is confirmed by direct laryngoscopy.

A more common complication of these nerves being stretched is the short-term development in some patients of a hoarse voice. Asking the patient to say "eeeeee" is a method of checking for this. The high-pitched note usually associated with this sound becomes deeper when the nerves have been slightly damaged. This is not a serious problem and the patient merely needs reassurance that the voice will return to normal.

Any swelling of the tongue or epiglottis may lead to airway obstruction. In practice this occurs in acute anaphylactic shock, which is precipitated by an allergic type of drug reaction. Although not common, it is a life-threatening condition and its management is described in Chapter 26.

INADEQUATE INSPIRATORY ACTIVITY

Another name for inadequate inspiratory activity is hypoventilation. The causes may be summarized as follows.

- Depression of the respiratory centre.
- Problems with the nervous reflex arc, which responds to changes in oxygen and carbon dioxide levels.
- Inadequate muscle activity.
- Restricted respiratory movement.

Hypoventilation is recognized by one, some or all of the following signs.

- Drowsiness.
- Unconsciousness.
- Respiratory rate less than 10 breaths each minute.
- Low tidal volume.
- Peripheral dilatation.
- Falling SaO_2.
- Constricted pupils (confirms opiate cause).

The main objective is to support ventilation and oxygenation until the cause, if possible, can be corrected and this may include intubating and ventilating the patient. Only after oxygenation is corrected should treatment of the cause of hypoventilation be considered. This will vary with the cause and will be discussed below.

DEPRESSION OF THE RESPIRATORY CENTRE

Depression of the respiratory centre is probably the commonest cause of hypoventilation. As explained in Chapter 7, the main stimulus to inspiration is firstly carbon dioxide and secondly hypoxia. Apart from the general sedative effect, opioids such as morphine desensitize the chemoreceptors to carbon dioxide, an increase of which normally results in greater respiratory effort. Hypoventilation persists until stimulation recurs at a higher level of carbon dioxide. The rise in the partial pressure of carbon dioxide is dose dependent.

Opioid overdose is diagnosed by a slow respiration rate of about eight or less and these breaths are not necessarily shallow but sighing in nature. The tidal volume of each inspiration is often satisfactory but because the rate is decreased, the minute volume is greatly reduced. Initially hypercarbia develops and this may be followed by hypoxia. Patients who receive excessive amounts of opioid have pinpoint pupils. This is easily recognized and is a valuable aid to diagnosis.

Opioid-induced respiratory depression should be reversed using a specific opioid antagonist (naloxone) or a respiratory stimulant (e.g. doxapram). Naloxone works very quickly but only lasts a short time (15–25 minutes). It will also reverse the beneficial effects of the opioid and therefore the dose should be titrated to produce the optimum effect with the minimal dose. In spite of this, the patient may well be in pain for a short time. Because the opiate has a much longer life than naloxone, there is a risk that respiratory depression will recur. If this happens, it is safe to give more naloxone but usually, when the naloxone wears off the remaining opiate is sufficient to reestablish pain relief but not to cause depression of the respiratory centre. It is therefore important that the patient remains in the recovery area until any chance of recurrence of the respiratory depression has passed.

Doxapram is a respiratory stimulant, which does not reverse all the effects of the opiate. Its action is to stimulate peripheral chemoreceptors, thereby increasing respiratory rate and depth.

Local anaesthesia with sedation is a useful technique as an alternative to anaesthesia or in cases of minor surgery. Benzodiazepines, such as midazolam and diazepam, are often used as the sedative. The response is unpredictable and respiratory depression may easily occur. Flumazenil is a benzodiazepine antagonist that is used to antagonize the unwanted side effects of these drugs. Like naloxone, it has a rapid action but a short half-life and therefore similar precautions must be taken.

By depressing the respiratory centre, the volatile agents may also be responsible for a decrease in minute volume. In a similar way a drug overdose by the patient may depress the respiratory centre sufficiently to cause hypoventilation and, because of the depressant effects of anaesthesia, this may become apparent after an anaesthetic given, for example, to facilitate stomach lavage.

Patients with severe respiratory disease depend on hypoxia and not carbon dioxide levels to drive their respiratory function. If these patients are given added oxygen the hypoxic drive will cease and hypercarbia will result. The patients will appear to be oxygenated but will lose consciousness from carbon dioxide narcosis. Treatment is by controlled oxygen therapy and is described below.

Intraoperative hyperventilation results in a fall in the partial pressure of CO_2 and therefore the chemoreceptors are not stimulated to initiate the normal drive for respiration. This problem is self-rectifying because as the patient's carbon dioxide tension increases due to hypoventilation, the normal respiratory drive returns. Some anaesthetists prefer to facilitate this by adding 5% carbon dioxide to the fresh gas flow.

PROBLEMS WITH THE REFLEX ARC

Any condition that adversely affects neural transmission may decrease the tidal volume and cause hypoxia and hypercarbia. Usually it is a combination of already decreased neural function exacerbated by anaesthesia, especially if muscle relaxants are used. Examples are multiple sclerosis and motor neurone disease.

Patients with an unstable cervical spine are at risk from spinal injury during positioning for surgery. Transection of the cervical spinal cord above C3–4 will sever the nerve supply to the diaphragm and the patient will be paralysed and unable to breathe. Examples of such potential problems include rheumatoid arthritis and traumatic cervical injury.

The brainstem may be damaged after a cerebral vascular accident or head injury and therefore fail to respond in the normal way. Anaesthesia may further increase an already raised intracranial pressure to such an extent that coning of the brain through the foramen magnum occurs and the end result may be a respiratory cardiac arrest.

Treatment of all these conditions is supportive until such time as the respiratory function improves.

INADEQUATE MUSCLE ACTIVITY

If muscle relaxants are not fully reversed the voluntary muscles of respiration do not function adequately and the tidal volume is reduced. This will lead to hypercarbia and, depending on the degree of residual paralysis, hypoxia. Although the problem is usually recognized before the anaesthetist hands over the patient to the recovery staff, this is not always the case and the patient's condition may deteriorate in the recovery area. For this reason the differential diagnosis is discussed here and not in Chapter 26.

Muscle relaxants are used if it is necessary to intubate the trachea. Once this is accomplished, the relaxant may be allowed to reverse (spontaneous respiration) or the patient may be kept paralysed by incremental doses (IPPV). The indications for the use of muscle relaxants are discussed elsewhere. Recovery staff must ascertain whether or not the muscle relaxants have worn off or their effects have been reversed to such an extent that the patient is safe to return to the ward. (If non-depolarizing muscle relaxants are used, complete reversal is not achieved until sometime later, except in the case of suxamethonium and possibly atracurium, but it is sufficient to allow the patient to maintain the airway and to have an adequate respiratory function.)

The following signs may lead one to suspect incomplete reversal from the effects of muscle relaxant.

- Absent or inadequate respiration.
- 'Seesaw' respiration.
- Tracheal tug.
- Abnormal twitching movements.

- Inability to respond to simple commands such as 'Lift your head off the pillow', 'Cough' and 'Squeeze my hand'.

Patients who have experienced being fully conscious but completely paralysed say that it is a most terrifying experience. Not only is this traumatic to the patient but it may also be a cause of litigation. It is most important, therefore, to ensure that a patient who is incompletely reversed remains anaesthetized until such time as adequate muscle activity returns.

The management of incomplete reversal is dependent on ventilatory support and the treatment of the cause. If the patient has regained consciousness they should be reassured that this condition is transient and that normal muscle tone will return naturally. However, if there is significant paralysis they should be reanaesthetized. Patients need to be kept warm because hypothermia may prolong muscle relaxation.

Non-depolarizing muscle relaxants block the acetylcholine receptors on the motor endplate and this prevents acetylcholine from initiating an electrical response leading to muscle contraction. This is a competitive reaction between the relaxant and the acetylcholine and is reversed by using an anticholinesterase called neostigmine. Neostigmine acts by preventing the breakdown of acetylcholine, thus allowing its concentration to increase so that it can compete favourably at the receptor sites in the neuromuscular junction. Thus potential reversal problems will occur if:

1. Too large a dose of relaxant has been given.
2. Too little time has elapsed between the last dose of relaxant and giving the reversal agent. If an operation finishes before reversal is achievable it is better to wait. Five or 10 minutes delay at this stage is better than 30–60 minutes later on because the reversal agent was given too early.
3. Too little reversal agent (or, less commonly, too much) has been used.
4. Insufficient cholinesterase is produced by the body (liver disease).
5. There is abnormal acetylcholine and/or receptors (myasthenia gravis).

It is important to differentiate the genuine failure of reversal from other conditions that may produce hypoventilation such as opiate overdose, electrolyte imbalance and residual volatile agents. A peripheral nerve stimulator is essential for this purpose. In all cases, time is the best healer but a half dose of neostigmine given after about 30 minutes may be useful. (Atracurium is metabolized in the body and therefore additional reversal agent is not indicated.)

If the patient fails to recover muscle tone they may have the condition known as myasthenia gravis in which the acetylcholine receptors are abnormal. Treatment is again supportive but the patient will need to be transferred to the ICU.

Depolarizing muscle relaxants, e.g. suxamethonium, first stimulate the muscle receptors of the motor endplate and then block them. Thus patients 'twitch' when they are given this drug, before they become paralysed. The enzyme pseudocholinesterase breaks down the suxamethonium but its metabolite is still weakly active. Although the patient reverses from the relaxant the motor endplate is changed as a result of the drug's action. In practice, it is as though a very small dose of non-depolarizing relaxant had been used. Excessive incremental or large doses of suxamethonium may therefore result in a failure of reversal. This is known as secondary suxamethonium apnoea or dual block. Theoretically, this block could be reversed by neostigmine but in practice, it is better to keep the patient ventilated and anaesthetized until the problem resolves naturally.

Another cause of prolonged apnoea is called a mixed block. This can occur when a non-depolarizing relaxant is given after suxamethonium and a non-depolarizing block follows the initial depolarizing block.

Suxamethonium apnoea is due to an abnormality or absence of the enzyme pseudocholinesterase. (A similar secondary condition may occur in patients with liver disease.) It is an inherited condition affecting about one in 2000 individuals.

Treatment is again supportive with prolonged ventilation until the effect of the suxamethonium wears off. The infusion of two units of fresh frozen plasma provides donated pseudocholinesterase which is able to break down the suxamethonium, but this is rarely indicated.

The problem and further management are explained to the patient and at a later date pseudocholinesterase levels are measured in the patient's blood and that of close family members. Subsequently an outpatient visit may be used to confirm the diagnosis to the patient and identify any family members who are at risk.

RESTRICTED RESPIRATORY MOVEMENTS

Pain is a significant cause of restricted respiratory movements in patients who have had high abdominal or thoracic surgery, e.g. cholecystectomy. The site of the operation makes deep breathing painful, which in turn results in shallow inspiration leading to hypercarbia, hypoxia and sputum retention, all of which contribute to patient morbidity. This is also exacerbated by the inability to cough. The use of epidural analgesia has significantly improved the pain management in patients undergoing this type of surgery. In addition, patients whose chest or diaphragmatic movements are restricted may benefit from being in a semiprone or sitting position. Morbidly obese patients need to be upright in order to prevent the abdominal contents from splinting the diaphragm.

The presence of a haemothorax or pneumothorax may restrict lung function and may be traumatic or postsurgical in origin. Whatever the cause, once confirmed by radiography, if lung function is compromised they require chest drainage.

OXYGEN THERAPY

Atmospheric air contains about 21% oxygen and this is normally sufficient to provide the body with all the oxygen it needs. As previously stated, anaesthesia and surgery compromise the cardiorespiratory system and as a result, higher inspired oxygen percentages are needed to maintain adequate oxygenation, both during and after surgery.

DIFFUSION HYPOXIA

During anaesthesia the anaesthetic gases, the lungs and the blood are in equilibrium. When the mask is removed at the end of anaesthesia the alveoli rapidly fill with a mixture of nitrogen, oxygen, carbon dioxide and water. There is, however, a large amount of nitrous oxide remaining within the blood and tissues. Because nitrous oxide is 34 times more soluble in blood than is nitrogen circulating nitrous oxide diffuses out of the blood and into the alveoli, thereby occupying space which would otherwise be taken up by inspired oxygen. So rapid is this process that the volume of gas expired is greater than that inspired and both oxygen and carbon dioxide are washed out of the lungs. The falling partial pressure of carbon dioxide reduces the

respiratory drive and the decreased oxygen tension may lead to hypoxia, which is especially dangerous in those patients who are elderly or critically ill. (If a 25:75 anaesthetic mixture of oxygen and nitrous oxide is used, up to 1500 ml of nitrous oxide will be expired in the first minute. The figures for the second and third minutes are 1200 ml and 1000 ml respectively.) This process usually lasts about 10–15 minutes after discontinuing the nitrous oxide and for this reason it is wise to give all patients oxygen in the recovery room for at least half an hour following general anaesthesia.

OXYGEN THERAPY

The concentration of oxygen in room air may not be sufficient to prevent or correct postanaesthetic hypoxia. There are a number of oxygen delivery devices that are suitable for use in the recovery area. Most work on the principle that, if rebreathing is to be prevented, the volume of gas delivered must be greater than the patient's peak inspiratory flow rate. Superficially this may appear to be very wasteful but in practice this is achieved by air entrainment or by the use of a reservoir bag.

Both fixed performance and variable performance masks work on the Venturi principle. If a gas passes through a constriction (injector) the flow rate increases but the pressure decreases. Thus gas from another source can be sucked in (entrained) at the site of the constriction and in this case the gas is room air. The concentration of oxygen delivered will depend on the size of the injector jet and the amount of air entrained.

The fixed concentration masks are only able to deliver a fixed concentration of oxygen. A range of masks with different injector sizes is therefore needed. The variable flow rates reflect the different entrainment ratios required for the delivery of approximately 40 litres/minute (Fig 24.1) but because the entrainment ratio remains constant, variation in the flow rate of the gas through the injector will not alter the percentage of oxygen delivered. It will, however, change the volume of gas available.

It is important not to obstruct the apertures in the mask as this will result in decreased entrainment and the

% Oxygen to be delivered	Entrainment ratio	Oxygen flow rate into mask	Total gas flow
24%	1 litre entrains 20 litres of air	2 litres/minute	40 litres/minute
28%	1 litre entrains 10 litres of air	4 litres/minute	40 litres/minute
35%	1 litre entrains 5 litres of air	8 litres/minute	40 litres/minute

Figure 24.1   Gas flows in the Ventimask™

delivery of a higher percentage of oxygen. The Ventimask™ is an example of a fixed concentration mask. Variable performance masks such as the Hudson Multivent™ have the ability to alter the amount of gas entrained through an orifice of fixed size by means of a variable aperture controlled by a sleeve. Thus the oxygen flow rate will determine the final oxygen percentage delivered. Much larger flow rates will be required for the higher oxygen concentrations and to overcome this, two sizes of injector are supplied with each mask. If concentrations of 24–30% oxygen are needed an injector with oxygen flow rate of about 3 litres/minute is used while final concentrations of 35–60% oxygen utilize flows of 6 litres/minute.

The MC™ (Mary Catherall) mask is lightweight, reasonably cheap and suitable for the average patient in recovery. The mask oxygen is diluted by air drawn in through the holes in the mask and a fresh gas flow of 5 litres/minute provides a concentration of about 40% oxygen. The actual concentration depends on how well the mask fits the patient, the patient's size and the tidal volume.

Nasal cannulae use low flow rates to deliver 25–30 % oxygen but they are unreliable in mouth-breathing patients. They may, however, be beneficial in patients who are reluctant to use a facemask.

Tracheostomy masks work in the same way as facemasks but are shaped to fit over the tracheostomy tube.

The T-piece consists of corrugated tubing attached directly onto an endotracheal tube, laryngeal mask or tracheostomy tube with an expiratory limb of the same material. Fresh, humidified oxygen with a flow of 8–10 litres/minute passes along the tube and exhaled air is washed out of the expiratory limb by the fresh gas supply. It is recommended that the volume of the expiratory limb should be about 150 ml. If it is too short the patient may inspire room air with the fresh gas and receive a lower than expected inspired oxygen concentration. If it is too long rebreathing of expired air may occur because the flow rate would not be high enough for the length of the tubing. The advantage of a T-piece system is that there is no resistance to expiration.

The Mapleson C circuit is sometimes referred to as a "Water's circuit" but this is not strictly true because of the absence of a carbon dioxide-absorbing canister. It is used for patients who are being artificially ventilated. When it is used on a spontaneously breathing patient, care should be taken, that the flow rate is between 10 and 15 litres per minute; lower flow rates will result in rebreathing of carbon dioxide.

CONTROLLED OXYGEN THERAPY

The stimulus to breathing in patients with severe chronic respiratory disease is not hypercarbia but hypoxia. If these patients are given sufficiently high concentrations of oxygen they will therefore stop breathing and gradually become comatose due to high levels of carbon dioxide. If the oxygen concentration is reduced the hypoxic drive returns, the patient recommences breathing and consciousness returns. Controlled oxygen therapy refers to the management of the inspired oxygen concentration in such a way as to ensure that the patient's respiratory drive is maintained. If, therefore, 28% oxygen does not stimulate respiration the percentage of inspired oxygen is reduced to 24%. Normally 24 or 28% inspired oxygen given postoperatively will improve oxygenation without depressing the respiratory drive.

PULMONARY FUNCTION AND GASEOUS EXCHANGE

The importance of pulmonary function and gaseous exchange is considered in Chapter 7. Generally speaking, anaesthesia and surgery do not have a major impact unless there is significant pulmonary collapse, pneumothorax, haemothorax or pulmonary oedema.

CARDIOVASCULAR STABILITY

No matter how efficient the lung function and gaseous exchange, unless the blood is able to carry oxygen to the tissues the patient will not survive. Assessment of cardiovascular stability is therefore a vital part of the recovery process. The oxygen-carrying capacity of the blood depends on the efficiency of the heart, the volume of blood in the circulation (cardiac output) and the concentration and saturation of the oxygen-carrying haemoglobin.

Before returning to the ward, the patient's vital signs should be monitored closely to ensure that they remain within normal limits, taking into account the patient's usual status and the drugs and techniques employed during the operation. Most drugs used in anaesthesia will depress the cardiovascular system to some degree and it is not unusual for patients to have a lower than normal blood pressure and heart rate but the overall picture depends on the physiological condition, the current drug therapy and pain status of the patient.

In recent years there has been a significant increase in the use of monitoring equipment in recovery rooms but it should be remembered that the best monitors we have are our senses. Monitoring equipment can aid diagnostic processes but there is no substitute for close, continuous observation of the patient's condition. Similarly, machines can only record what they sense and monitors that are incorrectly positioned or set up produce worthless information. If, however, that worthless information is recorded it may be of considerable embarrassment in a subsequent court of law. Recovery records must be both accurate and easy to read.

A point worth stressing is that when assessing cardiovascular status, blood pressure and heart rate are inextricably linked and it is, therefore, generally pointless to record or report a fall in blood pressure without also mentioning the rate and nature of the pulse. Although the body attempts to maintain cardiovascular stability, this is not always possible. Thus it is important to be aware of the relationship between blood pressure and cardiac output. This is best described as follows.

1. Cardiac output = blood pressure/peripheral resistance.
2. Cardiac output = stroke volume x pulse rate.
3. In turn, the stroke volume is dependent on the force of myocardial contraction and the amount of blood returning to the heart (the venous return).

There is always more than one scenario for any given set of circumstances and it is the skill of the clinical team as a whole that identifies and treats the cause of the problem but the basis of that skill is a sound knowledge of physiology. Previous history is most important and, therefore, the events in theatre may play a vital role in the diagnosis. Let me illustrate this with a few examples.

- A high blood pressure with a high pulse rate may indicate pain, anxiety or possible fluid overload but it could also be due to a phaeochromocytoma, which is a rare adrenaline-secreting tumour. However, the most likely cause will be pain and the patient may well confirm this on direct questioning.
- A high blood pressure with a low pulse is one of the signs of raised intracranial pressure but it is more common in patients with poorly controlled hypertension, which is treated with β-blocking drugs. Knowledge of current medication and the preoperative blood pressure will quickly solve the problem.
- A low blood pressure with a rapid thready pulse indicates hypovolaemia but this may be due to blood or fluid loss, septicaemia or an acute allergic reaction. In this case the first-line treatment is the same and the final diagnosis may be delayed.
- A low blood pressure with a low pulse rate may result from depression of the cardiac regulatory centre by drugs but could also be drug-induced bradycardia superimposed on hypovolaemia. Differentiation is most important.

These are just some of the potential problems associated with the cardiovascular system and show the importance of linking blood pressure with pulse rate but at the same time 'looking at the patient as a whole and not the hole in the patient'. The commonest postoperative cardiovascular complication is hypovolaemia, with the risk of deterioration into shock. Hypovolaemia (literally low blood volume) results from a number of factors, although the predominant cause is uncorrected intraoperative blood loss.

Preoperative fasting and evaporation from open operation sites, especially during major abdominal surgery, may contribute to and aggravate hypovolaemia. Early signs of mild hypovolaemia are increasing pulse rate, pallor and, if recorded, reducing urine output. If it is being measured, central venous pressure (CVP) will fall. Arterial pressure may not drop because compensatory mechanisms such as increased cardiac effort and vasoconstriction will be initiated in an attempt to maintain the blood pressure. Children will maintain blood pressure until hypovolaemia is well advanced and then there will be a precipitous fall. The venous pressure is almost totally dependent upon volume and, therefore, variations in blood volume are detected by CVP changes in advance of a measurable fall in blood pressure.

Treatment of hypovolaemia is aimed at the increasing circulatory volume. In mild cases, a crystalloid such as sodium chloride or compound sodium lactate is sufficient but with more severe blood loss colloid preparations, plasma substitutes or bloodproducts, e.g. Human Albumin Solution or blood, are more appropriate. Transfusion with crossmatched blood is given to provide red cells and maintain the oxygen-carrying capacity of the blood. Blood samples are not usually taken in the recovery area but the measurement of blood urea and electrolytes, haemoglobin and clotting factors may sometimes be indicated. Low blood pressure may respond to the simple act of raising the patient's legs, which increases the venous return and the preload on the heart. This in turn can improve cardiac output and blood pressure.

The pulse may be slow due to the effects of drugs, particularly neostigmine, which can cause severe bradycardia and must always be given with atropine or glycopyrrolate. The actions of neostigmine and atropine may be asynchronous, resulting in a temporary bradycardia. Time or further doses of atropine can be used to resolve the situation.

A rapid pulse rate may be due to anxiety, pain or drugs such as infiltrated adrenaline or topical cocaine. Pain-induced tachycardia should resolve when adequate pain relief is given. Tachycardia caused by local anaesthetic agents, such as cocaine used in nasal surgery, will settle in time and usually requires no treatment unless the tachycardia is thought to be potentially life threatening. This could occur if a large amount of local anaesthetic has been inadvertently injected intravenously but this should have become apparent well before the patient arrived in the recovery area.

ECG monitoring is now an integral part of the recovery room activity and is mandatory following major surgery, in patients with a history of heart problems or following an intraoperative cardiovascular critical incident. Recovery staff must therefore be familiar with the appearance of at least a normal ECG and have the ability to recognize the more common abnormal rhythms, which should be reported to the medical staff.

FLUID THERAPY

Not only will the anaesthetist prescribe pain relief and oxygen therapy but they also indicate the type and rate of postoperative fluid administration. This will consist of the immediate fluid management while in recovery and the longer term fluid regime for use on return to the ward.

It is not always easy to predict what fluid a patient will need immediately after a major surgical procedure and recovery staff should have a flexible approach to fluid management until the patient's condition has stabilized. This will obviously depend upon the age, the physiological status of the patient and the type of surgery performed. All fluids given to the patient in recovery should be clearly documented on the fluid balance chart, especially if they were not originally prescribed.

Before returning the patient to the ward, the fluid therapy should be legibly written on the prescription sheet and the recovery staff should be able to explain it in a logical and concise manner to the ward nurse and ascertain that they also understand it. Any fluids which are likely to run out should be replaced before the patient leaves the recovery area and all intravenous lines that are not in use should be shut off. If there are several infusions in place, e.g. peripheral, CVP, arterial and irrigation, each should be clearly labelled together with any additions to the fluid.

Finally, it is important to ensure that all connections are firmly in place and that the cannula will not become disconnected or pulled out from the vein, as sometimes happens in children and confused patients. This is essential because if there is active bleeding and vasoconstriction, resiting of the infusion could be difficult.

OXYGEN CARRYING CAPACITY

Finally, we need to consider how much haemoglobin is needed to carry sufficient oxygen to the tissues. Traditionally a haemoglobin concentration of less than 10 g/100 ml of blood was thought to be unacceptable. In fit healthy patients a lower level is acceptable but of more importance is the amount of that haemoglobin which is saturated with oxygen. This again stresses the importance of postoperative oxygen therapy.

PAIN RELIEF

Pain relief is fully dealt with in Chapter 22 and will not therefore be covered in detail in this chapter. One of the main concerns of the recovery staff is to assess and manage pain relief so that the patient is comfortable and more or less pain free on return to the ward. It is, however, important that the recovery personnel reassure patients who have had local anaesthetic procedures. The effect of bupivacaine may last several hours and the patient may become concerned as to the cause of the apparently long-lasting numbness.

GENERAL CONSIDERATIONS

Waking up from general anaesthesia can be a strange and frightening experience. The recovery staff need to be aware of and sensitive to the needs and feelings of each patient and to treat each one with empathy and individualized consideration. The sense of hearing often remains acute when patients appear to be unconscious and when emerging from anaesthesia, hearing may even be enhanced. The recovery room should therefore have a peaceful ambience and staff should speak quietly and gently.

Disorientation is common and one of the roles of recovery staff is to reorientate patients as to time and place, reminding them where they are and why they are there.

SURGICAL CONSIDERATIONS

Most of this chapter has concentrated on the recovery of patients from anaesthesia but the early recognition of potential surgical problems is equally as important.

DRESSINGS AND DRAINS

Signs of bleeding invariably precede hypovolaemia and subsequent hypotension. One of the first indications may be excessive oozing through the surgical dressings or greater than expected bleeding into the drains. Although initially this may be understandable, if it persists the surgeon must be told and the patient should not be allowed to leave the recovery area until the surgeon has seen the patient. In the meantime the rate of intravenous fluid therapy should be increased. If not already set up, an IV infusion should be established before vasoconstriction makes the procedure difficult. Observing the degree of blood staining in the irrigation fluid leaving the bladder helps to assess bleeding after prostatectomy.

If underwater seal drains are *in situ*, they should swing freely with respiration so that any excess air may bubble off. It is most important that they should be securely clamped before the patient is moved from the operating table to the trolley or if there is a likelihood of the drain being raised above the level of the patient's chest. Equally the drain should be unclamped and allowed to swing freely while the patient is in the recovery area and on return to the ward, but these drains must always be lower than the patient to prevent any of the drainage returning to the patient's chest.

Some surgeons now advocate that chest drains should not be clamped – even when lifted, because there is a risk of creating a tension pneumothorax which outweighs the risks of fluid entry into the pleural space.

Nasogastric tubes may also be thought of as drains and bleeding via these tubes may indicate a problem in gastric and upper intestinal tract surgery. Nasogastric tubes weaken the effect of the gastrooesophageal sphincter and therefore make regurgitation of stomach contents more likely and this is accentuated by an increase in intragastric pressure. The increase in pressure is also the basis of vomiting and both may be decreased if the intragastric pressure can be reduced. One way of doing this is to allow the tube to drain freely and if the pressure does tend to increase there will be a movement of fluid up the tube and into the drainage bag. Free-draining nasogastric tubes also allow assessment of postoperative gastric fluid loss.

Tourniquets should be deflated before the patient leaves theatre but rubber tourniquets placed around single digits may sometimes be missed. One of the duties of the recovery staff is to assess the integrity of the circulation after tourniquets have been removed. Occasionally the circulation may have been compromised, e.g. during surgery for Dupuytren's contracture and supracondylar fracture of the humerus, but it is not uncommon for dressings, splints and plasters to be applied too tightly and thus restrict the blood flow to a digit or limb. If this is not identified permanent ischaemic damage may occur.

When handing patients over to the care of the ward staff, the recovery staff must be confident that the patient is free from the immediate postoperative dangers previously described and is safe and comfortable. A full and recorded explanation of the operation and postoperative care is given to the receiving ward nurse, together with instructions for the patient's continuing care. Recovery from anaesthesia is a potentially hazardous time for patients, requiring careful observation and prompt action to prevent or treat problems. Recovery staff need to know what to do, when to do it and when and where to seek help in order to enable patients to begin their postoperative recuperation in an atmosphere of safety and dignity.

25

FUNDAMENTALS OF EMERGENCY AND OBSTETRIC ANAESTHESIA

T. Ryan

Emergency surgery must be undertaken before an injury or a disease becomes life-threatening. As a consequence, general anaesthesia may have to be administered in circumstances which would be considered unacceptable in elective work. Uniquely, in obstetric anaesthesia even elective cases must be managed as if they were emergencies because of the danger of regurgitation of stomach contents due to the increased intragastric pressure resulting from the pregnant uterus. This chapter discusses the problems encountered in emergency and obstetric anaesthesia and indicates how the risks can be reduced to a minimum.

PREOPERATIVE ASSESSMENT AND RESUSCITATION OF THE EMERGENCY PATIENT

The outcome of any emergency surgical procedure will be influenced to a greater or lesser extent by the factors listed in Box 25.1. The preoperative health of a patient is obviously important when considering the impact that the new emergency problem will have upon their postoperative well-being. In the early 1960s, the American Society of Anesthesiologists introduced a classification system that graded patients according to their overall general condition (Box 25.2). This can be a useful indicator of potential problems both intra and postoperatively which may not be directly related to the pathology underlying the need for emergency surgery.

The previous physical health of the patient and the site and nature of the proposed operation combine to indicate and influence the needs of the patient both intraoperatively and often, more importantly, postoperatively, in order to maintain cardiovascular and respiratory stability. These needs can range from simple

---

ASA 1	A normal healthy patient
ASA 2	A patient with mild systemic disease
ASA 3	A patient with severe systemic disease which limits activity but which is not incapacitating
ASA 4	A patient with incapacitating systemic disease which is a constant threat to life
ASA 5	A moribund patient not expected to survive 24 hours with or without operation

Box 25.2 ASA Status

---

analgesia to elective ventilation and physiological manipulation using fully invasive monitoring apparatus in an intensive care unit.

Fluid losses can occur from a variety of sources and in principle they should be replaced by similar fluids, so that in haemorrhage the major need is for blood, in burns for plasma and in intestinal losses, electrolyte-containing solutions. In extreme circumstances, however, almost any fluid can be used in an attempt to maintain the intravascular circulating volume and tissue profusion of the vital organs.

There is no doubt that the experience and training of the entire theatre team will have a major impact upon the outcome of any emergency operation. Without the necessary practical abilities, theoretical knowledge is of little value.

INDUCTION OF ANAESTHESIA FOR EMERGENCY SURGERY

Once the resuscitation or stabilization of the patient's condition has been achieved to the point where no further improvements could be expected without unnecessarily wasting time, induction of anaesthesia can commence. Most often, this will be done in the anaesthetic room but in critical cases it may be more appropriate on the operating table in theatre, with the surgeon scrubbed and ready to make his incision. (A typical example of the latter situation would be the ruptured aortic aneurysm). It must be remembered that great care is needed in the administration of most anaesthetic drugs in those who may already have an unstable cardiovascular system and therefore reduced doses are best given slowly to avoid any unnecessary problems.

Wherever induction of anaesthesia takes place, however, the items listed in Box 25.3 should be

---

1. The age and previous physical health of the patient
2. The nature and site of the proposed operation
3. Preoperative fluid losses, tissue damage, and their correction
4. Cardiovascular and respiratory stability
5. The experience and expertise of the entire operating team

Box 25.1 Factors Influencing Postoperative Outcome

instantly available. In addition, and perhaps most importantly, the presence of an appropriately trained, experienced and dependable assistant to the anaesthetist is not only essential but mandatory. Without such a person present, the induction of anaesthesia cannot be allowed to proceed.

The most urgent need following the induction of anaesthesia is to secure and protect the patient's airway. The combined effects of the physical insult of the pathology involved, fear, fluid losses, opiate administration and possible patient non-cooperation through depressed levels of consciousness make it impossible to assume that the stomach has fully emptied of its food and acid contents. As a result, regurgitation of those stomach contents and their aspiration into the lungs must always be considered probable, rather than possible, unless precautions are taken to prevent such an occurrence. For all emergency surgical procedures therefore, the so-called Rapid Sequence Induction (Box 25.4) *must* be employed.

During elective surgery, neuromuscular block will usually be achieved using long-acting drugs that take several moments to produce good intubating conditions. Whilst waiting for the block to be complete, the patient's oxygen saturation can easily be maintained by ventilation through a facemask and Geudel airway. With emergency cases, however, this option is not acceptable as some of the ventilated gas would inevitably pass into the stomach, exacerbating any tendency for its contents to regurgitate back up the oesophagus.

Suxamethonium, a neuromuscular blocking agent not without several potentially undesirable side effects, does however possess the unique ability to produce good intubating conditions within 30 seconds of its intravenous administration. As yet, it has no rival to its role in the rapid sequence induction. Even though suxamethonium is the fastest acting relaxant drug, there still remains the brief period where no sponta-

---

1. Intravenous access
2. A fully tilting trolley or table
3. Suction apparatus
4. Full monitoring equipment
5. Cuffed endotracheal tubes of varying sizes
6. A difficult intubation box
7. An emergency drug box
8. A mechanical ventilator

Box 25.3 Essential Needs Prior to Induction of Emergency Anaesthesia

---

1. Preoxygenation
2. The use of suxamethonium for neuromuscular block
3. Cricoid pressure (Sellick's Manoeuvre)
4. The use of a cuffed endotracheal tube

Box 25.4 Essentials of the Rapid Sequence Induction

---

neous breathing or ventilation can take place and should any difficulty be encountered at intubation, the patient's oxygen saturation could fall to dangerously low levels. In order to protect against this problem, preoxygenation is used to provide the patient with increased reserves of oxygen supplies. This is achieved, with a cooperative patient, by encouraging four or five maximum inspirations of 100% oxygen via a close-fitting face mask immediately prior to the administration of the induction agents and the suxamethonium. In those patients who are uncooperative or with a reduced level of consciousness, increased levels of inspired oxygen for as long as possible prior to induction is the only alternative. The aim in all circumstances is to achieve the maximum oxygen saturation level which is possible.

Assuming that regurgitation will start to occur as soon as induction and neuromuscular blockade have commenced, precautions must now be taken to prevent any stomach contents from entering the patient's airway. The application of cricoid pressure by the trained assistant must begin at the same instant that the induction agents are given. Also known as Sellick's Manoeuvre (named after the anaesthetist who first described its use and function), this entails the application of pressure by the thumb and first two fingers of one hand downward upon the cricoid cartilage of the supine patient, thereby compressing the oesophagus between the semirigid trachea and the rigid cervical vertebrae, effectively sealing of the lumen of the oesophagus. To be successful, counter pressure should, at the same time, be applied by the assistants other hand cupped behind the patient's neck. Because Sellick's Manoeuvre is a two-handed procedure, all the necessary requirements of the anaesthetist must already have been prepared and be close to hand before its application. These needs must include the contents of the difficult intubation box and the emergency drug box.

If regurgitated material leaks past the cricoid pressure points, tilting the table down will ensure their passage downwards and out of the mouth, aided by suction, rather than into the lungs. Under no circumstances should the cricoid pressure be released until a cuffed endotracheal tube has successfully been passed into the trachea, a good seal achieved and the anaesthetist is confident that the airway has been secured.

Occasionally, however, the anaesthetist will find it impossible to achieve successful intubation and, in the best interests of the patient, will decide to abandon any further attempts. It is at this point that a previously agreed failed intubation drill must be implemented (Box 25.5). It must be emphasized once again that in these circumstances the cricoid pressure must be maintained until the anaesthetist is confident that the patient's own protective cough reflex has returned. Although cricoid pressure is an invaluable component of the rapid sequence induction technique, it must never be used in an attempt to prevent active vomiting as opposed to passive regurgitation as this could result in the rupture of the oesophagus.

Once the anaesthetist has secured the safety of the airway and taken control of the patient's respiration, the operation may proceed and attention can be turned towards the remainder of the patient's overall condition.

MAINTENANCE OF EMERGENCY ANAESTHESIA

The needs of the patient both intraoperatively and postoperatively can now be considered in the light of the pathology being dealt with and the preexisting physical status of the patient (Box 25.6).

An accurate assessment of fluid balance must be undertaken and every effort made to replace all losses with similar fluids. (The pregnant uterus may obstruct the inferior vena cava and result in the supine hypotensive syndrome. This may be corrected by tilting the patient slightly to one side.) It is the degree of such losses and their likelihood of continuing which most influence the decision to use invasive monitors of blood pressure and central venous pressure. In the

---

1. Turn the patient to the left lateral position
2. Tilt the table steeply head down
3. Apply a facemask delivering 100% oxygen
4. Use gentle assisted ventilation when circumstances permit
5. Await return of the patient's own respiration
6. Maintain cricoid pressure throughout

Box 25.5 Failed Intubation Drill

---

1. Fluid losses and their replacement
2. The need for non-invasive or invasive monitoring
3. The maintenance of body heat
4. The prevention of infection
5. Postoperative care

Box 25.6 Intraoperative Considerations in Emergency Surgery

---

absence of these invasive techniques errors may be made in the volumes of replacement fluids administered which could result in either the under-perfusion of vital organs or else the overloading of the circulation and resultant cardiac failure.

Not only must fluid replacement be as accurate as possible, it should also be delivered at body temperature since hypothermia, probably already present to some degree in most cases, can otherwise be greatly exacerbated. (see Chapter 19). Hypothermia produced during surgery can occur from a variety of sources and, if severe enough, can have lasting effects on the function of some organs. In addition to warming all intravenous fluids, inline breathing filters can prevent loss of body water and heat the dry gases used for ventilation by humidifying. A warming mattress will reduce losses via the operating table and covering all exposed surfaces will reduce heat losses to the air in theatre. It should be remembered that infants and small children have much greater surface areas in relation to body mass than do adults and that, with an already increased basal metabolic rate, their heat losses are very much faster (see Chapter 18).

Failure to maintain body heat will become more obvious once the patient has emerged from the anaesthetic when the involuntary reflexes perceive the need to retain what heat is still present and peripheral shutdown accompanies the diversion of blood supplies to the vital organs. Shivering, metabolic acidosis and failure to eliminate drugs and waste products can then lead to excessive strain upon the overworked myocardium, inducing further hypoxia and tissue damage.

Just as hypothermia can pose immediate postoperative threats, so too can infection in the first few hours and days. In such circumstances, it is not surprising that postoperative infections are much more frequent following emergency surgery. Hypoxia, haemorrhage, damage to tissues and acidotic conditions are superb breeding grounds for bacteria of all kinds and whilst the administration of appropriate antibiotic cover is essential, attention to the principles of infection control by all members of the multidisciplinary team cannot be overemphasized, as poor practice at this stage can jeopardize the patient's postoperative recovery for weeks to come.

RECOVERY FROM EMERGENCY ANAESTHESIA

As surgery comes to an end, decisions have to be taken with regard to the continuing postoperative care of the patient. No matter what the individual pathology, the principles listed in Box 25.7 must apply to every patient.

---

1. Adequate oxygenation
2. Accurate fluid balance
3. Adequate and appropriate analgesia
4. The correction and continued avoidance of hypothermia
5. The avoidance of infection risks

Box 25.7 Postoperative Needs

Depending upon the individual circumstances, these needs may be achieved by a variety of means ranging from oral fluids, simple analgesics and no supplemental oxygen to admission to an intensive care unit for elective ventilation, full invasive monitoring and pharmacological support. The ultimate choices will depend upon the patient's general condition and experience of previous similar cases. If no elective ventilation is deemed necessary each patient should be extubated only when their own protective cough reflex has returned and their overall neuromuscular powers are considered to be adequate. All extubations should be performed with the patient in the left lateral, head-down position, with suction apparatus to hand in order to prevent any possible regurgitated or vomited material reaching the lungs.

Following extubation, the period spent in the recovery area must be used to establish adequate oxygen saturation levels, pain relief and warming and to ensure that no immediate postoperative problems, especially haemorrhage, go unnoticed. Only when all these conditions have been met can the patient be considered safe to leave the care of the multidisciplinary team.

26

IDENTIFICATION AND MANAGEMENT OF ANAESTHETIC EMERGENCIES

R. Wenstone

An anaesthetic emergency is usually an unexpected crisis event, which may lead to the imminent death of the patient. Crises may easily develop into panic scenarios affecting all theatre workers, both medical and non-medical, and it is therefore important that not only the anaesthetist but the assistant to the anaesthetist has a clear understanding of how these events may be managed.

MASSIVE BLOOD LOSS

BLOOD VOLUME

The blood volume of an adult is approximately 7ml/kg of body weight (about 8–9ml/kg in children). Thus the circulating blood volume of a 70kg patient is about 5 litres. This is not significantly increased in obesity as this calculation is based on ideal body weight.

RECOGNITION

The initial problem in the management of haemorrhage is its recognition. Blood loss during a major vascular procedure, for example, may be immediately obvious but this is not always the case and bleeding may often be occult, i.e. hidden. This may occur during minimal access surgery (such as transanal endoscopic procedures) or following trauma (with unrecognized bleeding into one or more body compartments, e.g. abdomen, retroperitoneal space, soft tissues of the thighs, etc.). Obviously definitive management of the patient will depend on identification of the source of blood loss.

Uncontrolled haemorrhage causes loss of both circulating blood volume and oxygen-carrying capacity and finally leads to hypotension and hypoxic cellular damage. The body has developed compensatory mechanisms that try and prevent this. Blood loss of up to about 15% of circulating volume (i.e. about 700 ml) may produce no change in blood pressure and only a mild reflex tachycardia but with further uncorrected haemorrhage (up to about 1500 ml), tachycardia will become obvious. However, although systolic blood pressure may be maintained, vasoconstriction may cause a rise in diastolic pressure with a consequent fall in pulse pressure (i.e. the difference between systolic and diastolic pressures gets smaller).

It is also important to realize that the ability to compensate for blood loss is reduced in elderly or frail patients, in those with significant coexisting diseases and in patients treated with antihypertensive drugs. In these individuals blood pressure will start to fall after a relatively small haemorrhage. In addition, compensatory features, such as tachycardia, may be easily masked or misinterpreted in the anaesthetized patient. If haemorrhage continues blood pressure will inevitably start to fall, as will urine output. At the same time haemoglobin oxygen saturation may decrease due to greater intrapulmonary shunting. This is because, as blood pressure falls, an increasing proportion of blood passing through the lungs fails to reach ventilated alveoli and therefore is unable to be fully saturated with oxygen. Children tend to maintain blood pressure at the expense of blood volume and decompensation occurs later and is more rapid than in the adult.

VENOUS ACCESS, EQUIPMENT AND MONITORING

Adequate venous access is essential to enable the rapid transfusion of fluids. Normally at least two peripheral venous cannulae of size 16 gauge or larger will be needed and some form of pressure infuser to increase the rate of transfusion is very useful in these circumstances. Transfused fluids should always be warmed prior to infusion in order to minimize the complications of hypothermia (see 'temperature' below). The use of blood filters has not been proven to be of any benefit and has the disadvantage of reducing the rate of infusion.

Increasingly, hospitals are using some form of blood salvage (autotransfusion) technique and it is important to know how to set up the necessary equipment as quickly as possible.

In the initial stages of transfusion central venous access is not essential but does offer the advantage of allowing the siting of an additional large-bore cannula (including, for example, a Swan Ganz introducer sheath or a dialysis line). If blood loss continues or recurs central venous pressure (CVP) monitoring would be useful to assess volume status of the patient. It is preferable to monitor the CVP with a pressure transducer rather than the traditional, but more cumbersome, fluid-filled manometer so that changes can be assessed continuously. Increasingly, anaesthetists are inserting a pulmonary artery (PA) flotation (Swan Ganz) catheter in cases where excessive blood loss can be predicted, particularly in patients with significant heart disease. A PA catheter may also be useful in the continuing and postoperative management of such patients following massive transfusion.

TRANSFUSION

The first priority is to restore circulating blood volume. An appropriate solution to use initially is 0.9% saline (NaCl). Glucose 5% is not useful in these circumstances because once the glucose is metabolized, free water remains, most of which is then distributed within the cells. The same applies to dextrose-saline (4% dextrose in 0.18% saline). Some clinicians feel that Hartmann's solution (also called Ringer's lactate) is inappropriate as it contains potassium and lactate (both of which are already likely to be raised in the patient requiring a large transfusion). In addition, packed red cells may clot when mixed with Hartmann's solution in a giving-set. There is debate as to whether crystalloid or colloid is preferable for the replacement of blood loss. Colloids include the dextrans, modified gelatins, starches, albumin and other blood products. No particular advantages are apparent but about three times as much crystalloid is needed compared to colloid to replace a given blood loss. This means that the patient will be more oedematous at the end of the resuscitation period if crystalloid is used. In summary, 'It's not what you do but the way that you do it'.

In the future other solutions such as hypertonic saline, perfluorocarbons or modified haemoglobins may be more widely available. Although all these solutions can restore circulating volume, none of them (with the exception of perfluorocarbons and modified haemoglobins) can increase oxygen-carrying capacity. Indeed, they will all tend to produce a reduction in haemoglobin due to dilution. In the case of large blood loss, therefore, blood transfusion is always required.

USE OF BLOOD

Normally fully crossmatched blood should be used. Whole blood is of most use but more commonly, packed red cells are supplied. Un-crossmatched group O Rh-negative blood is very rarely necessary because, in the event of a dire emergency, it should still be possible for the transfusion laboratory to provide group-specific blood. This subject is discussed more fully in Chapter 21.

COMPLICATIONS OF MASSIVE TRANSFUSION

Hypothermia

Bank blood is stored at about 4°C and will therefore cause a rapid lowering of body temperature if not warmed prior to transfusion. Hypothermia exacerbates any tendency to coagulopathy (see below) and further impairs the ability of haemoglobin to release oxygen in the tissues. Cold blood also contains higher levels of free potassium and has a higher viscosity, making it harder to infuse rapidly. Blood should always therefore be warmed prior to infusion. Blood salvage techniques tend to reduce the drop in temperature associated with

transfusion. Numerous types of blood warmers, of varying efficiency, are available and it is worth noting that their efficiency may vary with the speed of transfusion.

Biochemistry

Massive transfusion tends to cause a rise in serum potassium (K^+) and a fall in both serum magnesium (Mg_2^+) and calcium (Ca_2^+). Additionally, stored blood has a lower pH (i.e. is more acidic) than normal and will tend to produce a metabolic acidosis. (However, the transfusion of blood containing citrate as an anticoagulant may lead to a late metabolic alkalosis after the citrate has been metabolized). Stored blood also contains lower levels of 2,3-DPG (see Chapter 21) within the red cells. Consequently, the oxyhaemoglobin dissociation curve is shifted to the left (this also occurs in hypothermia), i.e. haemoglobin has an increased affinity for oxygen and therefore becomes less efficient at unloading oxygen in the tissues. This may contribute to a metabolic acidosis.

Coagulation

Transfused blood contains virtually no clotting factors or functioning platelets and patients may therefore develop a fall in platelet numbers (thrombocytopenia). Existing clotting factors become diluted (dilutional coagulopathy) and this is reflected in a rise in the prothrombin time (PT) and partial thromboplastin time (PTT). Any tendency to such a coagulopathy will be exacerbated by hypothermia and by hypocalcaemia. In addition, the patient who has suffered significant or prolonged hypotension may also develop a disseminated intravascular coagulopathy (DIC), causing a further deterioration of coagulation and complicating management. Traditional rules-of-thumb regarding the transfusion of platelets, clotting factors, fresh frozen plasma or cryoprecipitate after a particular number of transfused units of blood are unhelpful and should not be used. If at all possible, it is far more preferable to base the replacement of clotting factors on laboratory investigations. A similar consideration applies to the use of calcium salts. The problem of coagulopathy is not removed by the use of blood salvage equipment; indeed, this may even exacerbate it if significant quantities of heparin are transfused back into the patient.

Incompatibility

The risk of an acute haemolytic reaction when blood has been fully crossmatched (and given to the correct patient) is very small (about one in 10,000). However, if un-crossmatched group-specific blood is transfused this risk increases to about one in 1,000. It is important to realize that many of the classic features of a transfusion reaction, such as pyrexia, dyspnoea, chest pain, and nausea, will be masked in the unconscious, anaesthetized patient. Features such as hypotension, tachycardia and coagulopathy may incorrectly be ascribed to the general condition of the patient and rashes may not be noticed under the surgical towelling. Obviously the use of autotransfusion will eliminate problems of compatibility.

Other problems

Overtransfusion leading to volume overload or an excessively high haemoglobin concentration may occur, particularly where surgical control of bleeding is gained quickly and when CVP monitoring is not employed. The risk of air embolus should be borne in mind, particularly when rapid infusion devices are being used and there is much activity around the patient. This is particularly important when central venous lines are used. Blood is always a potential source of infection (to health-care workers as well as the recipient) but this is not likely to impact on the decision to use blood in these circumstances. The same considerations apply to other blood products.

ASPIRATION OF GASTRIC CONTENTS

BACKGROUND

The actual incidence of aspiration of gastric contents into the lungs is not known. Studies have shown that 'silent' aspiration may occur in up to one in five of all general anaesthetics but clearly the majority of these are not clinically significant. When significant aspiration does occur mortality is of the order of 5%. In addition, the risk of lung damage is said to increase if aspirated material has a pH of 2.5 or less. The volume of aspirated fluid necessary to produce lung injury is probably twice the usually quoted 25ml as recent evidence suggests it is 0.8 ml/kg. It is, however, closely dependent on the pH of the aspirate, fluid with a higher pH being less destructive.

RISK FACTORS

Certain factors are known to increase the risk of regurgitation or reflux of gastric contents, that must occur before aspiration is possible. These include:

- Recent ingestion of food or blood (oropharyngeal or gastric haemorrhage).
- Bowel obstruction or ileus.

- Raised intraabdominal pressure (e.g. obesity).
- Previous gastric surgery.
- Hiatus hernia with reflux oesophagitis.
- Long-standing peptic ulcer disease (pyloric obstruction).
- Delayed gastric emptying due to trauma, pain or drugs (e.g. opiates).
- Decreased lower oesophageal sphincter tone due to drugs (e.g. opiates, anticholinergic drugs, volatile agents).
- Pregnancy.
- Presence of nasogastric tube.
- Reduced level of consciousness for any reason.
- Old age.
- ASA grade 4E or 5E.

Many patients will have more than one of these risk factors. Although elective procedures are never carried out in patients who have recently eaten, some of the other risk factors cannot be eliminated. The usual approach in the 'at-risk' patient who requires a general anaesthetic is to use drugs to reduce gastric pH and volume, if possible, and to employ a rapid sequence induction technique (cricoid pressure or Sellick's manoeuvre). It is also important to remember that regurgitation and aspiration may occur at any time, not only during induction (even if cricoid pressure is used) but also during maintenance of anaesthesia (if the airway is not protected) or during reversal, emergence or recovery. Thus patients who are likely to aspirate should be recovered in the left lateral position if at all possible.

RECOGNITION THAT ASPIRATION HAS OCCURRED

The signs of aspiration listed below may be immediate or delayed and not all will necessarily occur in the same patient.

- Laryngospasm results from irritation of the upper airway. It may present as stridor or complete obstruction.
- Airway obstruction may be due to laryngospasm but it may also be produced directly by the presence of solid material in the airway.
- Bronchospasm is precipitated by foreign material reaching the lungs. Its intensity may be apparent from the severity of wheezing. In extreme cases the flow of gases into or out of the patient is so low that there may be no wheeze at all but great difficulty in ventilation. Bronchospasm may be particularly severe in asthmatic patients or those taking β-blocking drugs.
- Tachypnoea (an abnormally fast rate of breathing) may occur in the spontaneously breathing patient.
- Obvious severe coughing may be provoked but this would not occur in the paralysed patient.

- Tachycardia may sometimes occur but may be masked in the patient taking β-blocking drugs or be misinterpreted as due to other causes.
- Hypotension is sometimes reported.
- A fall in haemoglobin oxygen saturation (as determined on a pulse oximeter). This arterial desaturation may be due to many of the above features and, if severe enough, cyanosis may become apparent.

ASPIRATION PNEUMONITIS

This is sometimes called Mendelson's Syndrome (after its original description in obstetric patients in 1946) and is the result of aspirated material reaching the lungs. The features may include pulmonary oedema, bronchospasm and hypoxaemia and may eventually lead to respiratory failure and hypotension. Shadowing or infiltrates develop on the chest X-ray (CXR), usually bilaterally, but may initially be most pronounced in the area corresponding to the apex of the right lower lobe. Bacterial pneumonia or an acute lung injury (acute respiratory distress syndrome, ARDS) may supervene.

MANAGEMENT OF ASPIRATION

The patient should be positioned headdown and as much material as possible should be removed from the oropharynx while keeping the patient adequately oxygenated. Endotracheal intubation is likely to be required in all but the most minor of cases although continuous positive airway pressure (CPAP), provided by a special circuit and facemask, may be suitable for some patients. Further amounts of foreign material may be removed by suction following intubation.

Bronchospasm may respond to the use of a volatile agent such as halothane (although this may be limited due to resultant hypotension) but nebulized or, in severe cases, intravenous bronchodilators (such as salbutamol or aminophylline) may be required. Very refractory cases (i.e. those which are not helped by these measures) may respond to the direct tracheal instillation of salbutamol or even adrenaline. Occasionally inotropic support is required.

In the past, the use of intravenous steroids (e.g. hydrocortisone or methylprednisolone) has been recommended but there is no evidence of any beneficial effect and their use may contribute to the development of a subsequent bacterial pneumonia. So-called prophylactic antibiotics are also no longer recommended as no positive advantage can be demonstrated and their use appears to predispose to the subsequent growth of resistant organisms. Many anaesthetists recommend the early use of fibreoptic bronchoscopy to facilitate the removal of solid foreign material. Whilst this may be of benefit its use may worsen hypoxaemia and therefore is not suitable in unskilled hands. If signs such as wheeze or hypoxaemia or CXR changes have not developed within two hours, serious sequelae are unlikely; on the other hand, the most severe cases of aspiration will require a period of mechanical ventilation and support on an intensive care unit.

HYPOXAEMIA

BACKGROUND

Hypoxaemia, which means an abnormally low oxygen tension (pressure) in arterial blood, is a relatively common intraoperative and postoperative problem. The widespread use of pulse oximeters to measure haemoglobin oxygen saturation (SpO_2) has made the detection of hypoxaemia much easier, certainly before cyanosis has occurred. This is particularly true in anaemic patients, in whom the presence of hypoxaemia is even more difficult to detect (cyanosis requires about 5 g/dl of unsaturated haemoglobin before it is clinically detectable). Many anaesthetic emergencies may cause hypoxaemia and examples include aspiration of gastric contents, failed intubation, malignant hyperthermia or any other event associated with hypotension or cardiovascular collapse, e.g. anaphylaxis and cardiac arrest. These are discussed elsewhere.

CAUSES AND MANAGEMENT OF HYPOXAEMIA

Hypoventilation

In a patient breathing spontaneously, marked hypoventilation, in addition to producing serious carbon dioxide retention, may lead to a falling SpO_2. This will obviously occur rapidly if the patient becomes apnoeic. Hypoventilation or apnoea are not normally difficult to detect but do need to be distinguished from airway obstruction.

The three main causes of hypoventilation are excessive opiate analgesics, insufficient analgesia (in upper abdominal and chest surgery, pain may prevent effective inspiration) and inadequate reversal of muscle relaxants.

Treatment depends on the cause. Respiratory depression can be reversed using the specific antagonist naloxone or a respiratory stimulant such as doxapram. Pain may be controlled using analgesics or regional and local anaesthetic blocks.

Failure to reverse muscle paralysis may be due to an excessive dose of relaxant or the muscle paralysis may have been reversed too soon after the last drug increment. Occasionally, it may be due to myasthenia gravis, an inherited condition in which the neuromuscular acetylcholine receptors are abnormal. Time is the best corrector of failure of reversal and premature pharmacological interference often prolongs the process. True failure of reversal only occurs in the presence of normal electrolytes and pH, and in the absence of respiratory depression due to analgesics or volatile agents.

Airway Obstruction

Airway obstruction may occur at any stage of anaesthesia including postoperatively, in recovery. Normally it is readily recognized; for example, there may be exaggerated movements of the patient's chest or abdomen. Appropriate positioning of the head, neck and jaw or use of artificial airways usually resolves the problem.

Low inspired oxygen concentration (FiO$_2$)

This is now an infrequent cause of hypoxaemia as newer anaesthetic machines have a link between the oxygen and nitrous oxide flow meters, preventing the administration of an hypoxic gas mixture. However, the problem may still occur when using older machines or when the anaesthetic machine can supply air (or carbon dioxide) that may dilute the fresh flow delivered to the patient. It is also possible for cylinders to empty and pipeline supplies to fail or to have been crossed over during servicing. In the very rare event of there being doubt as to the integrity of the gas supply, the patient should be hand ventilated from a free-standing oxygen cylinder.

It is for these reasons that the Association of Anaesthetists has recommended that the oxygen concentration of the fresh and inspired gas should be monitored at all times.

Problems with the Anaesthetic Circuit (Breathing System) or Endotracheal Tube.

Circuit disconnections may occur at any time and obviously in a ventilated patient this would be disastrous if it were unrecognized. The use of disconnection alarms is therefore mandatory. It is also possible for circuits to become obstructed, endotracheal tubes (ETT) may become dislodged or the oesophagus may have been accidentally intubated. The cuff of an ETT may herniate, thus obstructing the lumen, but the ETT may also kink or become blocked with secretions. This situation may mimic bronchospasm (see below) and if there is any doubt about the patency of an ETT (e.g. after checking by passing a suction catheter down it) it should be removed, the patient ventilated by bag and mask and the tube replaced with another one.

Pressure-limiting valves or unidirectional flow valves on a circle system may malfunction and, depending on which valve jams and in what position, i.e. open or closed, the result may be immediate obstruction or a massive increase in dead space, leading to rebreathing. Obstruction should be detectable by the use of pressure alarms in the circuit and rebreathing by monitoring end-tidal carbon dioxide (ETCO$_2$).

Laryngospasm

Laryngospasm is usually easily recognized by its typically noisy respiration in a struggling patient recovering from anaesthesia. It is usually triggered by the presence of irritating material such as saliva or blood but may also occur due to aspiration (see above). Frequently, the spasm breaks rapidly and spontaneously and all that is required is to keep the patient well oxygenated with 100% oxygen. Sometimes a small dose of, for example, a benzodiazepine may help. Very rarely, reestablishment of anaesthesia and a neuromuscular blocking agent will be required. Laryngospasm may also occur during induction of anaesthesia, in which case it normally responds to deepening anaesthesia.

Bronchospasm

Bronchospasm may occur in any patient but is more common in those with preexisting asthma, chronic obstructive airway disease (COAD) or following a recent upper respiratory tract infection. It may be a feature of other problems such as pulmonary oedema, anaphylaxis, pneumothorax, aspiration or the effects of drugs (e.g. induction agents, neuromuscular blocking agents, opiates), laryngoscopy, intubation or reversal. In the spontaneously breathing patient there may be an audible wheeze. In the intubated patient ventilation may suddenly become difficult or a rise in airway pressure may be noted. Wheezes (rhonchi) may be heard on auscultation but in severe cases, however, there is so little gas flow in and out of the patient that no sounds will be heard and this is the so-called silent chest.

Slow hand ventilation, sometimes with 100% oxygen, may be needed to maintain oxygenation. Bronchospasm may respond to withdrawing the ETT slightly if it is close to the carina but also deepening anaesthesia with a volatile agent or intravenous agents can help.

There is a risk of producing hypotension in such patients as the high airway pressures already impair venous return and hence cardiac output. Inhaled or intravenous β-agonists, such as salbutamol, are usually helpful in treating bronchospasm but sometimes intravenous aminophylline is used although toxic levels are easily reached in a patient already taking theophyllines. Many anaesthetists also give intravenous hydrocortisone in these circumstances and some have found a role for ketamine. In extreme cases a patient will respond only to the administration of adrenaline either intravenously or sometimes by direct instillation into the trachea via the ETT.

Pneumothorax

Pneumothorax may occur spontaneously in patients, for example those with bullous lung disease which occurs in COAD and emphysema, but is more common after invasive procedures such as supraclavicular brachial plexus block, placing central venous lines (especially via the subclavian route) or in patients with recent rib fractures. It is much more likely to occur in ventilated patients than in spontaneously breathing patients as the former will have higher airway pressures. Surgeons may accidentally produce a pneumothorax during laparoscopic surgery or abdominal surgery if dissecting close to the diaphragm, e.g. during a nephrectomy. Obviously some surgery, e.g. thoracic, of necessity produces a pneumothorax and this should not be a problem if drains are functioning correctly when the chest is closed. During anaesthesia a preexisting pneumothorax will increase in size as nitrous oxide diffuses into it much faster than the less soluble nitrogen can diffuse out. Hypoxaemia results from the subsequent lung collapse and hence the establishment of massive ventilation/perfusion mismatch and shunt.

The first sign of a pneumothorax may be desaturation, but in a ventilated patient a rise in airway pressure is noted together with reduced movement of one side of the chest, hypotension and tachycardia (sometimes it may cause bradycardia). Examination usually reveals reduced air entry and a resonant percussion note because of the presence of air in the pleural cavity on the affected side. If a tension pneumothorax develops, compression and displacement of mediastinal viscera occurs which will ultimately cause cardiovascular collapse and death.

The management of all but the smallest pneumothorax includes the use of a drainage procedure. In addition, for the reason noted above, administration of nitrous oxide should be stopped. If tension pneumothorax is suspected X-ray confirmation is not sought as delay in treatment could be fatal. In a ventilated patient a large-bore cannula (e.g. 14 gauge) should be inserted on the affected side, which should immediately relieve the problem. This should then be followed unhurriedly by the insertion of a chest drain connected to an underwater seal.

Pulmonary Oedema

Pulmonary oedema describes the excessive presence of fluid within the lung alveoli. This obviously impairs gas exchange and hence leads to hypoxaemia. Pulmonary oedema may occur at any time during anaesthesia but is more common postoperatively.

Broadly speaking, there are two main causes: hydrostatic and non-hydrostatic. In addition, there are some less easily classified causes of pulmonary oedema such as that occurring after relief of airway obstruction, reexpansion of a lung or in association with neurosurgery or head injury.

Hydrostatic pulmonary oedema is typically due to either fluid overload or pump failure i.e. poor cardiac function. It may therefore be precipitated by excessive transfusion of fluids, a sudden increase in venous return (e.g. head-down or lithotomy position) or anything that produces a deterioration in cardiac status (e.g. dysrhythmia, myocardial ischaemia or infarction, valvular disease or cardiac tamponade).

Non-hydrostatic pulmonary oedema is caused by excessive permeability of the alveolar capillary membrane and is one of the components of acute lung injury or acute respiratory distress syndrome (ARDS), which result from such conditions as sepsis, pancreatitis, anaphylaxis and pulmonary aspiration.

The first signs may be desaturation, dyspnoea or presence of pink, frothy fluid within the ETT. Crackles and often wheezes are usually heard on chest examination. Whatever the cause, the initial management requires an increase in the FiO_2. More definitive treatment may include intubating the trachea and ventilating with PEEP and drugs such as nitrates, inotropes, antiarrhythmics, or diuretics. Precise therapy will depend on identifying and managing the underlying cause and monitoring with a pulmonary artery (Swan Ganz) catheter may well be needed.

Pulmonary embolism

Pulmonary embolism may be due to air, gas, clot (thromboemboli), amniotic fluid or, very rarely, a foreign body. The end result is a blocking of blood flow within the right atrium, right ventricle, pulmonary artery or lung capillary bed, all of which may dramatically impair gas exchange and cardiac output.

Air or gas embolus may occur during the siting or use of central (or occasionally peripheral) venous lines, surgery around the head or neck (rarely breast, pelvic or thoracic surgery) or during insufflation of the abdomen or chest during minimal access surgery. Only about 50 ml of gas is needed to completely occupy the right ventricle.

Air embolus may sometimes be immediately recognized (seen or heard) but may otherwise present as an altered respiratory pattern in a spontaneously breathing patient, dysrhythmias, hypotension, cyanosis, a sudden drop in end-tidal CO_2, a rise in CVP or, in massive cases, cardiac arrest. Very rarely auscultation will reveal the characteristic so-called millwheel murmur.

Management requires that the source of air is stopped. Open veins in the surgical field can be compressed, the area flooded with saline and the surgical field lowered to below the level of the heart. In order to reduce the entry of air into the heart the patient needs to be placed head and right-side down but this will not be possible if cardiopulmonary resuscitation is in progress. Nitrous oxide should be discontinued as it causes air emboli to expand (see above under Pneumothorax,) and 100% oxygen should be used. It may be possible to aspirate air from the right atrium or ventricle through a central line (or, in extremis, directly through a needle introduced into the right ventricle).

Thromboembolism can occur intraoperatively and may present with similar signs to air embolus. It is more common in elderly patients and those who have cancer, obesity or who have had prolonged bedrest prior to surgery.

Myocardial infarction

Myocardial infarction may be the end result of a perioperative ischaemic episode or possibly it would have occurred irrespective of anaesthesia and surgery. Because the patient is anaesthetized the usual symptom of severe chest pain would be masked. Thus the patient may present with any of the features of cardiac damage such as arrhythmias, hypotension, heart failure and unexplained hypoxia. Rarely this may be the cause of perioperative cardiac arrest.

Treatment is largely symptomatic in the first instance and is aimed at restoring oxygenation and myocardial function by means of oxygen, diuretics or myocardial stimulants. Perhaps the most important factor is to think of the possibility during the differential diagnosis of hypoxia or hypotension.

PROBLEMS WITH LOCAL ANAESTHETICS

BACKGROUND

Local anaesthetics may be used as part of a local (topical, infiltration, nerve block) or regional (epidural or spinal) technique and problems due to local anaesthetics may therefore be related to the drug themselves or to the technique or site of application. Anaphylaxis to the commonly used local anaesthetic drugs of the amide group (lignocaine, prilocaine, bupivacaine and ropivacaine) is extremely rare but it may be more common with the less frequently used local anaesthetics of the ester class (procaine, cocaine). Anaphylaxis is discussed below.

Local anaesthetics are frequently used with adrenaline in order to produce vasoconstriction and delay absorption and therefore allow a greater duration of action. It is worth remembering, therefore, that problems may arise due to adrenaline rather than to the local anaesthetic itself. For example, the accidental use of local anaesthetic with adrenaline (or felypressin) for infiltration of, for example, fingers, toes, penis, nose or ears may result in ischaemia and consequent loss of tissue. Where local anaesthetic is accidentally given intravenously (see below), adrenaline may contribute to the problems by causing hypertension, myocardial ischaemia and dysrhythmias, which are more common in the presence of halothane than with the other volatile agents.

Some techniques may be associated with a particular risk of specific complications, e.g. pneumothorax (supraclavicular brachial plexus block), severe hypotension (spinal or epidural blocks) or vertebral artery puncture (interscalene brachial plexus block).

DRUG TOXICITY

All the local anaesthetics have a stated maximum dose that is safe to use. Because adrenaline delays the absorption of local anaesthetics this dose may be higher when adrenaline is used than when the drug is used by itself ('plain'). Problems may also occur at less than the maximum dose if the blood level of the drug rises very rapidly, e.g. the increased absorption of cocaine used in patients with acute allergic rhinitis may precipitate convulsions. Elderly, hypovolaemic, shocked or pregnant patients are also more susceptible to the toxic effects of local anaesthetic drugs. Toxicity is likely to occur if large quantities of local anaesthetic are used for infiltration, particularly if a higher concentration of the drug is used than is realized. All theatre staff therefore need to be aware of how much local anaesthetic is being used in a particular patient and how to calculate the maximum safe dose in milligrams from the concentration given on the bottle, which is expressed in percentage terms.

If an injection is accidentally given intravenously there is a rapid rise in blood concentration of the drug, which can cause the same adverse events. This may also occur when local anaesthetic is deliberately given intravenously for intravenous regional anaesthesia (Bier's block) if the occluding cuff is inadequately pressurized and therefore leaks or is deflated too early.

SIGNS OF TOXICITY

The most serious effects of exceeding the maximum dose of local anaesthetic in a patient occur in the central nervous and cardiovascular systems. Pallor, especially around the mouth, and sweating are said to be common signs.

Central nervous system toxicity is manifest by visual disturbances, tingling or numbness of the tongue, tinnitus, confusion, twitching, depressed conscious level and convulsions leading to respiratory failure.

Adverse effects within the cardiovascular system include myocardial depression leading to hypotension and dysrhythmias such as bradycardia, ventricular tachycardia, ventricular fibrillation or asystole. Cardiovascular problems are more common and more serious with bupivacaine and for this reason it is no longer used for Bier's blocks.

TREATMENT OF LOCAL ANAESTHETIC DRUG TOXICITY

Convulsions need to be controlled immediately and thiopentone, diazepam and midazolam have all been used safely to this effect. It may also be necessary to intubate the patient, in which case suxamethonium is usually recommended.

Cardiovascular resuscitation may require cardiac massage, which may need to be prolonged due to the binding of bupivacaine to the myocardium, defibrillation and very large doses of adrenaline and atropine. The drug treatment of choice to treat the ventricular fibrillation is bretylium; surprisingly, lignocaine has also been used but bretylium is more effective.

The local anaesthetic drug prilocaine, if used in excessive dosage, can cause haemoglobin to be converted by oxidation of its iron atoms into the less efficient oxygen carrier methaemoglobin. This gives the appearance of cyanosis and is spontaneously reversible. If necessary specific treatment requires the

use of intravenous methylene blue, which converts methaemoglobin back to haemoglobin.

ACCIDENTAL INTRA-ARTERIAL INJECTION

BACKGROUND

Certain drugs such as vasoconstrictors, if injected intra arterially, may cause intense spasm of the artery. Others, e.g. thiopentone, may cause pronounced injury to the inner wall of the artery by means of a chemical endarteritis. This may destroy the endothelium and sometimes the deeper layers of the vessel wall. Intense arterial spasm and thrombosis may occur, causing obstruction to blood flow and subsequent ischaemia. There is then a very real risk of loss of tissue, a finger or hand. As a rule no drugs should be injected via an arterial line and all intravascular lines should be clearly marked to prevent this happening.

RECOGNITION

Accidental injection into an artery in a patient who is awake is usually followed immediately by very intense pain at the site of injection, which radiates distally towards the fingers. Blanching of the skin may occur but there may be a delay in the onset of drug action. If the injection is undetected, e.g. the patient is anaesthetized, oedema, motor weakness and anaesthesia or hyperaesthesia of the affected area may develop within two hours. Thrombosis can still occur even if a pulse is palpable and later, gangrene or tissue loss may follow. The increasing use of arterial lines intraoperatively means that accidental injection into an artery may occur at any time and not just at induction of anaesthesia. Therefore, any drug, not just induction agents, may be involved. In addition, the problem may arise at sites other than the hand or forearm.

MANAGEMENT OF ACCIDENTAL INTRA ARTERIAL INJECTION

If there is any doubt injection of the drug should be stopped immediately but the needle or cannula should not be removed because this can then be used for the management of the problem. The recommended treatment is to flush the line with saline in order to dilute the drug and then inject the vasodilator, papaverine, to relieve any vascular spasm. Heparin may also be used in this way. It may be possible to carry out a brachial plexus or a stellate ganglion block to interrupt the sympathetic nerve supply to the upper limb and assist in producing vasodilatation.

ANAPHYLAXIS

BACKGROUND

Anaphylaxis is the sudden, life-threatening systemic reaction of a patient to a foreign substance. In anaesthetic practice this may be drugs (e.g. an induction agent, neuromuscular blocking agent or antibiotic), intravenous fluids (e.g. plasma expanders or X-ray contrast media), blood products or another material such as latex. The release of endogenous mediators, of which histamine is only one, causes vasodilatation and increased capillary permeability, leading to severe hypotension.

Typically but not invariably, the reaction occurs immediately or within 15 minutes after a substance is given intravenously but may be delayed for several hours if other routes are used. This may make latex allergy, for example, extremely difficult to diagnose. Patients with a history of multiple allergies are described as atopic.

Strictly speaking, there is a distinction between an anaphylactic reaction and an anaphylactoid reaction but the two are clinically indistinguishable, equally life threatening and the initial management of each is identical.

The best way to avoid anaphylaxis is by carefully obtaining a reliable history from the patient and referring to it, but this may not always be possible. It is also essential to realize that cross-sensitivity may exist between some drugs, foodstuffs or other substances. For example, patients who are allergic to penicillin will also be allergic to ampicillin and possibly imipenem and have about a 10% risk of reacting to cephalosporins as well. Some patients allergic to latex also give a history of allergy to avocados and bananas.

CLINICAL FEATURES

It is important to maintain a high index of suspicion whenever drugs are administered to a patient and this applies whether or not the drug has been administered previously. The features which may occur in a severe case are:

- Hypotension
- Bronchospasm
- Angioedema of face/eyes/tongue/larynx
- Pulmonary oedema
- Flushing
- Urticaria
- Itching
- Tachycardia
- Sense of doom
- Sweating

- Sneezing or coughing
- Dyspnoea
- Nausea/vomiting/diarrhoea.

It is important to note that not all of these features will necessarily be present in every patient although some are very common, such as hypotension and bronchospasm, which occur in 90% and 33% of cases respectively. Many of these features, however, may be masked in the unconscious or ventilated patient or may present differently.

MANAGEMENT OF ANAPHYLAXIS

Firstly the responsible drug or infusion must be stopped or, in the case of latex, the appropriate material removed. The specific management of the patient includes the use of adrenaline, intravenous fluids and oxygen.

In very minor cases simple bronchodilators or subcutaneous adrenaline (epinephrine) may suffice but in most cases intravenous adrenaline will also be needed. The drug is given in a dose of 3–5ml of a one in 10,000 (10 micrograms/ml) solution and must be repeated as often as necessary. This is the essential part of the treatment of anaphylaxis because, as an α-agonist, it reverses peripheral vasodilatation, reduces oedema and urticaria and, as a β-agonist, it produces bronchodilatation, increases the contractility of the heart and reduces the release of histamine and similar substances from inflammatory cells. Sometimes an adrenaline infusion may be necessary.

Adequate venous access should be secured as soon as possible and fluid (either crystalloid or colloid) should be given rapidly. Large volumes may be required for adequate resuscitation in order to restore tissue perfusion. For the same reason 100% oxygen should be given and endotracheal intubation may be required to secure an airway. If severe laryngeal oedema has occurred cricothyroidotomy may be needed.

PROBLEMS IN THE MANAGEMENT OF ANAPHYLAXIS

By far the commonest problem in the management of this medical emergency is using too little adrenaline, too late. The risk of dysrhythmias with adrenaline has been greatly exaggerated and in one recent study the risk was less than 2% and none of these was life threatening.

OTHER THERAPIES

Antihistamines are of limited value because they can only prevent further histamine release. Similarly, there is no role for steroids in immediate therapy as their onset of action is too slow.

Aminophylline is occasionally useful as, in addition to its bronchodilator effect, it interferes with the action of histamine.

Glucagon may have a role in patients who are being treated with β-blocking agents because these individuals tend to be resistant to the beneficial effects of adrenaline.

MALIGNANT HYPERTHERMIA

BACKGROUND

Malignant hyperthermia (MH or malignant hyperpyrexia) is an inherited susceptibility of some patients to react to certain anaesthetic drugs by developing very high temperatures and other life-threatening biochemical changes. It is thought to be caused by a failure of the patient's muscle cells to control their intracellular levels of calcium. The drugs usually responsible are any of the volatile anaesthetic agents and suxamethonium. Untreated, the condition, once triggered, carries about an 80% mortality but even if treated, there is a mortality of about 5%.

A carefully obtained family history may make the anaesthetist suspicious that a particular patient is at risk. However, some patients who have MH have sometimes had uneventful anaesthesia in the past. Proof of a patient's risk depends on the results of testing a sample of muscle obtained at biopsy. Following such testing (using caffeine and halothane and called the invitro contracture test), 95% of patients can be labelled as MH susceptible (MHS) or MH non-susceptible (MHN). Sometimes the testing is inconclusive, in which case the patient is described as MH equivocal (MHE) but MHE patients are normally treated as though they are MHS. In the UK all this testing is carried out at the Leeds MH Investigation Unit.

When a patient is known to be MHS (or MHE) suitable precautions can be taken, such as using a regional or local technique. If general anaesthesia is required safe drugs must be used, known triggering agents avoided and additional monitoring employed. However, when an unexpected case of MH develops perioperatively the situation is life threatening.

CLINICAL FEATURES

Malignant hyperpyrexia is characterized by a rise in body temperature of more than 2°C/hr. The onset may be immediate but sometimes occurs after the patient reaches the recovery ward. Cyanosis or mottling of the skin may be noticed and the increase in metabolism causes a rise in carbon dioxide and other products of metabolism, tachypnoea, tachycardia,

sweating and hypertension. A severe acidaemia develops and at the same time damage to cells (rhabdomyolysis) produces hyperkalaemia, dark urine (due to myoglobinuria) and renal impairment. Sometimes generalized muscle rigidity or masseter (jaw muscle) spasm is seen. Many of these features produce severe dysrhythmias and frequently clotting abnormalities such as disseminated intravascular coagulation (DIC). Later hypoxaemia or hypotension may occur and cardiac arrest may be precipitated.

MANAGEMENT

When there is any suspicion that MH has been triggered, all potential triggering agents must be stopped immediately, MH-safe drugs used and a vapour-free system used to hyperventilate the patient with 100% oxygen. Surgery must be stopped as soon as possible. The only drug of specific value is dantrolene, which probably works by preventing intracellular levels of calcium from continuing to rise. Dantrolene must be made up from a dry powder with sterile water and given intravenously as soon as possible. Because it is very insoluble and large quantities may be required, a member of the theatre staff dedicated entirely to this role may be necessary.

At the same time efforts should be made to cool the patient by packing ice in the groins and axillae and giving cold intravenous saline (not Hartmann's because it contains potassium). Cold saline may also be used to cool body cavities, e.g. if the abdomen is open.

Sodium bicarbonate is used to correct the metabolic acidosis while insulin and 50% glucose are used to treat the hyperkalaemia. Mannitol promotes urine output and protects the kidneys from rhabdomyolysis.

Additional monitoring such as peripheral and core temperatures, arterial pressure, CVP, end-tidal $CO2$ and urine output, if not already sited, will be needed. Frequent measurement of blood gases, electrolytes, clotting and creatine kinase (CK) is also essential. Postoperatively the patient should be monitored and managed in an intensive care unit for 48 hours as further deterioration can occur.

RECOMMENDED READING

American College of Surgeons. 1990 *Advanced Trauma Life Support Student Manual*. Chicago:ACS.

Anon. 1994 Adrenaline for anaphylaxis. *Drug and Therapeutics Bulletin* 32: 19–21.

British National Formulary (Section 3.4.3, Allergic Emergencies).

MH Investigation Unit. 1993 *Malignant Hyperthermia:A Family Concern*. Leeds:M H Investigation Unit.

27

THE FUNDAMENTALS OF EMERGENCY RESUSCITATION

T.M. Hankin

INTRODUCTION

Resuscitation is the process by which an individual is brought 'back to life' or consciousness. Cardiorespiratory resuscitation is the process by which an individual's respiration and circulation may be temporarily supported to keep them alive long enough for the cause of the arrest to be treated, if this is possible. Ideally, all clinical personnel, both medical and non-medical, should be familiar with the principles and practice of cardiopulmonary resuscitation.

In the United Kingdom, the Resuscitation Council (UK) runs an excellent Advanced Life Support Provider course, which covers the principles and practice of life support in detail. This chapter provides an overview of the subject of resuscitation.

RECOGNITION AND ASSESSMENT

The importance of the recognition and assessment of the suspected cardiorespiratory arrest cannot be overstated. Failure to recognize and respond to the arrest wastes valuable time and reduces the chance of a successful outcome.

A *respiratory arrest* occurs when an individual stops breathing and becomes *apnoeic*. A *cardiac arrest* is when the heart fails to pump enough blood to maintain a pulse or blood pressure. If untreated, one always rapidly follows the other because, if breathing ceases, no oxygen enters the blood and the heart, brain and other vital organs are starved of oxygen. This hypoxia leads to the development of organ failure. Initially, because the brain has the greatest need for oxygen, it rapidly stops functioning properly and the patient loses consciousness. The brainstem is also affected and, shortly after, the heart ceases to beat effectively and the circulation fails, i.e. the blood pressure and pulse will be unrecordable. Without a circulation and the subsequent loss of tissue perfusion, damage to other vital organs will ensue.

If, on the other hand, the patient has a cardiac arrest the circulation fails first and the brain then becomes starved of oxygen-rich blood. Cerebral function is compromised and the patient rapidly becomes unconscious. Because the brain also contains the respiratory centre, which controls breathing, the breathing will become erratic and eventually stop. In this case, the respiratory arrest is secondary to a cardiac arrest.

Of all the vital organs which suffer injury following a cardiorespiratory arrest, the brain is the most vulnerable. Irreversible brain damage begins 3–4 min following a cardiorespiratory arrest. Not all parts of the brain, however, are damaged at the same rate.

HYPOXIC BRAIN DAMAGE

The two common patterns of hypoxic brain damage seen are:

1. Cortical death.
2. Brainstem death.

Cortical death is death of the cerebral cortex, which makes up the bulk of the brain. It contains the areas that control voluntary movement, interpret sounds, sights and smells, etc. and also the areas that relate to the higher functions, such as thought and consciousness. The cerebral cortex makes us what we are as human individuals and without it we enter a vegetative state (see below).

When clinicians refer to brain death, what is really meant is *brainstem death*. The brainstem is at the base of the brain and the cerebral cortex 'sits' on it. It contains the control areas for *vegetative* functions such as respiration, the gut and the circulation. It operates without the need for conscious effort. (That is why we do not die when we sleep.) Of all parts of the brain, it is the most resistant to hypoxic damage.

CORTICAL VERSUS BRAINSTEM DEATH

A significant number of patients who survive a cardiorespiratory arrest have sustained brain damage. If *only* the cerebral cortex is dead, they may live on for years in a persistent vegetative state, i.e. their body functions physiologically but they are unresponsive and have no awareness of their surroundings.

If their brainstem is dead, their basic bodily functions such as breathing have to be supported and in time their circulation will also fail. Doctors may perform a set of well-defined brainstem function tests and, if the patient's brainstem is proved to be dead, the patient can legally be pronounced as dead, even though the heart may still be beating. This is because, in time, these patients will *always* die.

CAUSES OF CARDIORESPIRATORY FAILURE

Any of the three main organ systems involved in cardiorespiratory failure may malfunction and lead to a cardiorespiratory arrest.

THE CENTRAL NERVOUS SYSTEM

Although the heart will continue to pump blood even though the brain has failed, the respiratory system cannot function in the presence of severe brain damage. This is because the brain contains the control centre for respiration (in the brainstem) and also a level of consciousness is required to maintain an airway.

Common causes of brain failure are:

- Direct trauma to the brain, producing unconsciousness or brain death.
- Depression of brain function by drugs (especially those used in anaesthesia or as a result of an accidental drug overdose), hypoxia or hypotension.
- Diseases of the brain, including strokes.

THE RESPIRATORY SYSTEM

The respiratory system includes the airway (mouth, tongue, oropharynx etc.), lungs and respiratory muscles.

Common causes of respiratory failure include the following:

- Airway obstruction by foreign bodies, the patient's own tongue or disease, such as anaphylactic shock and tumours, will rapidly lead to hypoxia and death.
- Lung problems such as lung disease or the collapse of healthy lung.
- Respiratory muscle weakness, which may be due to disease of the muscle or the nerves controlling them, e.g. Motor Neurone disease, or may be drug induced, such as occurs when muscle relaxants are used in anaesthesia.

THE CARDIOVASCULAR SYSTEM

Overall, heart disease is the commonest cause of cardiorespiratory arrests. Classically, this takes the form of a heart attack, or *myocardial infarction*, (death of heart muscle following obstruction of a coronary artery), due to ischaemic heart disease. Damage to the heart muscle causes it to become electrically unstable and a potentially fatal abnormal heart rhythm may develop.

Cardiac dysfunction may be secondary to other causes such as hypovolaemia or drugs. The causes of cardiorespiratory failure and arrest are often interrelated, as shown in the following example.

A patient with angina and emphysema undergoes a laparotomy for bowel surgery. Analgesic drugs and the tension and pain of a large abdominal wound depress his respiration. He becomes hypoxic despite oxygen therapy. The hypoxia worsens his angina and the consequent heart failure causes him to become hypotensive. This depresses his consciousness and worsens the respiratory failure, leading into a vicious circle, which may end in a cardiorespiratory arrest. Cardiorespiratory arrests, however, seldom occur without warning and these warning signs may be present or expected hours before the arrest occurs.

MANAGEMENT OF A CARDIORESPIRATORY ARREST

The principles of management of a cardiorespiratory arrest are universal and straightforward.

The *initial assessment* is undertaken when a patient acutely stops breathing, cannot be roused and/or has no palpable pulse. A diagnosis of cardiorespiratory arrest can then be made.

Following the initial assessment and confirmation that the patient has had an arrest, the management proceeds in a stepwise fashion known as *basic life support*.

BASIC LIFE SUPPORT

Basic life support follows a simple ABC and is the basis of cardiopulmonary resuscitation or CPR.

A- IS FOR AIRWAY

A clear airway must first be established, either by simple manipulation (e.g. jaw thrust), by the use of an airway adjunct (e.g. Guedel airway) or intubation.

> **WITHOUT A CLEAR AIRWAY, THE PATIENT CANNOT BREATHE AND WILL DIE.**

B- IS FOR BREATHING

Once an airway is established, the patient may breathe spontaneously or require assistance, either by 'mouth to mouth' (expired air ventilation) or by a self-inflating bag device.

> **WITHOUT VENTILATION, THE PATIENT WILL BECOME HYPOXIC AND THEIR CIRCULATION, IF ANY, WILL BE INEFFECTIVE.**

C- IS FOR CIRCULATION

Once breathing/ventilation is established, a circulation is needed to pump the oxygenated blood to vital organs. If a patient's circulation does not return once their airway and breathing have been attended to, it must be supported by external cardiac massage (closed chest compression).

> **WITHOUT THE CIRCULATION OF OXYGENATED BLOOD, THE PATIENT'S ORGANS WILL BEGIN TO DIE, BEGINNING WITH THEIR BRAIN**

The purpose of basic life support is to minimize any damage to vital organs and buy time for the patient before advanced life support begins.

ADVANCED LIFE SUPPORT

Advanced life support (ALS) is the process by which the cause of the arrest is determined and treated if possible, e.g. defibrillation for ventricular fibrillation and advanced airway techniques, such as tracheal intubation, employed if they are required. The aim of ALS is to stabilize the patient and minimize any further harm. The initial diagnosis is provided by the electrocardiogram, which should be obtained as soon as the facilities are available. An overview of the management of cardiopulmonary resuscitation is illustrated in Figure 27.1.

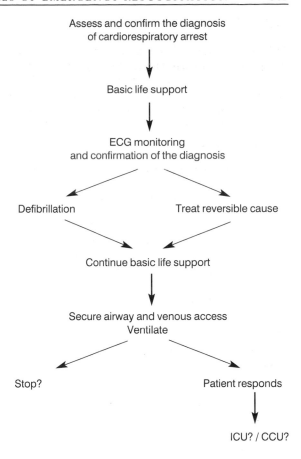

Figure 27.1 An overview of the management of a cardiorespiratory arrest

SOME SPECIFIC TYPES OF CARDIAC ARREST AND THEIR MANAGEMENT

ASYSTOLE

Asystole occurs when the heart comes to a standstill and ceases to pump blood. It has a very poor prognosis.

The single most important feature in the management of asystole is to ensure that the diagnosis is correct and is not a failure of either the ECG monitoring, such as a disconnected lead, or of interpretation.

Once the diagnosis is confirmed, management consists of CPR, with the addition of the drug adrenaline (epinephrine). Adrenaline is given to improve the effectiveness of the CPR. It does not *treat* the asystole. CPR is continued in the hope that the patient's heart will start to beat spontaneously, but it rarely does.

ELECTROMECHANICAL DISSOCIATION

Electromagnetic dissociation (EMD) occurs when the electrical activity of the heart is normal (as displayed on an ECG) but it fails to pump blood. It is also known as pulseless electrical activity (PEA).

The management of EMD is to continue CPR until the cause is determined and rectified if possible. Potentially reversible causes include:

- hypoxia
- hypovolaemia
- hyper/hypokalaemia
- hypothermia
- toxic disturbances
- thromboembolic episode
- tension pneumothorax
- cardiac tamponade.

PULSELESS VENTRICULAR TACHYCARDIA

When the ventricles of the heart are beating so fast they do not have time to fill with blood between beats, the condition is known as pulseless ventricular tachycardia. The heart therefore fails to pump out enough blood to maintain a circulation.

VENTRICULAR FIBRILLATION

Ventricular fibrillation causes the heart muscle to lose all its muscular coordination. In effect, the heart muscle 'shivers' and, because there are no effective muscle contractions taking place, no blood is pumped out from the heart.

The treatment of choice for both pulseless ventricular tachycardia and ventricular fibrillation is electrical defibrillation. It should be performed as rapidly as possible once the diagnosis is made because any delay diminishes the chance of successful conversion to a 'normal' sinus rhythm.

DEFIBRILLATION

Defibrillation is the passage of a large electrical shock current across an electrically unstable heart. By producing the synchronous depolarization of all the heart muscle cells, it briefly terminates unstable electrical activity and allows the heart's natural pacemaker tissue to take over and establish a normal rate and rhythm within the heart muscle.

The direct current defibrillator is basically a large capacitor that is charged to a predetermined voltage using a variable voltage step-up transformer, powered from the mains or from a rechargeable low-voltage battery. Output varies between 20 joules (used in children) and a maximum of 400 joules. The patient is usually given a number of shocks of increasing voltage until such time as a 'normal' rhythm is achieved or treatment is discontinued.

If defibrillation is used to treat an arrhythmia, the discharge must be synchronized to be released just after the occurrence of an R-wave on the ECG. Such a device is known as a *cardioverter* or *synchronized defibrillator*.

The surface area of the defibrillator paddles must be large enough to allow the necessary current to flow without burning the skin. Use of an electrically conductive jelly placed between the skin and the paddle will improve electrical contact. It will also reduce the likelihood of skin burns by ensuring that the total paddle surface is in electrical contact with the skin.

The paddle handles must be well insulated so that the user does not receive an electric shock. Similarly, it is also important that other members of staff stand well back before discharge commences. The large voltages used may be calculated from the formula:

$$E = CV^2/2,$$
where E = energy in joules
C = capacitance in farads
V = potential difference across the capacitor in volts.

Thus, to produce a charge of 400 joules, between 2000 and 9000 volts will be needed.

DRUGS COMMONLY USED IN RESUSCITATION

ADRENALINE

Adrenaline (epinephrine) is a naturally occurring sympathomimetic agent that is released when the sympathetic nervous system is stimulated. It increases the force of contraction of the heart and is therefore known as an *inotropic* agent. In addition, it also causes blood vessels to constrict, making CPR more effective.

ATROPINE

Atropine blocks the action of the neurotransmitter acetylcholine and is therefore known as an *anticholinergic* drug. It opposes the action of the vagus nerve on the heart and thereby increases the heart rate.

LIGNOCAINE

Lignocaine (lidocaine) is commonly used as a local anaesthetic agent, but it is also an anti-arrhythmic drug used to stabilize abnormal heart rhythms.

DRUGS LESS COMMONLY USED

SODIUM BICARBONATE

Sodium bicarbonate is an alkaline salt that is often used as an antacid. Patients who have had a cardiorespiratory arrest rapidly accumulate acid from cellular anaerobic respiration in their blood. Sodium bicarbonate was given to neutralize this acid but its use is no longer recommended. The best way to reduce acid in the blood is effective CPR.

CALCIUM

Calcium is now only used when specifically indicated, e.g. in hyperkalaemia.

PATIENT CARE FOLLOWING CARDIOPULMONARY ARREST

If a patient is successfully resuscitated from a cardiorespiratory arrest they often require further specialized medical care. This care is commonly continued in an intensive care or coronary care unit and is not only supportive in nature but enables physicians to invasively measure cardiac parameters that may be used in the treatment of these patients.

PROGNOSIS

The overall prognosis for in-hospital cardiorespiratory arrests is poor, with only 17.6% of such patients leaving hospital. Of those patients who survive the initial arrest but remain in a coma after six hours, only 15% go on to have an 'independent' existence.

These figures, however, are pooled and include all causes. Postoperative cardiorespiratory arrest generally carries a much better prognosis, usually because the causes are acute and reversible, e.g. acute airway obstruction in a sedated patient, and because they occur in areas where the clinical staff are highly trained and vigilant.

SUMMARY

Cardiorespiratory arrest is a common occurrence within hospitals, but much less common within the operating department. Despite its overall poor prognosis, rapid assessment and treatment do save lives.

> **ALL PATIENTS IN CARDIORESPIRATORY ARREST WILL DIE, UNLESS AN ATTEMPT AT RESUSCITATION IS MADE. RESUSCITATION MUST, HOWEVER, BE APPROPRIATE.**

This chapter merely provides an overview of resuscitation but there is no substitute for taking part in an ALS course. The algorithm produced by the Resuscitation Council as a guide to the management of cardiopulmonary arrest is reproduced in Appendix 5.

RECOMMENDED READING

Advanced Life Support Course Provider Manual, 3rd edn. Resuscitation Council (UK), London.

Appendix 1
ABBREVIATIONS USED IN THE TEXT

ADH	Antidiuretic hormone	MDA	Medical Devices Agency
ALS	Advanced Life Support	MED	Medical engineering department
ARDS	Adult respiratory distress syndrome	MH	Malignant hyperpyrexia
ASA	American Society of Anesthesiologists	ml	Millilitre
ASA grade	ASA patient fitness scale	mmol/l	Millimoles per litre – a measure of the concentration of ions etc.
AV node	Atrioventricular node		
B	Bar – a unit of pressure	mV	Millivolts
BAODA	British Association of Operating Department Assistants (now known as the Association of Operating Department Practitioners)	Na^+	Sodium ion
		NDMR	Non-depolarizing muscle relaxant
		NHS	National Health Service
		NSAI(D)s	Non-steroidal antiinflammatory (drugs)
BP	Blood pressure	O_2	Oxygen
°C	Degrees Celsius or Centigrade	ODA	Operating Department Assistant
CBI	Confederation of British Industry	ODP	Operating Department Practice/Practitioner
cm	centimetres	P	Pressure
CNS	Central nervous system	Pa	Pascal
CO	Cardiac output	PA	Pulmonary artery
CO_2	Carbon dioxide	PA_{gas}	Partial pressure of alveolar gas
COSHH	Control of Substances Hazardous to Health	Pa_{gas}	Partial pressure of arterial gas
		PCA	Patient-controlled analgesia
CPAP	Continuous positive airway pressure	PEEP	Positive end-expired pressure
CPR	Cardiopulmonary resuscitation	PFT(s)	Pulmonary function test(s)
CSF	Cerebrospinal fluid	Pgas	Partial pressure of a gas
CXR	Chest X-ray	pH	Hydrogen ion concentration (more acid = lower pH)
DIC	Disseminated intravascular coagulopathy		
DVT	Deep venous thrombosis	ppm	Parts per million
EBME	Electro-bioengineering department	PT	Thromboplastin time
ECF	Extracellular fluid	PTT	Partial thromboplastin time
ECG	Electrocardiograph/electrocardiogram	QA	Quality assurance
ENT	Ear, nose and throat	Q_t	Perfusion/unit time, i.e. cardiac output
ETT	Endotracheal tube	PVR	Pulmonary vascular resistance
ERV	Expiratory reserve volume	RV	Residual volume
Fd	Farad	SA	node Sinoatrial node
FEV_{10}	Forced expired vital capacity in 1 second	SIMV	Synchronized intermittent mandatory ventilation
F_{gas}	Fraction of gas in a mixture of gasses		
FRC	Functional residual capacity	SI	unit Système International d'Unités
H^+	Hydrogen ion	SVR	Systemic vascular resistance
H&S	Health and Safety	T	Temperature
HASAWA	Health and Safety at Work Act	TENS	Transcutaneous electrical nerve stimulation
HFJV	High-frequency jet ventilation		
HIV	Human immunodeficiency virus	TLC	Total lung capacity
Hg	Mercury	TUC	Trades Union Congress
HSC	Health and Safety Commission	VC	Vital capacity
HSE	Health and Safety Executive	V	a) Ventilation/unit time
ICF	Intracellular fluid		b) Volume
ICP	Intracranial pressure	V_A	Alveolar ventilation
IMV	Intermittent mandatory ventilation	V_{CO2}	Volume of carbon dioxide produced in 1 minute
IPPV	Intermittent positive pressure ventilation		
IRV	Inspiratory reserve volume	VIC	Vaporizer inside circuit
K	Kelvin – the unit of absolute temperature	VIE	Vacuum-insulated evaporator
K^+	Potassium ion	VOC	Vaporizer outside circuit
kPa	Kilopascal	V_{O2}	Volume of oxygen used in 1 minute
LA	Local anaesthetic	V_T	Tidal volume
MAC	Minimum alveolar concentration	v/v	Volume per volume
mb	Millibar	w/v	Weight per volume

Appendix 2

COMMONLY USED SYSTÈME INTERNATIONALE UNITS (SI UNITS)

Quantity	Symbol	SI unit name	SI unit symbol	Expression in SI units
Length	l	metre	m	
Mass	m	kilogram	kg	
Temperature	T	Kelvin	K	
	t	Celsius	^{0}C	
Time	t	second	s	
Electric current	I	ampere	A	
Amount of substance	n	mole	mol	
Area	A	square metre	m^2	
Volume	V	cubic metre	m^3	
Density	p	kg/cubic metre		kgm^{-3}
Specific volume		cubic metres/kg		m^3kg^{-1}
Concentration		mole/cubic metre		$mole/m^{-3}$
Molar mass	M	g/mole		$gmol^{-1}$
Speed/velocity	u, v	metre/second		ms^{-1}
Acceleration	a	metre/second/second		ms^{-2}
Force	F	newton		$kgms^{-2}$
Weight (+ gravity)	W	kilogram-force		$kg \times 9.81ms^{-1}$
Acceleration (gravity)	g	9.81 metres/second/second		$9.81ms^{-2}$
Pressure	p	pascal	Pa	Nm^{-2}
Work	U	joule	J	N m ' kgm^2/s^{-2}
Energy	U	joule	J	N m ' kgm^2/s^{-2}
Power	P	watt	W	$N ms^{-1} Js^{-1}$
Specific heat capacity		joule/kg/K		$Jkg^{-1}K^{-1}$
Electric charge	Q	coulomb	C	A s
Electric potential	V	volt	V	WA^{-1}
Electric resistance	R	ohm	Ω	VA^{-1}

Appendix 3

AN EXAMPLE OF A CARE PLAN

POTENTIAL NEEDS/POTENTIAL PROBLEMS	ACTION REQUIRED	EVALUATION
Preoperatively		
Anxiety due to nature of surgery:	A preoperative visit allows for explanation of what to expect post-operatively.	Preoperative visit the day before
1. fear of surgery/anaesthesia	It also gives an opportunity to introduce oneself to the patient.	
2. body image adjustment	Reassurance: escort patient to anaesthetic room and receive in recovery	Escorted patient to theatre
3. prognosis		
Perioperative and postoperative care		
Ensure patient safety before, during and after surgery until ready to return to the ward	Check patient identity and operation details	Checked
	Accompany patient through the department, ensuring comfort and safety	
	Correct, safe positioning	Patient safe
	Continuous monitoring of unconscious patient	Monitoring throughout
	Maintenance of sterile area for surgery	Complete
	Account for swabs, needles and instruments prior to skin closure	Complete
	Care of pressure areas with use of pressure	Checked in recovery – care given
Maintain clear airway	Maintain patient's airway by supporting angle of jaw	Not necessary
	Administer oxygen as prescribed	Oxygen for six hours
	Apply suction if necessary	Not necessary
	Observe respiratory rate and depth	Continuous observation
	Observe patient's colour	Continuous observation
	Monitor oxygen saturation levels	Continuous observation
Emotional support	Offer reassurance	Reassured
	Observe for signs of emotional distress	Appears calm
	Assess patient's emotional response to surgery	Appears calm
Assess levels of consciousness	Monitor patient for return of normal motor reflexes	Continuous monitoring
	Check: Cough reflex Pupil response	
	Hand grip Eyes open	
	Head lift Is patient awake?	
	Document observations	
Maintain fluid balance	Continuous intravenous infusion as prescribed	Intravenous infusion for 24 h
	Ensure patency of the infusion	
	Monitor and record urine output	
Prevent complications of surgery/anaesthesia	Maintain airway and observe for changes as above	
Shock/haemorrhage	Observe wound site for haematoma/swelling	Wound OK
	Monitor the output from drains and ensure patency	Minimal drainage
	Continue to monitor vital signs as above	Continual monitoring
	Reassure	

Pain	Record vital signs and action taken	Nursed upright in bed
	Maximize comfort by nursing in bed	
	Nurse upright to aid breathing as patient is a heavy smoker	
	Assess patient's experience of pain	
	Administer prescribed analgesia	Analgesia given intramuscularly
	Monitor effects of analgesia given in recovery or in theatre	Responded well to analgesia
	Continue to monitor respiratory rate and depth, pulse rate and BP	Continual monitoring
	Observe patient's physical and emotional responses	
	Adjust position to ensure comfort, taking into account the site of any suction drains	
Postoperative shaking	Maintain comfortable body temperature	Kept warm
	Disturb the patient as little as possible	Patient allowed to sleep
	Continue to administer oxygen and observe	No postoperative shaking
	Explain to patient that the shaking will pass	
	Encourage to relax and breath normally	

(with thanks to Ms Sheila Boyer)

Appendix 4d
CONSENT FORM

ST HELENS & KNOWSLEY HOSPITALS
MERSEYSIDE
CONSENT FORM FOR INVASIVE
CLINICAL PROCEDURE

ATTACH PATIENT LABEL OR PRINT DETAILS →	✦ _____ ✦ _____ Christian name(s) Surname ✦ _____ Address _____ Address ✦ __/__/____ ✦ _____ ✦ _____ Date of birth Sex Patient Registration Number

CONSULTANT IN CHARGE: ✦ _____

ALL SECTIONS MARKED (✦) AND (✖) MUST BE COMPLETED

(✦) – Sections to be completed by healthcare professional   **(✖)** – Sections to be completed by person giving consent

I ✖ **PRINT NAME**_____ being the patient/
the parent of the patient/the legal guardian of the patient/☐legal
advocate of the patient *(delete as appropriate)* referred to above, freely
consent to the procedure(s) of:

✦_____
PRINT CLEARLY, NO ABBREVIATIONS
_____.

☐Only a patient, or a parent or legal guardian of a child, may give consent in a legal sense. A *relative's assent* to a procedure on an unconscious or incompetent person *has no legal standing* but is taken as good practice. A "legal advocate" (identified as being a legally appointed representative, or advocate as demonstrated in a witnessed, written "living will") may give consent on the patient's behalf.

The **reasons** for, the **nature** of, the **benefits** of, the substantial
risks of, the **discomforts** of, the **alternatives** to, and the
consequences of not having, the procedure(s) written above have
been explained to me by ✦_____.
PRINT Healthcare Professional's name

IMPORTANT NOTES FOR A PERSON GIVING CONSENT

1. No guarantee can be given that any particular clinician will perform the procedure described above.
2. An anaesthetic agent will be given either as a local (LA) or general anaesthetic (GA), or on some occasions as a combination of the two. On occasions, a Regional Anaesthetic is used which numbs a specific part of the body e.g. a limb; a spinal anaesthetic is an example of this. On some occasions, a sedative (with LA) may be given that will make you drowsy but not asleep, so called "twilight sleep". Under GA, when you are asleep, your heart and blood pressure and other important factors will be monitored. Pain relief will be given during a GA. In some circumstances, particularly children, this may be given rectally as this is a very effective route to give pain relief. An anaesthetist will be available to answer questions and explain things to you about the anaesthetic.
3. Consent for the procedure(s) written above may be withdrawn at any time by the patient or the person giving consent.

CONTINUE OVERLEAF

CONSENT FORM

4. The named healthcare professional is there to explain things and help you to decide what is best for you. Do not be afraid to ask questions.

5. Occasionally during a procedure, an unexpected finding or disease may be discovered which if left untreated could have a potentially serious adverse effect on the patient's life. The Trust **assumes** that your consent is given to deal with any such findings, *however, you may indicate below any procedure you **do not want** performed*:

_____

_____

6. The healthcare professional taking your consent has experience, training and understanding of the proposed procedure and as such has identified below certain possible complications and substantial risks. These are not necessarily due to any failure of care on the part of the health professional, but exist by the nature of disease (some examples are: wound infections, risk of pregnancy after sterilisation and vasectomy, surgical complications, anaesthetic complications). The substantial risks are:

✦ _____

_____

_____

CONSENT
The signature below is evidence of my consent to the procedure(s) described overleaf and to an anaesthetic, and to my understanding of the above notes.

✖ _____   ✖ ____/____/____
         signature   *Today's date*

HEALTHCARE PROFESSIONAL'S SECTION

A. **Risks** (e.g.conception with vasectomy and sterilisation procedures and contraception; rectal suppository and analgesia; risks appropriate to surgery and anaesthesia;) **must** be **discussed and recorded** above.

B. **Patients have a legal right to withdraw or restrict consent** this must be respected without duress or prejudice being applied to the patient or legal guardian/representative. Time must be given to the patient and/or person giving consent for understanding and consideration of options.

> ✦ I believe myself to be an appropriately qualified and experienced person to explain the **reasons** for, the **nature** of, the **benefits** of, the **risks** of, the **discomforts** of, the **alternatives** to, and the **consequences of not** accepting the above described procedure(s) and have done so in such a way that I feel that the person giving consent clearly understands and is well informed.
> **(PRINT name, qualifications, department & grade)**
>
> NAME: _____   SIGNATURE: _____
>   *PRINT   Initials & Surname*
>
> QUALIFICATIONS: _____   DATE: ____/____/____
>
> DEPARTMENT: _____   GRADE: _____

SHK HN 170 5.98

Appendix 4b
PATIENT INFORMATION SHEET

**ST HELENS & KNOWSLEY HOSPITALS
AT WHISTON, ST HELENS & NEWTON SITES
MERSEYSIDE   L35 5DR
DEPARTMENT OF ORTHOPAEDICS & TRAUMA**

THE PROCEDURE IS CALLED: <u>TOTAL HIP REPLACEMENT</u>

YOUR CONSULTANT IS: _____
(Print Consultants Name)

THE CONTACT TELEPHONE NUMBER IS:_____

THE REASONS FOR THE PROCEDURE:

Your hip has become worn out over time due to arthritis and the normally smooth surfaces of the hip joint are roughened. This means that you are getting pain in your hip and are finding it more difficult to walk.

THE NATURE OF THE PROCEDURE:

This involves a major operation performed under a General or a Spinal Anaesthetic with a stay in hospital. A Spinal Anaesthetic means that local anaesthetic is injected around the nerves in your back which control the hip and legs so that, whilst you remain awake you are unable to feel from the waist down until the operation is over.

In the operating theatre, a cut is made in the skin over the thigh. The top end of the femur (called the femoral head) is removed exposing the socket of the hip joint (called acetabulum). The acetabulum is surgically prepared to accept the socket part of the hip replacement that is then fixed to the bone using either cement or screws.

The top of the shaft of the femur is then prepared to accept a metal stem with a ball end; this is the femoral part of the total hip replacement. The stem is fixed to the femur with cement or by a cementless technique that involves hammering the stem into the thighbone (called impaction fit). When such cementless methods of fixation are used, there is usually a special coating on the femoral part of the new hip to encourage bone to grow from the thighbone into the component to improve fixation.

The operation takes between 1 to 2 hours. After repair of the muscles and skin, a dressing will be applied to the wound. Often fine plastic tubes called drains will be placed into the wound and brought out through the skin. These drains connect to a bag or a bottle and remove any blood that might collect in the wound. These drains are normally removed between 24 and 48 hours after surgery.

After surgery you will spend a period of time in the Recovery Ward where your blood pressure and pulse will be measured to ensure you have recovered from the anaesthetic and then you will be taken back to your ward.

People are mobilised very quickly following hip replacement with the assistance of nurses, physiotherapists and physiotherapy aids. Generally people are up on crutches at 24 to 48 hours after surgery and get home between 8 and 14 days after surgery.

THE BENEFITS OF THE PROCEDURE:

The main benefit is to relieve the pain in your hip is because there is a "wearing away" of the hip joint. Although there may be an increase in your ability to walk, this is not the main aim of surgery.

CONTINUE OVERLEAF

THE RISKS OF THE PROCEDURE:

The general risks of your operation include bleeding into the wound, wound infection and a temporary inability to pass urine. This may require a catheter to be temporarily passed into the bladder for a few days. You will be lying on your back for a few days and there is a risk of developing pressure sores on the buttocks or heels, however the nurses will be taking precautions to avoid this problem. There is a risk of developing a chest infection or pneumonia, particularly if you are a smoker. If you smoke you should try to stop before your operation. There is also a risk of developing a clot in the veins of the leg (called a DVT) which could work loose and go the lungs which may be serious (called a Pulmonary Embolus). The risk of a Pulmonary Embolus is **less than** 1 in 100 (hundred) and various precautions are taken against it.

The specific risks of hip replacement include rare occasions when a patient's blood pressure can drop during the insertion of the cement. This is an uncommon occurrence these days, however, in very frail, elderly people such a complication can occur and may be fatal.

After surgery, it is possible for the hip to dislocate (the ball comes out of the socket). If this should happen, it is usual to give an anaesthetic to put the ball back in the socket and have a longer period in bed to allow the tissues about the new hip to heal. If this problem recurs, further surgery maybe necessary. A small number of people may develop an infection in the new hip that is probably only treatable by further surgery to replace the hip in one or two stages.

Young people who have high expectations of their artificial hip and who get a lot of use out of their artificial hip may actually wear the artificial hip out or loosen it. Such wearing or loosening will require future revision surgery.

THE DISCOMFORTS OF THE PROCEDURE:

Are the inevitable pains following any surgical procedure when skin, muscle and bone are operated upon. Generally, the pain is worse for the first two days, but the doctors caring for you will ensure you have good pain relief.

THE ALTERNATIVES TO THE PROCEDURE:

Tablets prescribed by your GP, physiotherapy or weight reduction may ease some of your hip pain, however, total hip replacement is so successful in treating severe pain this is the only reliable method of pain relief for this condition.

Other operations, which are occasionally used, include "Arthrodesis" where the hip is stiffened up, and "osteotomy" which involves breaking and resetting the femur or pelvis to alter the shape. Arthrodesis is generally only suitable for young patients as older people have wear and tear in other joints. Osteotomy does not always give good pain relief and can be a little unpredictable. In a very young patient osteotomy can be a sensible alternative to a total hip replacement if x-rays suggest an osteotomy will improve the shape of the hip. A drawback of osteotomy is that any future hip replacement may be more difficult to perform.

Everyone has a right to avoid surgery if they wish and in which case all that can be recommended is tablets for pain relief and a walking stick.

THE CONSEQUENCES OF NOT HAVING THE PROCEDURE:

The pain will not go away once arthritis is established in a joint and pain has arisen.

Appendix 5
CARDIAC ARREST SHEET

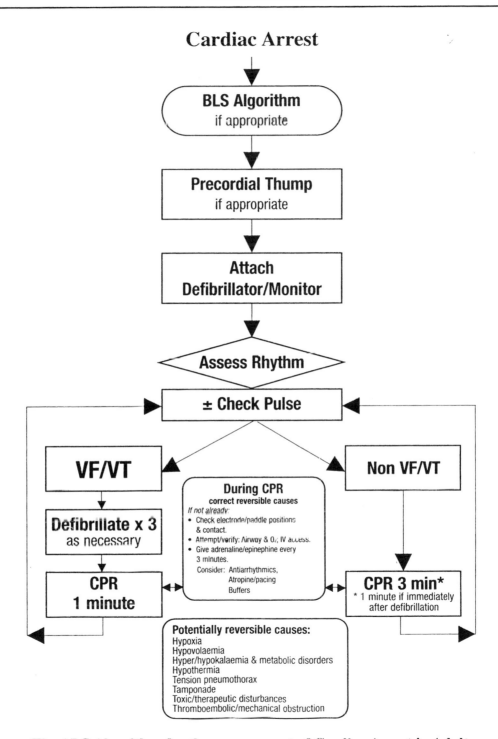

Resuscitation Council (UK)

Cardiac Arrest

BLS Algorithm
if appropriate

Precordial Thump
if appropriate

Attach
Defibrillator/Monitor

Assess Rhythm

± Check Pulse

VF/VT

Non VF/VT

During CPR
correct reversible causes
If not already:
- Check electrode/paddle positions & contact.
- Attempt/verify: Airway & O₂, IV access.
- Give adrenaline/epinephine every 3 minutes.
  Consider: Antiarrhythmics, Atropine/pacing Buffers

Defibrillate x 3
as necessary

CPR
1 minute

CPR 3 min*
* 1 minute if immediately after defibrillation

Potentially reversible causes:
Hypoxia
Hypovolaemia
Hyper/hypokalaemia & metabolic disorders
Hypothermia
Tension pneumothorax
Tamponade
Toxic/therapeutic disturbances
Thromboembolic/mechanical obstruction

The ALS Algorithm for the management of Cardiac Arrest in Adults
Note that each successive step is based on the assumption that the one before has not been successful

Index